AF539170

Women and Family Health

INTERNATIONAL ENCYCLOPAEDIA OF WOMEN - 4

WOMEN AND FAMILY HEALTH

By

Dr. Digumarti Bhaskara Rao

Reader and Research Director
R.V.R. College of Education
D-43 (277) S.V.N. Colony
Guntur – 522 006
Andhra Pradesh (India)

&

Mrs. Digumarti Pushpa Latha

Executive Member
Care Welfare Society
Guntur – 522 006
Andhra Pradesh (India)

DISCOVERY PUBLISHING HOUSE PVT. LTD.

NEW DELHI-110 002

WOMEN AND FAMILY HEALTH

Edition – 2016

ISBN: 978-81-8356-911-8 (Set)
ISBN: 978-81-7141-497-0

Women and Family Health

Published by:

DISCOVERY PUBLISHING HOUSE PVT. LTD.
4383/4B, Ansari Road, Darya Ganj
New Delhi-110 002 (India)
Phone: +91-11-23279245, 43596064-65
Fax: +91-11-23253475
E-mail: discoverypublishinghouse@gmail.com
sales@discoverypublishinggroup.com
web: www.discoverypublishinggroup.com

Printed at:
Infinity Imaging Systems
Delhi

Contents

FOREWARD

Women and men are equal in every human concern in this World. They are equally competing in almost all spheres of work and power and are equally achieving the set goals. Culture, economy and polity may be barriers to women in certain parts of the globe, still women are marching ahead with great conviction and confidence to keep themselves on par with their counter parts in every affair.

This International Encyclopaedia of Women is touching every area concerned to women. Volume 1 explains the status of the world's women, Volume 2 discusses the role of education in women's empowerment, Volume 3 discusses the challenges and advancement of women, Volume 4 outlines the family health, and Volume 5 presents the details of the international instruments applicable for the development of women.

This Encyclopedia will meet the requirements of planners, researchers, educationists and activists.

Dr. Digumarti Bhaskara Rao
Mrs. Digumarti Pushpa latha
R.V.R College of Edication
Nagarjuna University,
Guntur 522006 (India)

Acknowledgements

We are thankful to the United Nations and its various commissions, agencies, divisions and departments, the UNESCO, Paris, the UNESCO Institute for Education, Hamburg, the United Nations Centre for Human Rights, Geneva, the UNESCO, Dakar, the International Institute for Population Sciences, Bombay, the Organisation of African Unity; and the United Nations Information Centre, New Delhi for extending their kind cooperation in providing us with the necessary material on our request for the preparation of this International Encyclopaedia of Women.

Volume 1 of the Encyclopaedia contains the material taken from *The World's Women 1995: Trends and Statistics*, United Nations. We thank Prof. Ann Marie Erb-Leoncavallo, Associate Information Officer, Department of Public Information, United Nations, New York for sending the above cited material along with some other valuable documents with the necessary permission to cite material with due credit.

Volume 2 contains the material obtained from Carolyn Medel-Anonueva, ed., *Women, Education and Empowerment: Pathways Towards Autonomy*, UNESCO Institute for Education, Carolyn Medel-Anonueva, ed, *Women Reading the World: Policies and Practices of Literacy in Asia*, UNESCO Institute for Education, Namtip Aksornkool, *Daughters of the Earth,* UNESCO; Cynthia Guttman, *In Our Own Hands,* UNESCO; *The African Conference on the Empowerment of Women through Functional literacy and the Education of the Girl Child*, Kampala: We thank Prof. Cendrine Sebastiani, Publications Department, UNESCO Institute for Education; Prof. Francoise Pinzon, Global Action Programme on Education For All, UNESCO; The Organisers of the African conference on the Empowerment of Women for sending the material for use in our work.

Volume 3 contains the material obtained from *Worldwide Facts and Statistics About the Status of Women,* Committee for the '95 World conference on Women, *Women: Challenges to the Year 2000*, United

Nations; *Fourth World Conference on Women, The Advancement of Women: Notes for Speakers*, United Nations, etc. We are thankful to the concerned Personnel of United Nations Department of Public Information, New York, United Nations Information Centre, New Delhi; Committee for the '95 World Conference on Women, New York; and East- West centre, Honolulu for their kind material support.

Volume 4 contains the material obtained from International Institute for Population Science, *National Family Health Survey (MCH and Family Planning) India, 1992-93*, IIPS. We are thankful to the IIPS, Bombay, Government of India; East-West Centre, and Population Research Centres in India for their valuable cooperation.

Volume 5 contains the material taken from *The International Bill of Human Rights*, United Nations, *Discrimination Against Women: The Convention and The Committee*, UN Centre for Human Rights, Geneva, *Harmful Traditional Practices Affecting the Health of Women and Children*, UN Centre for Human Rights, *The Nairobi Foreword-Looking Strategies for the Advancement of Women*, United Nations (as adopted by the World Conference to Review and Appraise the Achievements of the United Nations Decade for Women: Equality, Development and Peace, Nairobi, Kenya, 15-16 July 1995), and *The Flatform for Action*, United Nations, We are thankful to the United Nations for using these international instruments on women.

We are also thankful to many scholars, researchers, teachers, administrators and friends working on women around the globe who helped us in gettings the necessary information and material on women to prepare this International Encyclopaedia of Women.

Dr. Digumarti Bhaskara Rao
Ms. Digumarti Pushpa Latha

Overview of the World's Women

Issues of gender equality are moving to the top of the global agenda but better understanding of women's and men's contributions to society is essential to speed the shift from agenda to policy to practice. Too often, women and men live in different worlds—worlds that differ in access to education and work opportunities, and in health, personal security and leisure time. *The World's Women 1995* provides information and analyses to highlight the economic, political and social differences that still separate women's and men's lives and how these differences are changing.

How different are these worlds? Anecdote and misperception abound, in large part because good information has been lacking. As a result, policy has been ill-informed, strategy unfounded and practice unquestioned. Fortunately, this is beginning to change. It is changing because advocates of women's interests have done much in the past 20 years to sharpen people's awareness of the importance of gender concerns. It is changing because this growing awareness has, by raising new questions and rephrasing old, greatly increased the demand for better statistics to inform and focus the debate. And it is changing because women's contributions—and women's rights—have moved to the centre of social and economic change.

The International Conference of Population and Development, held in Cairo in 1994, was a breakthrough. It established a new consensus on two fundamental points:

—Empowering women and improving their status are essential to realizing the full potential of economic, political and social development.

—Empowering women is an important end in itself. And as women acquire the same status, opportunities and social, economic and legal rights as men, as they acquire the right to reproductive health and the right to protection against genderbased violence, human well-being will be enhanced.

The International Conference on Population and Development drew together the many strands of thought and action initiated by two decades of women's conferences. It was also the culmination of an active effort by women's groups to lobby international forums for women's issues. At the United Nations Conference on Environment and Development in Rio de Janeiro in 1992, nongovernmental organizations pushed for understanding the link between women's issues and sustainable development. At the World Conference on Human Rights in Vienna in 1993, women's rights were finally accepted as issues of international human rights.

At the Population Conference and later at the World Summit for Social Development, held in Copenhagen in 1995, the terms of discourse shifted. Not only were women on the agenda—women helped set the agenda. The empowerment of women was not merely the subject of special sessions about women's issues. It was accepted as a crucial element in any strategy seeking to solve social, economic and environmental problems. And building on the advances made in the recognition of women's human rights at the World Conference in Vienna, women's human rights became a focus of the debate in Cairo. The rights approach, advanced by women's groups, was added to the core objectives of development policy and the movement for women's equality.

To promote action on the new consensus, this edition of *The World's Women* builds on the first, presenting statistical summaries of health, schooling, family life, work and public life. Each has to be seen in proper context, however. Yes, there have been important changes in the past 25 years and women have generally made steady progress, but it is impossible to make sweeping global statements. Women's labour force participation rates are up in much of the world, but down in countries wracked by war and economic decline. Girls' education is improving, but there are hundreds of millions of illiterate women and girls who do not complete primary schooling, especially in Africa and southern Asia.

It is also important to look at a range of indicators. Women's political participation may be high in the Nordic countries, but in employment Nordic women still face considerable job segregation and wage discrimination. Women's higher education may be widespread in western Asia, but in many of those countries there are few or no women in important political positions and work opportunities are largely limited to unpaid family about.

It is also important to look at a range of indicators. Women's political participation may be high in the Nordic countries, but in employment Nordic women still face considerable job segregation and wage discrimination. Women's higher education may be widespread in western Asia, but in many of those countries there are few or no women in important political positions and work opportunities are largely limited to unpaid family labour.

The World's Women presents few global figures, focusing instead on country data and regional averages (see the box on regional trends). There are myriad differences among countries in every field and *The World's Women* tries to find a meaningful balance between detailed country statements and broad generalization. Generalizations are primarily drawn at the regional and subregional levels where there is a high degree of uniformity among countries. For all the topics covered, *The World's Women* has tapped as many statistical sources as possible, with detailed references as a basis for further study. Specialized studies are used when they encompass several countries, preferably in more than one region, so as to avoid presenting conclusions relevant in only one country.

Indicators relevant to specific age groups are crucial to understanding women's situation. The Programme of Action of the International Conference on Population and Development identified equality for the girl-child as a necessary first step in ensuring that women realize their full potential and become equal partners with men. This edition of *The World's Women* responds to this concern by highlighting the experience of the girl-child. Evidence of prenatal sex selection and differences in mortality, health, school enrolment and even work indicates that girls and boys are not treated equally.

The experience of the elderly is more difficult to describe from the few available data. Although elderly people constitute a valuable component of societies' human resources, data on the elderly are insufficient for regional generalizations. Considering that the number of elderly are growing rapidly in all regions, this gap needs to be addressed.

Regional trends

Latin America and the Caribbean

* Fertility has declined significantly—dropping 40 per cent or more over the past two decades in 13 of the region's 33 countries. The total fertility rate has fallen from 4.8 to 3.2. But adolescent fertility remains high—13 per cent of all births are to mothers below age 20. In Central America, 18 per cent.

* Maternal mortality has declined in most countries of Latin America but the incidence of unsafe abortion in South America is the highest in the world.

* Literacy has reached 85 per cent or more across most of the region, and girls outnumber boys at both secondary and tertiary levels of education.

* Latin America's recorded labour force participation rate for women (34 per cent) is low, but in the Caribbean it is much higher (49 per cent).

* Latin America's and the Caribbean are as urbanized as the developed regions, with 74 per cent of the population in urban areas. But the rate of growth is much higher—2.5 per cent a year compared with 0.9 per cent—which strains housing, water and sanitation and other infrastructure.

Sub-Saharan Africa

* Minimal progress is seen in the basic social and economic indicators. Health and education gains have faltered in the face of economic crises and civil strife. Literacy remains the lowest in the world, 43 per cent of adult women and 67 per cent of adult men, and the difference between women's and men's literacy rates is the highest.

* Fertility is the highest in the world at about six children per woman.

* Women's labour force participation has dropped throughout the past two decades—the only region where this occurred.

* Urban areas are growing at a rate of 5 per cent a year, but with new housing and economic growth at a standstill, many live in poverty and squalor. Africa's urban migrants are predominantly male, shifting the sex ratio in rural areas to 106 women per 100 men.

* Estimated HIV infection rates continue to soar, and unlike any other region, the per centage of women infected with HIV is estimated to be as high if not higher than the per centage of men. In Uganda and in Zambia, the life expectancy of both women and men has already declined because of the disease, and eight other countries are beginning to see similar effects.

Northern Africa and western Asia

* In the past two decades, many countries in the region have invested in girl's education—bringing the primary -secondary enrolment ratio for girls to 67 in northern Africa (from 50 in 1970) and 84 in western Asia, and raising women's literacy to 44 per cent in the region. But women's illiteracy in northern Africa remains high, and girls' enrolment still lags behind boys."

* Women are entering the labour force in increasing number—up from 8 per cent in 1970 to 21 in 1990 in northern Africa and from 22 to 30 per cent in western Asia. Still, these numbers are the lowest in the world. Also low is women's share of decision-making positions in government and business.

* Marriage among girls aged 15--19 has declined significantly in northern Africa and to a lesser degree in western Asia—from 38 per

cent to 10 per cent in northern Africa and from 24 per cent to 17 per cent western Asia. Teenage fertility, however, remains fairly high.

* Fertility—which was traditionally high—has declined significantly in the past 20 years, especially in northern Africa. It remains high (with total fertility rates over 5) in several countries in western Asia. These countries also have low female literacy.

Southern Asia

* Many health and education indicators remain low. Although it has risen by 10 years in the past two decades, life expectancy remains lower in southern Asia than in any other region but sub-Saharan Africa—58 for both women and men. Equal life expectancies are also exceptional—in all other regions, women have an advantage of several years.

* One in 35 women dies of pregnancy-related complications. Maternal mortality has declined but still remains high.

* Nearly two thirds of adult women are illiterate and the per centage of girls enrolled in primary and secondary levels of schooling is far below all other regions except sub-Saharan Africa.

* Women continue to marry early—41 per cent of girls aged 15-19 are already married—and adolescent fertility remains high.

* More women are counted in the labour force but most are still relegated to unpaid family labour or low-paying jobs. Although women's representation at the highest levels of government is generally weakest in Asia, four of the world's 10 current women heads of state or government hold office in this region.

Eastern and South-eastern Asia

* Development indicators continue to improve. Infant mortality has declined significantly in south-eastern Asia in the past two decades.

* Literacy is nearly universal in most countries for men but not for women. However, girls and boys now have nearly equal access to primary and secondary education.

* Adolescent marriage rates in eastern Asia are the lowest in the world—only 2 per cent of women and less than 1 per cent of men aged 15-19 are married—and household size is shrinking.

* Eastern Asia reports the largest average decline in fertility, from 4.7 to 2.3, and its contraceptive use now exceeds that of developed regions. Fertility has also declined in south-eastern Asia, but is still generally higher than in eastern Asia.

* Women's participation in the labour force is as high as in developed regions—approximately 55 per cent.

Developed regions

* Basic health and education indicators generally indicate high levels of well-being but in eastern Europe some show signs of deterioration. Currently, women in 13 countries have a life expectancy of 80 years of more and 11 more countries are expected to reach that level after the year 2000. Men's life expectancy has increased little during the past two decades in eastern Europe, however, partly due to a rise in death rates for middle--aged men. Women's life expectancy in eastern Europe has increased much less than in other regions.

* Fertility continues to fall—from 2.3 in 1975 to 1.9 in 1995. But teenage pregnancy is relatively high in some countries—Bulgaria, the Republic of Moldova, Ukraine and the United States.

* Traditional family structure and size are changing. People are marrying later or not at all, and marriages are less stable. Remarriage rates have dropped—especially for women—and single parent families now make up 10—25 per cent of all families. The population is ageing and becoming increasingly female as it does.

* Women's labour force participation increased significantly for regions outside of eastern Europe from 38 per cent in 1970 to 52 per cent in 1990. In eastern Europe, where women's labour force participation was already 56 per cent in 1970, the increase was small (to 58 per cent).

* Women continue to earn less than men—in manufacturing, women's average wage is three quarters that of men's. And women and men tend to work in different jobs—women in clerical, sales and services, and men in production and transport. And men commonly do work which is accorded higher pay and status. For example, the majority of school administrators are men while most teachers are women, and the majority of hospital consultants are men while most nurses are women.

* Women work longer hours than men in the majority of these countries—at least 2 hours longer than men do in 13 out of 21 countries studied. Much of the unpaid work is done by women—for example, women contribute roughly three quarters of total child care at home.

Education for empowerment

In the Programme of Action of the International Conference on Population and Development, education is considered one of the most important means to empower women with the knowledge, skills and self—confidence necessary to participate fully in development processes. Educated women marry later, want fewer children, are more likely to use effective methods of contraception and have greater means to improve their economic livelihood.

Through widespread promotion of universal primary education, literacy rates for women have increased over the past few decades—to at least 75 per cent in most countries of Latin America and the Caribbean and eastern and south—eastern Asia. But high rates of illiteracy among women still prevail in much of Africa and in parts of Asia. And when illiteracy is high it almost always is accompanied by large differences in rates between women and men.

At intermediate levels of education, girls have made progress in their enrolment in school through the second level. The primary—secondary enrolment ratio is now about equal for girls and boys in the developed regions and Latin America and the Caribbean and is approaching near equality in eastern, south—eastern and western Asia. But progress in many countries was reversed in the 1980s, particularly among those experiencing problems of war, economic adjustment and declining international assistance—as in Africa, Latin America and the Caribbean, and eastern Europe.

In higher education enrolments, women equal or exceed men in many regions. They outnumber men in the developed regions outside western Europe, in Latin America and the Caribbean and western Asia. Women are not as well represented in other regions, and in sub—Saharan Africa and southern Asia they are far behind—30 and 38 women per 100 men.

The Framework for Action to implement the World Declaration on Education for All states that it is urgent to improve access to education for girls and women—and to remove every obstacle that hampers their active participation. Priority actions include eliminating the social and cultural barriers the discourage—or even exclude—girls and women from the benefits of regular education programmes.

Seeking influence

Despite progress in women's higher education, major obstacles still arise when women strive to translate their high—level education into social and economic advancement. In the world of business, for example, women rarely account for more than 1 to 2 per cent of top executive positions. In the more general category of administration and management including middle levels, women's share rose in every region but one between 1980 and 1990. Women's participation jumped from 16 to 33 per cent in developed regions outside Europe. In Latin America, it rose from 18 to 25 per cent.

In the health and teaching professions—two of the largest occupational fields requiring advanced training—women are well represented in many countries but usually at the bottom levels of the status and wage hierarchy.

Similarly, among the staff of an international group of agriculture research institutes, women's participation at the non—scientific and trainee levels is moderate, but there are few women at management and senior scientific levels.

The information people receive through news papers, radio and television shapes their opinions about the world. And the more decision—making positions women hold in the media, the more they can influence output—breaking stereotypes that hurt women, attracting greater attention to issues of equality in the home and in public life, and providing young women with new images, ideas and ideals. Women now make up more than half of the communications students in a large number of countries and are increasingly visible as presenters, announcers and reporters, but they remain poorly represented in the more influential media occupations such as programme managers and senior editors.

In the top levels of government, women's participation remains the exception. At the end of 1994 only 10 women were heads of state or government; of these 10 countries only Norway had as many as one third women ministers or subministers. Some progress has been made in the appointment of women to ministerial or subministerial positions but these positions are usually tenuous for them. Most countries with women in top ministerial positions do not have comparable representation at the subministerial level. And in other countries, where significant numbers of women have reached the subministerial levels, very few have reached the top. Progress for women in parliaments has also been mixed and varies widely among regions. It is strongest in northern Europe, where it appears to be rising steadily.

Missing from this summary is women's remarkable advance in less traditional paths to power and influence. The importance of the United Nations Decade for Women and international women's conferences should not be underestimated, for these forums enabled women to develop the skills required for exercising power and influence, to mobilize resources and articulate issues and to practise organizing, lobbying and legislating. Excluded from most political offices, many women have found a voice in non—governmental organizations (NGOs) at the grass roots, national and international levels. NGOs have taken issues previously ignored— such as violence against women and rights to reproductive health—and brought them into the mainstream policy debate.

Since the women's conference in Nairobi in 1985, many grass—roots groups have been working to create new awareness of women's rights, including their rights within the family, and to help women achieve those rights. They have set agendas and carved out a space for women's issues.

And as seen in recent United Nations conferences, NGOs as a group can wield influence broad enough to be active partners With governments in deciding national policies and programmes.

Reproductive health-reproductive freedom

With greater access to education, employment and contraception, many women are choosing to marry later and have fewer children. Those who wait to marry and begin child—bearing have better access to education and greater opportunities to improve their lives. Women's increased access to education, to employment and to contraception, coupled with declining rates of infant mortality, have contributed to the worldwide decline in fertility.

The number of children women bear in developed regions is now below replacement levels at 1.9 per women. In Latin America and in most parts of Asia it has also dropped significantly. But in Africa women still have an average of six children and in many sub—Saharan African countries women have as many or more children now than they did 20 years ago.

Adolescent fertility has declined in many developing and developed countries over the past 20 years. In Central America and sub—Saharan Africa, however, rates are five to seven times higher than in developed regions. Inadequate nutrition, anaemia and early pregnancies threaten the health and life of young girls and adolescents.

Too many women lack access to reproductive health services. In developing countries maternal mortality is a leading cause of death for women of reproductive age. WHO estimates that more than half a million women die each year in childbirth and millions more develop pregnancy—related health complications. The deteriorating economic and health conditions in sub—Saharan Africa led to an increase in maternal mortality during the 1980s, where it remains the highest in the world. An African woman's lifetime risk of dying from pregnancy-related causes is 1 in 23, while a North American woman's is 1 in 4,000. Maternal mortality also increased in some countries of eastern Europe.

Pregnancy and childbirth have become safer for women in most of Asia and in parts of Latin America. In developed countries attended delivery is almost universal, but in developing countries only 55 per cent of births take place with a trained attendant and only 37 per cent in hospitals or clinics. Today new importance is being placed on women's reproductive health and safe motherhood as advocates work to redefine reproductive health as an issue of human rights.

The Programme of Action of the International Conference on Population and Development set forth a new framework to guide government actions in population, development and reproductive health—and to measure and evaluate programmes designed to realize these objectives. Instead of the traditional approach centéred on family planning and population policy objectives, governments are encouraged to develop client—centered management information systems in population and development and particularly reproductive health, including family planning and sexual health programmes.

Fewer marriages—smaller households

Rapid population changes, combined with many other social and economic changes, are being accompanied by considerable changes in women's household and family status. Most people still marry but they marry later in life, especially women. In developing regions, consensual unions and other non-formal unions remain prevalent, especially in rural areas.

As a result of these changes, many women— many more women than men—spend a significant part of their life without a partner, with important consequences for their economic welfare and their children's.

In developed regions, marriage has become both less frequent and less stable, and cohabitations is on the rise. Marriages preceded by a period of cohabitations have clearly increased in many countries of northern Europe. And where divorce once led quickly to remarriage, many postpone marriage or never remarry.

Since men have higher rates of remarriage, marry at an older age, and have a shorter life expectancy, most older men are married, while many older women are widows. Among women 60 and older, widowhood is significant everywhere—from 40 per cent in the developed regions and Latin America to 50 per cent in Africa and Asia. Moreover, in Asia and Africa, widowhood also affects many women at younger ages.

Between 1970 and 1990 household size decreased significantly in the developed regions, in Latin America and the Caribbean and in eastern and south—eastern Asia. Households are the smallest in developed regions, having declined to an average of 2.8 persons per household in 1990. In eastern Asia the average household size has declined to 3.7, in south—eastern Asia to 4.9. In Latin American countries the average fell to 4.7 persons per household, and in the Caribbean to 4.1. In northern African countries household size increased on average from 5.4 to 5.7.

In developed countries the decline in the average household size reflects an increase in the number of one—person households, especially among unmarried adults and the elderly. In developing regions the size of the household is more affected by the number of children, although a shift from extended households to nuclear households also has some effect.

Household size remains high in countries where fertility has not yet fallen significantly—for instance, in some of the African and western Asian countries.

Work—paid and unpaid

Women's access to paid work is crucial to their self—reliance and the economic well—being of dependent family members. But access to such work is unequal between women and men. Women work in different occupations than men, almost always with lower status and pay.

In developing countries many women work as unpaid family labourers in subsistence agriculture and household enterprises. Many women also work in the informal sector, where their remuneration is unstable, and their access to funds to improve their productivity is limited at best. And whatever other work women do, they also have the major responsibility for most household work, including the care of children and other family members.

The work women do contributes substantially to the well—being of families, communities and nations. But work in the household—even when it is economic—is inadequately measured, and this subverts policies for the credit, income and security of women and their families.

Over the past two decades, women's reported economic activity rates increased in all regions except sub—Saharan Africa and eastern Asia, and all of these increases are large except in eastern Europe, central Asia and Ocean. In fact, women's labour force participation increased more in the 1980s than in the 1970s in many regions. In contrast, men's economic activity rates have declined everywhere except central Asia.

The decline in women's reported labour force participation in sub—Saharan Africa stands out as an exception—dropping from a high of 57 per cent in 1970 to 54 per cent in 1980 to 53 per cent in 1990.

In 1990 the average labour force participation rate among women aged 15 and over ranged from a high of 56—58 per cent in eastern and central Asia and eastern Europe to a low in northern Africa of 21 per cent. The participation rates of men vary within a more limited range of 72—83 per cent. Because so many women in developing countries work in agriculture and informal household enterprises where their contributions are underreported, their recorded rates of economic activity should be higher in many cases. The estimated increase in southern Asia—from 25 per cent of women economically active in 1970 to 44 per cent in 1990—may be due largely to changes in the statistical methods used rather than to significant changes in work patterns.

Although work in subsistence production is crucial to survival, it goes largely underreported in population and agricultural surveys and censuses.

Most of the food eaten in agricultural households in developing countries is produced within the family holding, much of it by women. Some data show the extent of women's unreported work in agriculture. In Bangladesh, India and Pakistan, government surveys using methods to improve the measurement of subsistence work, report that more than half of rural women engage in such activities as tending poultry or cattle, planting rice, drying seeds, collecting water and preparing dung cakes for fuel. Direct observation of women's activities suggests that almost all women in rural areas contribute economically in one way or another.

The informal sector—working on own -account and in small family enterprises—also provides women with important opportunities in areas where salaried employment is closed or inadequate. In five of the six African countries studied by the Statistical Division of the United Nations Secretariat, more than one third of women economically active outside agriculture work in the informal sector, and in seven countries of Latin America 15-20 per cent. In nine countries in Asia the numbers vary—from less than 10 per cent of economically active women in western Asia to 41 per cent in the Republic of Korea and 65 per cent in Indonesia.

Although fewer women than men participate in the labour force, in some countries—including Honduras, Jamaica and Zambia—more women than men make up the informal sector labour force. In several other countries, women make up 40 per cent or more of the informal sector

In addition to the invisibility of many of women's economic activities, women remain responsible for most housework, which also goes unmeasured by the System of National Accounts. But time—use data for many developed countries show almost everywhere that women work at least as many hours each week as men, and in a large number of countries they work at least two hours more than men. Further, the daily time a man spends on work tends to be the same throughout his working life. But a woman's working time fluctuates widely and at times is extremely heavy—the result of combining paid work, household and child—care responsibilities.

Two thirds to three quarters of household work in developed regions is performed by women. In most countries studied, women spend 30 hours or more on housework each week while men spend around 10 hours. Among household tasks, the division of labour remains clear and definite in most countries. Few men do the laundry, clean the house, make the beds, iron the clothes. And most women do little household repair and maintenance. Even when employed outside the home, women do most of the housework.

Efforts to generate better statistics

The first world conference on women in Mexico in 1975 recognized the importance of improving statistics on women. Until the early 1980s women's advocates and women's offices were the main forces behind this work. Big efforts had not yet been launched in statistical offices—either nationally or internationally.

The collaboration of the Statistical Division of the United Nations Secretariat with the International Research and Training Institute for the Advancement of Women (INSTRAW) —beginning in 1982—on a training programme to promote dialogue and understanding between policy makers and statisticians, laid the groundwork for a comprehensive programme of work.

By the time of the world conference in Nairobi in 1985 some progress was evident. The Statistical Division compiled 39 key statistical indicators on the situation of women for 172 countries, and important efforts at the national level included the preparation of *Women and Men* in Sweden, first published in 1984 and with sales of 100,000.

Since Nairobi numerous developments have stregthened and given new momentum to this work. The general approach in development strategy has moved from women in development to gender and development. The focus has shifted from women in isolation to women in relation to men—to the roles each has, the relationships between them and different impacts of policies and programmes.

In statistics the focus has likewise moved from attention to women's statistics to gender statistics. There now is a recognition, for example, that biases in statistics apply not only to women but also to men—in their roles as husbands and fathers and in their roles in the household. That recognition reaches beyonds the disaggregation of data by sex to assessing statistical systems in terms of gender. It asks:

—Do the topics investigated on statistics and the concepts and definitions used in data collection reflect the diversities of women's and men's lives?

—Will the methods used in collecting data take into account stereotypes and cultural factors that might produce bias?

—Are the ways data are compiled and presented well suited to the needs of policy makers, planners and others who need such data?

The first World's Women: Trends and Statistics, issued in 1991, presented the most comprehensive and authoritative compilations of global indicators on the status of women ever available. The book's data have informed debates at international conferences and national policy meetings and provided a resource to the press and others. Its publication greatly contributed to the understanding of data users and created, for the first time, a substantial global audience for statistical genderbased information. This audience has demanded, in turn, more and better data. The book also stimulated more work on the compilation of statistics and led to The World's Women 1995 being prepared as an official conference document for the Fourth World Conference on Women in Beijing in 1995.

As gender issues receive greater priority in the work programmes of international organizations, support to the Statistical Division of the United Nations Secretariat and to national efforts to improve this work have gathered strength at UNFPA, UNICEF, UNDP, WFP, UNIFEM and INSTRAW, among others, ILO, FAO, WHO, UNESCO and UNHCR are also rethinking statistical recommendations and guidelines in their work to better understand women's activities and situations, and products of this change are evident in The World's Women 1995.

The World's Women 1995 shows considerable development in the statistics available on women and men—and in ways of presenting them effectively. But it also points to important needs for new work—to be addressed in the Platform for Action of the Fourth World Conference on Women. Some problems identified by the first world conference—such as the measurement of women's economic contribution and the definition of the concepts of household and household head—are still unresolved. But significant improvements have been made in many areas. Data users know much more today than 20 years ago about how women's and men's situations differ in social, political and economic life. And consumers of data are also asking many more questions that are increasing the demand for more refined statistics. Still other areas not commonly addressed in the regular production of official statistics have only begun to be explored: the male role in the family, women in poverty and women's human rights, including violence against women.

Important in today's more in-depth approach are:

—Identification of the data needed to understand the disparities in the situation, contributions and problems of women and men.

—Evaluation of existing concept and methods against today's changed realities.

—Development of new concepts and methods to yield unbiased data.

—The preparation of statistics in formats easily accessible to a wide array of users.

None of this is easy—or without cost. Every step requires considerable efforts and expertise. All require integrated approaches that pull together today's often fragmented, specialized efforts and take a fresh look at methods and priorities—in, say, education, employment, criminal justice, business, credit and training. All require a broader, more integrated treatment of social and economic data. And all require special efforts to improve international comparability. But required above all—for true national, regional and global assessments of the social, political and economic lives of women and men—is agreement on what the key issues are and support for how to address them.

The objectives is always to produce timely statistics on women and men that can inform policy, refine strategy and influence practice. After two decades of efforts, improved gender statistics are doing much to inform policy debate and implementation. But to proved truly effective monitoring at all leaves requires continuity and reinforcing the dialogue between statisticians and the consumers of statistics—policy makers, researchers, advocates and the media.

1

INTRODUCTION

1.1 INDIA'S HISTORICAL BACKGROUND

India is one of the oldest civilizations with a kaleidoscopic variety of people and a rich cultural heritage. The river Sindhu gave India its name. In the language of the Aryans who invaded India from the northwest 2,000—3,000 years ago, the word "Indus" (which was given to the river Sindhu) meant "river" or "flood". It was first applied to the river, then to the land drained by the river, and finally to the whole country. Although it is impossible to give a full account of Indian history in a few paragraphs, an attempt is made here to briefly sum up the most important historical events that occurred both before and after India became an independent nation in 1947.

EARLY INDIA

A dark-skinned people, known as the Dravidians, are regarded as the aborigines of India, although the great variety of racial types found among the peoples is due to the many migrations into the sub-continent that have taken place during the past 5,000 or 6,000 years. In 1921, excavations in the Indus Valley at the sites of Harappa and Mohenjo Daro have shown that as early as 3000 B.C., India was the home of a civilized people, who lived in well-planned towns, practised agriculture, and were skilled craftsmen. Between about 1500 and 200 B.C., Aryan speaking tribes from Central Asia streamed into India through the Khybc er and other northwest passes. These groups eventually controlled the whole of northern India as far as the Vindhya belt of hills, pushing the original inhabitants further south in the process. They imposed their culture on the civilization they found there, and from the combined cultures arose the philosophy, religion, art, and letters that were the glory of ancient India. The Vedic texts reveal that the Aryans, in their efforts to maintain themselves in the rich plains of the Land of the Seven Rivers, waged incessant warfare on the non-Aryan tribes (the latter called *Dasa* or *Dasyu),* and extended their dominion as far as the Ganges delta to the east and along the coasts which flank the central plateau to the south. These events occupy the centuries of the growth of Vedic literature. Vedic texts refer to different tribes who achieved supremacy, the most important being the Bharatas and their descendants the Kuru-Panchalas, who later made Kurukshetra (Rohilkhand) the centre of the Brahmanic culture, and the clans of Videhas in north Bihar whose power came to an end only shortly before the rise of Buddhism (Renou, 1959).

The Buddhist texts mark a new shift of the centre of gravity toward the east, with the establishment of the kingdom of Magadha (south Bihar). Two of its rulers, Bimbisara and his son Ajatashatru, are contemporaries of the Buddha (whose Nirvana took place in 543 B.C.) and also of Mahavira. On the death of Ajatashatru, the dynasty relapsed into obscurity. The subsequent dynasty of the Nandas was overthrown by Chandragupta, who founded the first great Indian empire (of the Mauryas) around 320 B.C.

During the period when the Aryans were consolidating their hold on northern India, the heartland narrowly missed two other invasions from the northwest. The first was by the Persian king, Darius (521-486 B.C.), who annexed Punjab and Sindh to his empire. Not long afterwards (in 326 B.C.), Alexander the Great reached India in his epic march from Greece. However, his troops refused to march further than the Beas river, the easternmost extent of the Persian Empire he had conquered, and he turned back without extending his power into India itself.

It was Chandragupta who put an end to Greek rule, at least on the left bank of the Indus. At the same time, he overthrew the last of the Nandas and seized the throne at Pataliputra (Patna), consolidating his power over the whole of Northern India; With his grandson Asoka (around 260-221 B.C.), the Mauryan empire attained its greatest height. Asoka conquered Kalinga (Orissa) in a sanguinary war, and extended his power over a territory which eventually included all of India, except the extreme south and part of Afghanistan. Disillusioned by the bloodshed accompanying the war, Asoka embraced Buddhism and propagated the religion in many other Asian countries. Following the death of Asoka, the empire rapidly disintegrated and finally collapsed in 184 B.C.

A number of empires rose and fell following the collapse of the Mauryas. The successors of Alexander's kingdoms in the northwest expanded their power into the Punjab and this later developed into the

Gandhara kingdom. During the first century of the Christian era, the Kushana empire was established. The frontiers of this kingdom reached as far as the cities of Ayodhya, Banaras and Pataliputra. Kanishka, one of the Kushana kings, who set up his capital at Purushapura (Peshawar), is celebrated especially for having convened an important Buddhist council.

From 318 A.D., the great Gupta dynasty established itself in the region of Pataliputra. It assumed importance first with Chandragupta I, and later with his successor Samudragupta. Samudragupta reigned up to 380 A.D. and subdued almost the whole of India, either by direct annexation of principalities or by maintaining vassal states. His reign and those of his immediate successors saw the golden age of Indian civilization. Chandragupta II, surnamed Vikramaditya (380-413 A.D.), extended his domain still further by wars and alliances. His name has been made legendary by the memory of a magnificent court and the "nine jewels" which adorned it, among whom the poet Kalidasa is included. The Gupta empire disintegrated when the Huns invaded from Central Asia. Harsha Vardhana succeeded in establishing a stable empire at Kanyakubja (Kanauj), from 607 to 648 A.D., the last in pre-Muslim India. As a result of successful campaigns, he won recognition from the princes of north India. On the death of Harsha, disintegration proceeded still further.

The southern parts of India were not very much affected by the kingdoms that rose and fell in the north of the country, and the historical developments in this region took place more or less independently from the developments in the north. The south's prosperity was based upon its long-established trading links with other civilizations. The Egyptians and later the Romans traded by sea with the south of India and, later still, strong links were formed with Southeast Asia. Other outside influences which came to the south of India in this period included St. Thomas the Apostle who is said to have arrived in Kerala in 52 A.D.

The great empires that rose in the south included the Cholas, Pandyas, Cheras, Chalukyas and Pallavas. The Chalukyas ruled mainly over the Deccan region of central India, although at times their power extended further north. With a capital at Badami in Karnataka, they ruled from 550 to 753 A.D. before they were defeated by Rashtrakutas - only to rise again in 972 and continue their rule through to 1190. Further south, the Pallavas pioneered Dravidian architecture with its exuberant, almost baroque, style. In 850 A.D., the Cholas rose to power and gradually superseded the Pallavas. They too were great builders, and they carried their power overseas. Under the reign of Raja (985-1014

A.D.), they controlled almost the whole of southern India, the Deccan, Sri Lanka and parts of the Malay peninsula and the Sumatran-based Srivijaya kingdom.

India Under the Muslims

While the Hindu kingdoms ruled in the south and Buddhism was fading in the north, Muslim power was approaching India from the Middle East. Less than a century after the death of Prophet Mohammed, there were raids into the Sindh and even Gujarat by Arabs. Muslim power made itself strongly felt in the subcontinent with the arrival of Mahamud of Ghazni in Afghanistan. He raided northern India through the province of Lahore 15 times between A.D. 997 and 1026. It was not until 1192 that Mudim power arrived on a permanent basis. In that year, Mohammad of Ghori, who had been expanding his powers across the Punjab, moved into India and took control of Ajmer. The following year, his general, Qutb-ud-din, captured Varanasi and Delhi. After Mohammad Ghori was killed in 1206, Qutb-ud-din became the first of the Sultans of Delhi. Within 20 years the whole of the Ganges basin was under the control of the Delhi Sultanate.

Once again events took a different path in the south than in the north. The Aryan invasions never reached the south and the early Muslim invasions also failed to permanently affect events there. Between 1000 and 1300 A.D., the Hoysala Empire, with centres at Belur, Halebid and Somanathapur, was at its peak. This empire fell to a predatory raid by Mohammed Tughlaq in 1328, and then to the combined opposition of other Hindu kingdoms. Two other great kingdoms developed in the north Of modern-day Karnataka — one Muslim and one Hindu. With its capital at Hampi, the Hindu kingdom of Vijayanagar was founded in 1336. It was probably the strongest Hindu kingdom in India during the time the Muslim Sultans of Delhi were dominating the north of the country. Meanwhile, the Bahmani Muslim kingdom also developed, but in 1489 it split into five separate kingdoms at Ahamadnagar, Bijapur, Golconda, Bidar, and Berar. In 1520, Vijayanagar took Bijapur, but in 1565 the kingdom's Muslim opponents combined to destroy Vijayanagar in the epic battle of Talikota. Later the Bahamani kingdoms were to fall to the Mughals.

In the sixteenth century, a new conqueror, Babur the Mughal, overthrew the other Muslim powers of northern India. Originally from Turkestan, Babur led four expeditions through northwestern passes. In his fifth expedition, he defeated Sultan Ibrahim, the last Lodi king of Delhi, on the field of Panipat in 1526 and founded the Mughal Empire. His dominions extended over part of northern India. Akbar (1556-1605), the grandson of Babur, was the greatest of Mughal emperors. Up to this time the Mughal sway in India had been little more than a military occupation, but Akbar left to his son Jahangir (1605-27) a strong and well administered empire. For about a hundred years from the accession of Jahangir, the Mughal Empire was governed by a line of able and powerful rulers. In the reign of Shah Jahan (1627-58) the southern Muslim kingdoms of Bijapur and Golconda acknowledged the sovereignty of Delhi. In the reign of Aurangzeb (1658-1707), there was a gradual rise of the Marathas led by Sivaji (1627-80), who success fully resisted Mughal efforts to crush him and gradually extended his sway over southern India. The descendants of Sivaji in the second generation reigned only as pageant kings at Satara, and the real sovereignty passed to their Brahmin minister or Peshva, Balaji Vishvanath, who founded a dynasty seated at Poona. The Maratha power still grew, and by the middle of eighteenth century threatened every settled government from cape comorin to Bengal and Rajputana. In 1776, a terrible defeat on the field of Panipat by the Afghan invader of India, Ahmad Shah Durrani, drove them back, but the conqueror returned to his own country and the Marathas soon recovered their position.

India Under the British

The British were not the first European Power to arrive in India, nor were they the last to leave. In 1498, Vasco da Gama from Portugal arrived on the coast of modem-day Kerala, having sailed around the Cape of Good Hope. Pioneering this route gave the Portuguese a century of uninterrupted monopoly over Indian and Far Eastern trade with Europe. In 1510 they captured Goa, the Indian enclave they controlled until 1961, 14 years after the British had left India.

In 1612, the British made their first permanent inroad into India when they established a trading post at Surat in Gujarat. In 1600, Queen Elizabeth I granted a charter to a London based trading company giving them a monopoly on British trade with India. For 250 years British power was exercised in India not by the government but by the East India Company which developed from this initial charter. British trading posts were later established at Madras, Bombay and Calcutta.

The British and Portuguese were not the only Europeans in India. The Dawnes and Dutch also had trading posts. In 1672 the French established themselves at Pondicherry, an enclave that they, like the Portuguese in Goa, held even after the British had finally departed.

The stage was set for over a century of rivalry and violent contest between the British and French for control of Indian trade. In 1756,

Siraj-ud-daula, the Nawab of Bengal, attacked Calcutta and outraged the British. A year later, Robert Clive retook Calcutta. In the Battle of Plassey, he defeated Siraj-ud-daula and his French supporters, thus not only extending British power but also curtailing French influence. The victory ushered in a long period of unbridled profiteering by members of the East India Company until its powers were taken over by the British Government in the nineteenth century.

India at this time was in a state of flux due to the power vacuum created by the disintegration of the Mughal Empire. The Marathas were the only power to step into this gap. In the south where the Mughal influence had never been so great, the picture was confused by the strong British-French rivalries, with one ruler consistently played off against another. Tipu Sultan of Mysore fought a series of wars with the British. In the fourth Mysore war in 1799, Tipu was killed at Srirangapatnam and the British power took another step forward. The long running British struggle with the Marathas was finally concluded in 1803.

By the early nineteenth century, India was effectively under British control. The British followed a policy of divide and rule with great success and negotiated distinctly one-sided treaties giving them the right to intervene in local states if they were "inefficiently" run. Even under the British, India remained a patchwork of states, many of them nominally independent but actually under strong British influence. This policy of maintaining "princely states" continued right through to independence. The British interest in trade and profit resulted in the expansion of iron and coal mining; the development of tea, coffee and cotton growing; the construction of the basis of today's vast Indian railway network; the commencement of irrigation projects which revolutionized agriculture; the establishment of a post and telegraph network; and a well-developed and smoothly functioning government and civil service structure (Roberts,1967).

There was, however, a price to pay for these achievements. Cheap textiles from the new manufacturing industry of Britain flooded into India, virtually crippling the local cottage industries. The British outlawed sati, the Hindu custom of a wife burning herself on her husband's funeral pyre, but they encouraged the system of zamindars. These absentee landlords eased the burden of administrative and tax collection for the British, but contributed to an impoverished and landless peasantry in parts of India. The British also established English as the local language of administration. While this may have been useful in a country with so many different languages and still fulfils an important function in nationwide communication, it did keep the new rulers, to varying degrees, at arm's length from the Indians.

In 1857, less than half a centuly after Britain had taken firm control of India, they had a serious setback, because of the "Indian Mutiny". The Mutiny was never really co-ordinated and soon died out. It was following this Mutiny that the East India Company was wound up and administration of the country was handed over to the British government.

Two parallel developments during the latter part of the nineteenth century paved the way for the independent India: of today. First, the British slowly began to hand over power and bring more people into the decision making process. At the same time, Hinduism underwent a resurgence under reformers like Raja Ram Mohan Roy, Ramakrishna Paramahamsa, Swami Vivekananda and Sri Aurobindo. With the turn of the century, opposition to British rule began to take on a new light. The Indian National Congress, which had been established to give India a degree of self-rule, began to push for independence, under the leadership of Mahatma Gandhi. Mahatma Gandhi adopted a policy of passive resistance, or satyagraha, to British rule. The central pillar of his achievement was to broaden the scope of the independence struggle from the middle classes to the peasants and villagers. After the Second World War, when the Labour Party won the British elections, the drive for India's independence was strengthened. However, there was a divide within India along purely religious lines with the Muslim League, led by Muhammad Ali Jinnah, seeking a separate Muslim nation. Nevertheless, India finally achieved independence with a declaration by Lord Louis Mountbatten, the then viceroy, at midnight on 15 August 1947.

Independent India

With India's independence, the country was divided into two parts: India and Pakistan. Pakistan had an eastern and western region divided by India. Following partition, the greatest exodus in human history took place east and west across the Punjab. Trainloads of Muslims, fleeing westward, were held up and slaughtered by Hindu and Sikh mobs. Hindus and Sikhs fleeing to the east suffered the same fate. By the time the Punjab chaos had run its course, over 10 million people had changed sides and at least 250,000 people had been killed. An additional million people changed sides in Bengal. The final stages of Independence witnessed one last tragedy on 30 January, 1948, with the assassination of Mahatma Gandhi, who ·was deeply disheartened by Partition and the subsequent bloodshed.

The first Indian government, headed by Prime Minister Jawaharlal

Nehru, had to face a number of other problems the country had inherited from the British apart from the partition of India. One of these was the princely states, large and small, numbering about 362. The British had renounced their treaty rights and had advised all to join one or the other of the two new states. By independence, all but Hyderabad, Kashmir, Junagadh and Travancore had joined either India or Pakistan. Sardar Vallabhbhai Patel, who is known as the Iron Man of India, was largely instrumental in persuading these princely states to join the Indian Union.

Nehru's prescription against poverty was industrialization, and he established the National Planning Commission with himself as the first chairman. The Planning Commission drew up a succession of five-year plans for national development. Another major development during Nehru's time was the reorganization of state boundaries on linguistic lines in 1956. However, Bombay remained a single state with both Marathi and Gujarati speaking populations and Punjab had both Sikhs and Hindus. Within four years, however, Bombay was split into Gujarat and Maharashtra. Six years later, Punjab was divided into Punjab and Haryana.

A border war was also fought with China in 1962 in the North-East Frontier Agency (NEFA) and Ladhakh, which resulted in the loss of Aksai Chin and smaller areas in the NEFA. Following the death on Nehru in 1964, Lal Bahadur Shastri was elected as the Prime Minister of India. During his 19 months in office three issues arose: the first was a food shortage caused by a bad harvest and the growing population; the second was the Hindi crisis of early 1965, stemming from the proclamation of Hindi as the sole national language; and the third came from Pakistan. In 1965, there were clashes with Pakistan over Kashmir.

Indira Gandhi, daughter of Jawaharlal Nehru won the election in 1966, and she led India to victory in a war against Pakistan in 1971, which culminated in the emergence of Bangladesh as an independent democratic country. She faced serious opposition and unrest in 1975 which she countered by declaring a state of emergency. In the 1977 general election, Indira Gandhi and the Congress Party were defeated by the Janata Party. The new government fell apart in late 1979 and the 1980 election brought Indira Gandhi back to power with a larger majority than ever. In 1984, Mrs. Gandhi was assassinated. Rajiv Gandhi, Indira's son, was soon swept into power with an overwhelming majority and enormous popular support.

Despite his initial lack of interest in politics, Rajiv Gandhi ushered in new and pragmatic policies. Foreign investments and the use of modern technology were encouraged, import restrictions were eased and many new industries were set up. Following the November 1989 elections, Rajiv Gandhi's Congress Party, although the largest single party in Parliament, was unable to form a government in its own right. A new National Front Government, made up of five parties, headed by V.P. Singh, formed the next government. However, the new government did not last long, and fresh elections were announced.

During the election campaign tour of Tamil Nadu, Rajiv Gandhi was assassinated in a bomb blast by a supporter of the Tamil Tigers active in Sri Lanka. P.V. Narasimha Rao assumed the leadership of the Congress Party and led it to victory at the polls. With the new government, the economy was given a new boost in 1992 when the finance minister, Manmohan Singh, introduced. many reforms as part of an economic liberalization policy. Due to the failure of Congres Party in elections, an United Front government come in to existence at center under the primeministerhsip of H. D. Dewgouda in 1996 and in 1997 Mr. I. K. Gujral succeded Mr. H. D. Dewgowda.

Throughout history, even the mightiest of India's ancient civilizations did not ecompass all of the modern India, and today India is still as much a country of diversity as unity. Yet a national consciousness has developed, and ever since Independence, India has remained the world's largest democracy.

1.2 Geographic Features

Physical Characteristics

India lies between 8⁰ 4' 28" and 37⁰ 17' 53" north latitude and 68" 7' 53" and 97⁰ 24' 47" east longitude. With an area of 3,287,263 square kilometres, India accounts for 2.4 per cent of total world area. India is bounded by China, Nepal and Bhutan in the north; Afghanistan, Pakistan and the Arabian Sea in the west; Sri Lanka and the Indian Ocean in the south; and the Bay of Bengal, Bangladesh and Myanmar (Burma) in the east. India presents contrasting landscapes of mountains, hills, plateaus and plains which are at different stages of evolution. The country can be divided physiographically into regions of the Himalayas, the Great Plains, the Central Highlands, the Peninsular Plateau and the Coastal Plains (Office of the Registrar General and Census Commissioner, 1988).

The Himalayas are the highest mountain system in the world and are the youngest in age, extending over 2,500 km from east to west and from 150 km to 400 km in width. From the foothills, the Himalayas rise rapidly northward to over 8,000 metres, with snow clad peaks which give rise to several perennial rivers. From north to south, the Himalaya region can be divided into three sections: the Great Himalaya, the Lesser Himalaya and the Outer Himalaya (the Siwaliks). The Great Himalaya consists of the highest mountain peaks, which are generally capped with snow. Mount Everest (8,848 m), Kanchenjunga (8,598 m), Nanga Parbat (8,126 m), Nanda Devi (7,817 m), Kamet (7,756 m) and Chomo Lhari (7,314 m) are some of the highest peaks in this section. The Lesser Himalaya mountains, south of the Great Himalaya, have heights of 2,000 to 3,000 metres. The zone of the Siwalik range lies between the Lesser Himalaya in the north and the Great Plains in the south. It extends for more than 2,400 km from the Indus Gorge in the northwest to the river Brahmaputra in the northeast, almost parallel to the Himalayan are. The height of the mountains rarely exceeds 1,300 metres. Some flat valleys known as Duns are found between the Siwaliks and the Himalayas. These valleys are filled with deep deposits of silt and rocks brought by the swift-flowing rivers from the Himalayas. Dehra Dun is one of the major examples of such Duns.

The Great Plains, one of the most productive and densely populated lowlands in the world, extend from the Ganga delta and the Brahmaputra valley in the east to the semi-arid plains of Rajasthan in the west. These plains occupy an area of 652,000 square kilometres and are filled with alluvium of varying thickness. This vast depression, an arm of the sea that has been filled up with sediment brought down by the Indus, Ganges and Brahmaputra, and their tributaries, is constantly being replenished by silt transported by rivers and spread over the land during floods. The Great Plains are bordered in the north by two narrow belts: (i) a piedmont plain, known in Punjab as Bhabar, composed of coarse pebbles mixed with finer and extremely pervious detritus, where the smaller Himalayan rivers disappear underground, and (ii) a marshy tract, terai, where the hidden rivers reappear on the surface and cause floods. The Great Plains can further be divided into the Arid Plains of Rajasthan, the Punjab Plain and the Ganga Plain. The arid plains of Rajasthan are drained by the only river in the region, the Luni. There are a number of salt lakes in this region, such as Sambhar, Didwana, Pachpadra, and Lunkaransar Tal. The Punjab Plain, which extends from the west of Yamuna in the southeast to Ravi in the northwest, is buried under alluvium brought by the Satluj, Beas and Ravi rivers. This plain is flat and has an elevation between 200 and 240 metres above sea level. A considerable part of the Ganga Plain is occupied by the states of Uttar Pradesh, Bihar and West Bengal. The Yamuna forms the western boundary of this plain and joins the Ganga at Allahabad in Uttar Pradesh. To the north of the Ganga, the alluvial tract is subdivided into Rohilkhand in the west and Avadh in the east. Further east in Bihar, the plain is divided into two distinct sections — the north and the south.

The Central Highlands lie between the Great Plains and the Deccan Plateau. About half of Madhya Pradesh, one-third of Rajasthan and a small portion of Uttar Pradesh lie in this zone. It forms a compact block of mountains, hills and plateaus with valleys and basins of major and minor rivers. A major part of this region is forested. To the north of the Narmada Valley extends the Malwa Plateau which is bordered by the Aravalli Hills to the west and northwest. The Aravallis are crossed by several seasonal rivers and streams. Toward the south, the Malwa Plateau is bounded by the Vindhyas.

South of Narmada is the Peninsular Plateau, the largest physiographic unit, which faces the Bay of Bengal in the east and Arabian sea in the west. The maximum height of the plateau is 1,000 metres in the south but it hardly exceeds 500 metres in the north. The western Ghats (Sahyadri Hills) stand majestically along the Arabian Sea. The western Ghats are continuous, running north to south, occasionally intercepted by a few gaps or passes, such as Bhorghat, Thalghat and Palghat. There are many rivers which originate from the western slope and many others from the eastern slope. The Eastern Ghats form the eastern boundary of the Deccan tableland. There are a series of hillocks of various heights separated from one another by big gaps usually occupied by rivers from the Western Ghats and Satpuras. The whole tableland is drained by a number of rivers, the most important of which are the Godavari, Bhima, Krishna, Koyna, Tungabhandra, Cauvery, Mahanadi and Damodar.

The Deccan Plateau is surrounded by low lying Coastal Plains to the west and the east known as the western and eastern coasts, respectively. The eastern coastal plain may be divided into two sections, upper and lower. The lower section consists of deltas of rivers while the upper section consists mostly of plains lying in the upper reaches of the rivers.

The entire subcontinent is drained by numerous rivers which generally fall into two broad groups: the rivers of Himalayan origin and those flowing in the peninsula. The rivers which originate from the snow clad peaks and mountain ranges of the Himalayas are perennial whereas those originating in the peninsula at relatively lower altitudes are mostly rainfed. The most important river systems and basins in the country are: the Sindhu System, the Ganga System, the Mahanadi System, the Godavari System, the Krishna System, the Cauvery System, the Sabarmati System, the Sahyadri River System, the Pennar-Palar Basin, the Tapi-Purna Basin and the Narmada Basin.

Climate, Rainfall and Seasons

Nowhere else in the world is the monsoon climate so well marked as in the Indian sub-continent, and in no other region of similar size do so many people depend for their prosperity on climatic conditions (Stembridge, 1963). In most parts of India there are three seasons: the cold season (winter) from October to March; the hot season (summer) from April to mid-June; and the rainy season from mid-June to October. However, the country as a whole has no real winter, and the term 'cold' is a relative one. From October to January temperatures decrease, while air pressures increase from the south to the northwest of India, which is the centre of a high-pressure system. Toward the end of October, the winter monsoon winds start blowing over India from the high-pressure areas over the land toward the areas of low pressure over the sea. Except where they have crossed the sea, they are dry winds. The northeast winds, which gather moisture as they pass over the Bay of Bengal, bring rain to the southeast of India during the winter. Most parts of India receive little rain during the cold season. As the sun moves northward toward the Tropic of Cancer, temperatures rise and pressures diminish. During the hot season, the heat is intense and by the beginning of June it is almost unbearable in the plains. The southwest of India receives some rain in April and May, as does Assam, where it is of great importance for the tea crop; but with these exceptions the rainfall throughout India during the hot season is negligible.

Toward the end of May winds blowing from the south and west cause violent storms, with heavy showers, which are repeated every few days. These storms herald the southwest monsoon — the rain-giver of India — which arrives about the middle of June, when rain descends in torrential downpours accompanied by thunder and lightning. The southwest monsoon owes its origin to the very high summer temperatures over northwest India. Here the heated air rises and winds from the Indian Ocean are drawn in. The rotation of the earth causes these winds to circulate in a counter-clockwise direction, so that the winds come from the southwest over the Western Ghats, from the south in Bengal, and from the southeast in the Ganges Basin. During the monsoon season, heavy rain is experienced all over India except in the northwest. Exceptionally heavy rain is experienced in those areas in which the monsoon winds, blowing directly from the sea, rise suddenly over the mountain ranges, e.g., the Western Ghats, the Himalayas, and the Khasi Hills. The southwest winds, blowing across the Arabian sea, cause heavy rain on the windward slopes of the Western Ghats and the strip of the Malabar Coast at their base, both of which have over 2,000 mm of rain per annum. But the Deccan Plateau, on the leeward side of the Western Ghats, receives only moderate rainfall (about 1,000 mm per annum), while the belt near the eastern foot of the Ghats, lying in the rain shadow of the mountains, has 800 mm or less a year. Southwest monsoon winds blowing across the Bay of Bengal cause extremely heavy rainfall (over 2,000 mm per annum) on the windward slopes of the mountains in Assam and other northeastern states. Cherrapunji, in the Khasi Hills, and nearby areas have the heaviest recorded rainfall in the world, an average of more than 11,000 mm.

Thornthwaite (1933) has divided the country into six microclimatic regions, namely Perhumid, Humid, Subhumid, Dry, Semi-arid and Arid. According to the criteria developed in 1972 by the Irrigation Commission and the Central Water Commission, 122 districts are identified as drought-affected. It is also estimated that an area of about 1.3 million square kilometres is affected by inadequate and erratic rainfall which accelerate drought conditions. These areas cover 41 per cent of the total geographical area of the country, directly affecting one- third of the population, especially in 13 major states (Office of the Registrar General and Census Commissioner, 1988).

Western India, covering Rajasthan and the Rann of Kachch in Gujarat, is generally arid. This part of the country experiences a severe deficiency of water throughout the year. Rainfall evaporates as fast as it comes with the result that there is no retention of any moisture in the soil at any time of the year. The low ground water table results in a relatively scanty vegetation, mostly scrub. Another important area liable to frequent drought lies in the states of Punjab, Haryana, semi-arid Rajasthan, western Uttar Pradesh and Maharashtra, Karnataka, Andhra Pradesh and Tamil Nadu. Subsistence in these areas is based on irrigation. To the immediate east of this semi-arid belt, a large dry area spreads over large parts of Uttar Pradesh, Bihar and some parts of northern Madhya Pradesh, Maharashtra, Andhra Pradesh, Karnataka and the Tamil Nadu coast. Due to the nature of the soil surface, the water-holding capacity is marginally favourable for good cropping. A similar type of climatic region occurs in a narrow belt in the rain-shadow area of Sahyadri.

Sub-humid conditions are experienced over large parts of the country covering the states of Madhya Pradesh, Bihar, West Bengal and Orissa. The major rainfall occurs in the period from June to October due to the southwest monsoon while the winter rains supply moisture for winter crops. Within this belt, some areas in Kalahandi and Phulabani districts in Orissa have a scarcity of water due to the rough topography. The drought in West Bengal is caused mostly by inadequate irrigation and untimely rainfall.

In the humid climatic regions of the country, water deficiency is either negligible or quite small. The perhumid regions lie along the west coast of India, south of Goa and over the northeastern states excluding Arunachal Pradesh and the Brahmaputra valley. This type of climate also prevails over the hilly parts of Himachal Pradesh, Jammu and Kashmir and Uttar Pradesh .

1.3 Area and People

Area and Administrative Divisions

India, a union of states, is a Sovereign Socialist Secular Democratic Republic with a parliamentary system of government. The Republic is governed by the Constitution, which was adopted by the Constituent Assembly on 26 November 1949. The Constitution, which envisages a parliamentary form of government, is federal in structure with unitary features. The President of India is the constitutional head and executive of the Union. Real executive power rests in the Council of Ministers with the Prime Minister as the head. The Council of Ministers is collectively responsible to the House of the People (Lok Sabha). Similarly, in the states, the Governor is head of the executive branch, but principal decision making power lies with the Council of Ministers headed by the Chief Minister. The Council of Ministers of a state is collectively responsible to the state legislative assembly. Union Territories are administered by the President acting through an Administrator appointed by him. There is a strict division between the activities handled by the states and by the national government. The police force, education, agriculture and industry are reserved for the state governments. Certain other areas, including health and family welfare, are jointly administered by the two levels of government.

For administrative purposes, India is divided into 32 units including 25 states, 6 Union Territories, and the National Capital Territory of Delhi, which are further divided into 466 districts. The administrative units below the district level are generally known as *tahsils* in northern states, *taluks* in southern states and sub-divisions/Community Development Blocks/Police Stations in the eastern states and Union Territories.

Geographically, Madhya Pradesh is the biggest state accounting for 13.5 per cent of the total area of the country. Other large states, in order of sizes are Rajasthan, Maharashtra, Uttar Pradesh and Andhra

Pradesh. The smallest state is Sikkim (which is the only state where the NFHS was not conducted), preceded by Tripura, Nagaland, Manipur and Meghalaya. Uttar Pradesh, which is fourth in land area, stands first in the country in population size accounting for 16 per cent of the total population of India. The next largest states in terms of population size are Bihar, Maharashtra, West Bengal, Andhra Pradesh and Madhya Pradesh.

People, Culture, Religion and Language

Many countries are heterogeneous with respect to ethnic origins, languages, religions, geography and traditions, but none can match the vast scale and diversity to be found in India. The country has been called an "ethnological museum"; it is a land with a huge variety of races, religions and languages. Looking at India's cultural scene, one is generally struck by two contradictory features: the existence of diversity and unity at the same time. The endless variety is striking and often incongruous. There are wide variations in modes of dress, speech, physical appearance of the people, customs, standards of living, food, climate, and geographical features. There is no one spoken language or alphabet; more than a dozen languages and scripts appear on Indian currency notes. There is no typical Indian diet or type of dress. It is quite easy to tell the difference between the shorter Bengalis of the east, the taller and lighter-skinned people of the centre and north, the Kashmiris with their distinctly central Asian appearance, the Tibetan people of Ladakh, Sikkim and the north of Himachal Pradesh, and the dark-skinned Tamils of the south. Cultural differences between Indians even in the same state, district or city are as wide as the physical differences between the various parts of the country (Kosambi, 1981). Despite these regional variations, the government has managed to successfully establish an Indian ethos and national consciousness.

Change is inevitably taking place as modern technology reaches further and further into the fabric of society, yet it is often said that village India remains essentially the same as it has for thousands of years. So resilient are its social and religious institutions, that India has either absorbed or rebuffed attempts to radically change them. Even in fast-paced modern cities like Bombay, Madras, Calcutta, Bangalore and Delhi, what appears to be a complete change of ttitude and lifestyle is only surface gloss. Underneath, the age-old verities, loyalties and obligations still strongly influence people's lives.

Hindi in the Devanagari script is the official language of the Union. About 225 languages are spoken on the subcontinent, but there are only about 15 major languages. The main languages are either derived from Sanskrit or belong to the Dravidian family. The former include Hindi, widely spoken in north India, Bengali used in West Bengal, Urdu, Punjabi, Marathi and Gujarati. The Dravidian languages (Tamil, Telugu, Kannada and Malayalam) are common in the south of India. English is understood by many educated people.

Religion is inextricably intertwined with every aspect of life in India. There are large numbers of Buddhists, Jains, Muslims, Christians, and Sikhs but the dominant religion of the people is Hinduism. India was the birthplace of two of the world's greatest religions (Hinduism and Buddhism), and of the Jain and Sikh religions. It is also home to one of the world's few remaining communities of Parsis, adherents of the faith of Zoroastrianism. In 1991, there were about 102 million Muslims in India, making India one of the largest Muslim countries in the world, much larger than any of the Arab Middle East nations. Christians number about 20 million, Sikhs 16 million, Buddhists 6 million, and Jains 3 million (Office of the Registrar General and Census Commissioner, 1995).

Hinduism has a number of holy books, the most important of which are the four Vedas Divine Knowledge) which are the foundations of Hindu philosophy. The *Upanishads* delve into the metaphysical nature of the universe and the soul. The *Mahabharata* (Great War of the Bharatas), an epic poem containing 100,000 stanzas, tells the story of the warrior princes called the Kauravas and the Pandavas, two branches of the royal clan of Kurus who lived in northern India thousands of years ago. No one is quite certain when the epic was composed, but scholars, who give various estimates between 3000 and 1500 B.C., all agree that the Mahabharata is one of the oldest literary works known to mankind. The *Bhagavad Gita* is a famous episode of the *Mahabharata* where Krishna related his philosophies to Arjuna. The *Ramayana,* another great epic that is the mark of India's culture, consists of 24,000 verses, divided into seven cantos. It tells in the bardic style of epic lore, the story of Rama, prince and later king of Kosala. For centuries, both the *Ramayana* and the *Mahabharata* have been known throughout the length and breadth of India as an inexhaustible treasure-house of anecdotes, proverbs and sayings that have formed a continuous oral tradition. They have provided a powerful and universally identifiable source for themes in Indian literature, art, drama, dance, and song.

The caste system is one of Indian society's unique characteristic features. Historically, Indian society has been under the grip of the caste system, segregating the population into thousands of non-associating groups parted from each other by traditional barriers, which forbid common social interaction and intermarriage. The origin of the caste system is uncertain but basically it seems to have been developed by the Brahmins or priest class in order to make their own superior position more permanent. Later it was probably extended by the invading Aryans who felt themselves superior to the indigenous pre-Aryan Indians. Eventually the caste system became formalized into four distinct castes, each with distinct rules of conduct and behaviour. At the top are the Brahmins who are the priests and the traditional arbiters of what is right and wrong in matters of religion and caste. Next come the Kshatriyas, who are soldiers and administrators. The Vaisyas are the artisan and commercial class and the Sudras are the farmers and the peasant class. These four castes are said to have come from Brahma's mouth (Brahmins), arms (Kshatriyas), thighs (Vaisyas) and feet (Sudras). Beneath the four major castes is a fifth group, the untouchables. Today the caste system has been considerably weakened but it still has considerable power, particularly among the less educated and in rural areas.

More than 50 million Indians belong to tribal communities which are distinct from Hindu caste society. These *Adivasis*, as they are known in India, have origins which precede the Vedic Aryans and even the Dravidians of the south. For thousands of years they have lived more or less undisturbed in the hills and densely wooded regions which were regarded by others as unattractive areas for habitation. Many still speak tribal languages and follow ancient customs which are foreign to both Hindus and Muslims.

1.4 Economy

Since Independence, India has made enormous strides but faced enormous problems. The mere fact that India has not, like many Third World countries, succumbed to dictatorships, military rule or wholesale foreign invasion is a testament to the basic strength of the country's government and institutions. The British left the Indian economy with deep marks of stagnation. A very large proportion of the national income (around 60 per cent) originated in agriculture, and a much smaller proportion (around 15 per cent) in mining, manufacturing and the construction sector (Agrawal, 1991). The national government responded to the situation with a concerted and co-ordinated attack, in the form of Five Year Plans, starting in 1951. While short-term problems were surmounted during the 5-year period of the First Plan, the long-term problem of overcoming lost economic growth continued to be tackled by successive plans. In this process, quite a few advances have been made. The face of the Indian economy as it is today is not only much changed, but it is qualitatively a lot different from that in 1951. The presence of large stocks of foodgrains, a high investment rate, and sizeable foreign reserves are symbolic of these achievements. Despite periodic setbacks, the process of economic liberalization is well underway. There is a considerable (but inadequate) amount of capital stock, which can be of great help in rapidly adding to the productive capacity of the economy. An industrial class is quickly growing, and industries have expanded to the stage where India is one of the world's top 10 industrial powers. India has important heavy industries, such as iron, steel and textiles, as well as a large manufacturing base and a growing reputation for computer software development. All these were nonexistent some 40 years ago.

A paradox of the Indian situation is that despite overall economic growth, a large proportion of the population continues to live a miserable life, often falling far short of even minimum calorie needs. According to the estimates of the Planning Commission, 29.9 per cent of the population in 1987-88 (33.4 per cent in rural areas and 20. 1 per cent in urban areas) lived below the poverty line[1]. However, the Expert Group[2] estimated that 39.3 per cent of the country's population (39. 1 per cent in rural areas and 40. 1 per cent in urban areas) was below the poverty line in 1987-88 (Government of India, 1994). The average per capita income is Rs. 5,529 per annum for 1991-92 (Central Statistical Organization, 1993). The majority of the poor live in rural areas and belong to the categories of landless labourers, small and marginal farmers, fishermen, rural artisans and backward classes and backward tribes. These people have either no assets or assets with very low productivity, few relevant skills and either no regular full-time jobs or very low paid jobs. The Indian economy also suffers from large inequalities. In rural areas, land continues to be highly inequitably distributed. Small and marginal farmers (with operational holdings of less than 2 hectares) constitute over three-quarters of the landholders, but own only 29 per cent of the land. Large farmers (with operational holdings of over 10 hectares) constitute only 2 per cent of the landholders, but own more than 20 per cent of the land (Agarwal, 1991). In the urban areas, the distribution picture is less fully known, but inequalities are perpetuated by large-scale tax evasion and the generation of "black money". Underemployment and unemployment are another standard feature of urban economic life.

India is rich in natural and human resources. These resources have, however, not been exploited fully and are capable of greater utilization. India's economy is still predominantly agricultural, but since Independence, a concerted effort has been made to diversify the economy.

Agriculture

Agriculture is the largest and most important sector of the Indian economy. Agriculture contributed 51 per cent of the country's Gross Domestic Product in 1950-51 but in 1992-93 its ontribution was 26 per cent (Centre for Monitoring Indian Economy, 1994). Yet agriculture is the source of livelihood for over 70 per cent of the population in the country. For some time after Independence, India depended on foreign aid to meet its food needs, but in the last 30 years production has risen steadily, mainly due to the expansion of irrigated land and the increasing use of high-yield seeds, fertilisers and pesticides. India now has large grain stockpiles and is a net exporter of food grains.

The main crops are rice (with an annual yield of 75 million tonnes) and wheat (55 million tonnes), but cash crops such as cotton, tea and coffee dominate the export market. Rice, which occupies one-third of the cultivated area of India, is grown on the lowlands which have abundant supplies of water. Because rice produces large yields per acre, and because two crops of rice can often be produced annually along with one other crop on the same plot of ground, the density of population in the rice-growing districts is very high. Wheat is grown chiefly in the drier districts of the centre and the northwest. Millet is the chief food crop in those parts of India which are not wet enough for the cultivation of rice or fertile enough for the cultivation of wheat. Oil seeds, such as groundnuts and linseed, are widely cultivated on the Deccan Plateau and on the eastern coastal plain. Cotton is cultivated on irrigated land in Punjab and on the so called "black-cotton soil" of the Deccan. India is the world's largest producer of tea with annual production of around 700 million kg, of which over 200 million kg is exported. Virtually all Indian tea is grown in Assam, West Bengal, Kerala and Tamil Nadu.

There are three main crop seasons: Kharif, rabi and summer. Major kharif crops are rice, jawar, bajra, maize, cotton, sugarcane, sesame and groundnuts. Major rabi crops are wheat, jawar, barley, gram, linseed, rapeseed and mustard. Rice, maize and groundnuts are also grown in summer season.

The average annual per capita food grain production in the country in 1988-91 was 204 kilograms. The compound annual rate of growth of food grain production from 1970-73 to 1988-91 was 2.7 per cent (Centre for Monitoring Indian Economy, 1992).

Industry

The progress of industrialization since Independence has been a striking feature of India's economic development. The process of industrialization, launched as a deliberate policy under the Industrial Policy Resolution of 1956 and vigorously implemented under the Five Year Plans, involved heavy investments in building up capacity over a wide spectrum of industries. As a result, industrial production multiplied by about five times over the last 40 years. The industrial structure has been widely diversified covering broadly the entire range of consumer, intermediate and capital goods. The progress India has made in the field of industrialization is clearly reflected in the commodity composition of India's foreign trade in which the share of imports of manufactured goods has steadily declined. On the other hand, industrial products, particularly engineering goods, have become a growing component of India's exports. The rapid strides in industrialization have been accompanied by a corresponding growth in technological and managerial skills for efficient operation of sophisticated industries and also for planning, designing and constructing such industries. India's major industries include iron and steel, cotton textiles, jute, sugar, cement, paper and petrochemicals. Major iron and steel plants are located in Jamshedpur, Rourkela, Bhilai and Durgapur.

India has ample supplies of coal and more than enough iron ore and manganese to supply her growing iron and steel industries. The chief iron mining areas lie along the Bihar-Orissa border, where manganese is also mined. The major coal fields are found in the Damodar Valley of Bihar and West Bengal. Bauxite is mined along the Bihar-Madhya Pradesh border, gold in the Kolar gold mines in Karnataka, and mica in northern Bihar and Tamil Nadu.

Traditional handicrafts, made in the villages, provide employment for large numbers of people. Of these cottage industries, cotton-spinning and weaving are the most important. Silk and wool are also manufactured. Other handicrafts include pottery, leather goods, and metal goods.

In 1990, there were nearly 22 million enterprises employing more than 60 million people. About three-fourths of these enterprises were run entirely by family members without engaging any hired labour. Of the remaining six million establishments, only about a quarter or 1.5 million were industrial enterprises (Centre for Monitoring Indian Economy, 1994).

The public sector has played an important role in Indian industry. Expansion of the Public sector was undertaken as an integral part of the Industrial Policy in 1956. Government industrial operations extend from basic capital goods like steel, coal, copper, zinc and other minerals to heavy machinery, drugs and chemicals, fertilisers, and consumer goods such as textiles, hotel services, and watches. The privatization wave that swept the world in the late 1980s has not bypassed India. The Industrial Policy of 1991 limited the role of the public sector to essential infrastructure and defence and Opened up more areas to the private sector. To provide a larger scope to the private Sector, a number of changes in policy have been introduced with regard to industrial licensing, export-import policy, technology upgradation, fiscal policy, foreign equity capital, removal of controls and restrictions, and rationalization and simplification of fiscal and administrative regulations. A more congenial environment has also been established for foreign capital to seek avenues of direct foreign Investment (Datt and Sundharam, 1995).

1.5 Basic Demographic Indicators

Trends in basic demographic indicators for India are presented in Table 1.1. According to the 1991 Census, India's population is 846.3 million, including the projected population of 7.7 million for Jammu and Kashmir, where the 1991 Census was not held. India is the second most populous country in the world, accounting for 16 per cent of the worlds population. Between 1981 and 1991 the population increased by 23.9 per cent. In absolute terms, the population of India increased by 163 million during the same period, which is more than the total population of Japan. The per cent increase in population during 1981-91 was slightly lower than the per cent increase during 1971-81, which was 24.7 per cent. The average annual exponential growth rate also decreased from 2.22 per cent during 1961-71 to 2.14 per cent during 1981-91.

Population density per km2 increased from 177 in 1971 to 230 in 1981 and further to 273 in 1991. Nearly three-fourths (74 per cent) of the population live in rural areas. In 1991, the sex ratio of the population (number of females per 1,000 males) was 927, which is slightly lower than the sex ratio in 1981. According to the Sample Registration System (SRS) for 1992 36 per cent of the population are children under age 15 and 4 per cent are elderly (age 65 and above). The proportion of the population age 0-14 years declined from 42 per cent in 1971 to 36 per cent in 1992, indicating a decline in fertility during the period.

Table 1.1

Trends in basic demographic indicators

Trends in basic demographic indicators, India, 1971-91

Index	1971	1981	1991
Population	548,159,652	683,329,097	846,302,688
Per cent population increase (previous decade)	24.8	24.7	23.9
Density (Population/km^2)	177	230[a]	273[a]
Per cent urban	19.9	23.7	26.1
Sex ratio	930	934	927
Per cent 0-14 years old	42.0	39.6[b]	36.0[c]
Per cent 65+ years old	3.3	3.8[b]	3.9[c]
Per cent Hindu	82.7	83.1[a]	82.0[d]
Per cent Muslim	11.2	10.9[a]	12.1[d]
Percent Christian	2.6	2.5[a]	2.3[d]
Per cent Sikh	1.9	2.0[a]	1.9[d]
Per cent scheduled caste	14.6	15.8[a]	16.7[a]
Per cent scheduled tribe	6.9	7.8[a]	8.0[a]
Per cent Literete[e]			
Male	45.9	53.5	64.1
Female	22.2	28.5	39.3
Total	34.4	41.4	52.2
Crude birth rate	36.9	33.9	29.2[c]
Crude death rate	14.9	12.5	10.1[c]
Exponential growth rate	2.22	2.20	2.14[c]
Total fertility rate	5.2	4.5	3.6[c]
Infant mortality rate	129	110	79[c]
Life expectancy			
Male	50.5[f]	52.5[g]	57.7[h]
Female	49.0[f]	52.1[g]	58.1[h]
Couple protection rate	10.4	22.8	43.5[i]

[a]Excludes Assam and Jamnu and Kashmir.

[b]Excludes Assam.

[c]1992, SRS.

[d]Excludes Jammu and Kashmir.

[e]Based on the population age 5 and above for 1971 and 1981 and the population age I and above for 1991.

[f]1970-75

[g]1981-85

[h]1986-90

[i]1992, provisional

Source: Office of the Registrar General (1982, 1985, 1992, 1993a, 1994), Office of the Registrer General end Census Commissioner (1972, 1974, 1976, 1984b, 1987, 1995), Ministry of Health end Family Uelfare (1989, 1991, 1992a).

The religious composition of the population has not changed much during 1971-91, although there has been a slight increase in the proportion Muslim during this period. Persons from scheduled castes and scheduled tribes[3] constitnted 17 and 8 per cent of the population, respectively, in 1991.

According to the 1991 Census, the literacy rate in India for persons age 7 years and above was 52 per cent (64 per cent for males and 39 per cent for females). The literacy rate increased one and a half times from 34 per cent in 1971 to 52 per cent in 1991, but it is still very low, especially for females. Although the improvement in literacy has been more pronounced for females than males in relative terms, the absolute gap in literacy between males and females remained almost the same during the period 1971-91.

According to estimates derived from the SRS in 1992, India has a crude birth rate of 29.2 per 1,000 population, a crude death rate of 10. 1 per 1,000 population, a total fertility rate of 3.6 per woman, and an infant mortality rate of 79 per 1,000 live births. The crude birth rate has declined slowly but steadily, from 36.9 per 1,000 population in 1971 to 29.2 per 1,000 in 1992. The total fertility rate fell from 5.2 to 3.6 children per woman between 1971 and 1992, a decline over 30 per cent. The crude death rate also declined, from 14.9 per 1,000 population in 1971 to 10.1 per 1,000 in 1992. The infant mortality rate showed a substantial decline (39 per cent) from 129 per 1,000 live births in 1971 to 79 per 1,000 in 1992. Estimates of life expectancy shows that female life expectancy increased by about 9 years from 49 years in 1970-75 to 58 years in 1986-90. The increase in male life expectancy during this period was 7 years. During the last two decades, the sex differential in life expectancy has reversed; females in India now live slightly longer than males, the pattern observed in most populations.

The couple protection rate (defined as the percentage of eligible couples effectively protected against pregnancy) is 43.5, based on 1992 estimates prepared by the Department of Family Welfare, Government of India. The percentage of couples effectively protected against pregnancy increased steadily from 10 per cent in 1971 to 44 per cent in 1992.

1 .6 Health and Family Welfare Policies and Programmes

The general health condition of the people of India was very poor before Independence with a crude death rate of 22.4 per 1,000, an infant mortality rate of 162 per 1,000 live births, and an expectation of life at birth around 26 years. Nearly half the total number of deaths were among children under 10 years. India was a reservoir of smallpox and endemic diseases such as leprosy, filariasis, guinea worms and hookworms. Sanitary conditions in both urban and rural areas were very poor. The provision of protected water supplies and drainage, and preventive and curative services was totally inadequate (Government of India, 1946). The health services and programmes were based on the recommendations of several committees convened by the government from time to time. The first such committee, the Health Survey and Development Committee popularly known as the Bhore Committee), was set up in 1943 and submitted its recommendations in 1946. After Independence, the Health Survey and Planning Committee (the Mudaliar Committee), set up in 1959, worked within the broad framework provided by the Bhore Committee. Subsequently, three other committees were set up to review the various aspects of health care services in India: the Multipurpose Workers Committee (the Kartar Singh Committee) in 1972, the Committee on Health Services and Medical Education (the Srivastava Committee) in 1974, and the Krishnan Committee in 1984.

An important development took place when the country adopted the National Health Policy in June 1981. This development may be viewed as an outcome of the Declaration of Health Issues at the International Conference on Primary Health, jointly sponsored by the World Health Organization and UNICEF at Alma Ata in 1978 (World Health Organization and UNICEF, 1978). Delivery ofhealth services is mainly governed by the National Health Policy, which was approved by Parliament in 1983. Although the National Health Policy places a major emphasis on ensuring primary health care to all by the year 2000, it nevertheless identifies certain areas which need special attention. These areas are: (1) nutrition for all segments of the population, (2) the immunization programme, (3) maternal and child health care, (4) the prevention of food adulteration and maintenance of the quality of drugs, (5) water supply and sanitation, (6) environmental protection, (7) school health programmes, (8) occupational health services, and (9) prevention and control of locally endemic diseases. Active community participation has been considered to be one of the most important supportive activities for the successful implementation of the health programmes.

After India became a signatory to the Alma Ata Declaration of 1978, thereby committing the country to the goal of "Health for All" by 2000 A.D., the government started to concentrate on the development of the rural health infrastructure. This was done to provide health care services to the rural population, which had, by and large, been neglected. Family welfare services, including maternal and child health schemes, are offered though the existing network of Primary Health Centres (PHCs), sub-centres, and referral centres called Community Health Centres (CHCs), and also through Village Health Guides and Traditional Birth Attendants at the village level. According to the present infrastructure plan, there is one sub-centre for every 5,000 population, one PHC for every 30,000 population and one CHC for every 100,000 to 120,000 population. In tribal and hilly areas, one sub-centre is planned for every 3,000 population and one PHC for every 20,000 population. As of March, 1992, there were 20,719 Primary Health Centres and 131,464 sub-centres, providing health and family welfare services to the rural population (Government of India, 1994). In cities and towns, the health and family welfare services are provided through a network of government or municipal hospitals and dispensaries, and urban family welfare centres. Private hospitals, clinics and dispensaries also play a major role in providing these services in urban areas.

India was the first country to have an official family planning programme, which was initiated in 1952. However, even during the preindependence period, a birth control movement was started by a number of social activists including R.D. Karve, Dr. A.P. Pillai, Lady Cowasji Jehangir, Shakuntala Paranjape and others. A review of the eight development plans adopted since 1951 indicates that family planning as a measure of population control has been given a high priority in each five year plan (Bhende and Kanitkar, 1994). However, greater emphasis was given to family planning only after the Third Five Year Plan. Only Rs. 6.5 million were allocated to family planning in the First Five Year Plan, compared with Rs. 50 million in the Second Plan, and Rs. 250 million in the Third Plan. Planned expenditures increased more than ten-fold during the Fourth Plan (to about Rs. 2,777 million).

Since its inception, the programme has been the responsibility of the Ministry of Health. It is a centrally sponsored and financed programme implemented by the states. The programme began with the creation of a Family Planning Cell in the Planning and Development Section of the Director General of Health Services in 1952. In 1966, a full-fledged Department of Family Planning was established within the Ministry, which was redesignated as the Ministry of Health and Family Planning, and a minister of cabinet rank was placed in charge.

The national family planning programme at first adopted a clinical approach. The extension approach was introduced in 1963. This involved educating the population to bring about changes in the knowledge, attitude and behaviour of the people with regard to family planning. The approach identified several conditions needed for accelerating the adoption of family planning by the people: group acceptance of a small family norm, knowledge about different methods of family planning, and easy availability of family planning supplies and services. However, before giving a fair trial to the extension approach, the integrated approach was adopted in 1966. With this, the family planning programme formed an integral part of maternal and child health and nutrition services. It was expected that the change in policy would find wider acceptance.

The Indian family planning programme emphasized the rhythm method during its initial stages. Diaphragms and contraceptive jelly and later on foam tablets were also promoted as methods of family planning. The intra-uterine contraceptive device (IUD) was introduced into the programme as a method of family planning in 1965. In 1968, the Social Marketing Programme for condoms was introduced, under which condoms or Nirodhs are made available at a highly subsidized price. The camp approach was adopted to promote surgical methods of birth control during the early 1970s. In this same period, a community-oriented service network was developed, in which family planning services were offered as a part of the overall package of health services. The mother and child care approach, which commenced in 1977-78, is still continuing. A Programme of Social Marketing of Oral Pills was started in 1987. In 1992, the National Child Survival and Safe Motherhood (CSSM) Programme was introduced to implement a package of services combining immunization with mother and child health care interventions (Ministry of Health and Family Welfare, 1992b).

The national family planning programme has had several ups and downs. The biggest setback to the programme was during 1975-77, the period of the National Emergency. There was a sudden increase in the number of sterilizations carried out, from 2.67 million in 1975-76 to 8.26 million in 1976-77. With the change in government in 1977, a new National Population Policy was adopted and the welfare approach to the population issue was re-emphasized. The family planning programme was redesignated as the family welfare programme, and the Community Health Volunteer (CHV) Scheme was introduced.

The programme promotes responsible parenthood with a two-child family norm (regardless of the sex of the children), through the voluntary use of contraceptive methods and a variety of maternal and child health schemes (Ministry of Health and Family Welfare, 1991). Messages on the small family norm are conveyed to the masses through motivational and educational means. Imaginative use of mass media and interpersonal communication are used to increase the awareness and remove sociocultural barriers to family planning (Ministry of Health and Family Welfare, 1992a).

The long-term national demographic goal is to achieve replacement-level fertility (Net Reproduction Rate of 1.0) by 2016. As a part of this goal, the country aims to reduce the crude birth rate to 21 per 1,000, the crude death rate to 9 per 1,000, and the infant mortality rate to below 60 per 1,000 live births, and to increase the effective couple protection rate (the percentage of eligible couples effectively protected through any family planning method) to 60 per cent. In addition, the recently introduced National Child Survival and Safe Motherhood Programme accelerates the goal for infant mortality and introduces additional health goals. The programme aims to reduce infant mortality from 80 to 75 by 1995 and 50 by 2000, reduce the child mortality rate (at ages 1-4) from 41 to less than 10 by 2000, reduce the maternal mortality rate from 400 to 200 per 100,000 live births by 2000, eliminate tetanus among neonates by 1995, prevent 95 per cent of deaths due to measles and reduce measles cases by 90 per cent, prevent 70 per cent of deaths due to diarrhoea and reduce diarrhoea cases by 25 per cent and prevent 40 per cent of deaths due to acute respiratory infection by 2000 (Ministry of Health and Family Welfare, 1992b).

NOTES

1 The Task Force on "Minimum Needs and Effective Consumption Demand" constituted by the Planning Commission in 1979 defined the poverty line as per capita monthly expenditure of Rs. 49.09 in rural areas and Rs. 56.64 in urban areas at 1973-74 prices, corresponding to the per capita daily calorie requirement of 2,400 in rural areas and 2,100 in urban areas. For subsequent years, the poverty line has been adjusted because of price changes, using the price indices which are implicit in the private consumption expenditure series reported in the National Accounts Statistics. The corresponding levels at 1987-88 price levels are Rs. 131.80 in rural areas and Rs. 152.13 in urban areas.

2 The Planning Commission constituted an Expert Group in 1989 to consider the methodology and computational aspects of the proportion and number of poor in the country. The Expert Group, while retaining the concept of the poverty line as recommended by the Task Force, suggested a change in the price deflator to update the poverty line in later years.

3 The Government of India has identified certain castes as socially and economically backward and, recognizing the need to protect them from social injustice and all forms of exploitation, the Constitution of India has conferred on them special protection. Scheduled castes refer to such castes, nraces or tribes or parts of groups within such castes, races or tribes as are declared to be scheduled castes by the President of India by public notification. Scheduled tribes refer to such tribes or tribal communities or parts of or groups within such tribes or tribal communities as are declared to be scheduled tribes by the President of India by public notification (Office of the Registrar General and Census Commissioner, 1984b). A total of 1,090 castes and 573 tribes have been declared as scheduled in 1991 (Office of the Registrar and Census Commissioner, 1992).

2

SURVEY DESIGN AND IMPLEMENTATION

2.1 OBJECTIVES OF THE NFHS

The primary objective of the (National Family Health Survey) NFHS is to provide national-level and state-level data on fertility, nuptiality, family size preferences, lanowledge and practice of family planning, the potential demand for contraception, the level of unwanted fertility, utilization of antenatal services, breastfeeding and food supplementation practices, child nutrition and health, immunizations, and infant and child mortality. The NFHS is also designed to explore the demographic and socio-economic determinants of fertility, family planning, and maternal and child health. This information is intended to assist policymakers, administrators and researchers in assessing and evaluating population and family welfare programmes and strategies. The NFHS used uniform questionnaires and uniform methods of sampling, data collection and analysis with the primary objective of providing a source of demographic and health data for interstate comparisons. The data collected in the NFHS are also comparable with those of the Demographic and Health Surveys (DHS) conducted in many other countries[1].

2.2 QUESTIONNAIRES

Three types of questionnaires were used in the NFHS: the Household Questionnaire, the Woman's Questionnaire, and the Village Questionnaire. The overall content and format of the questionnaires were determined in a Questionnaire Design Workshop held in Pune in September, 1991. The workshop was attended by representatives from all the, Population Research Centers, PRCs, the Consulting Organizations,

Ministry of Health and Family Welfare, (MOHFW), International Institute for Population Sciences, (IIPS), other Indian organizations, USAID, and the East-West Center/Macro International. The contents and design of the questionnaires were based broadly on the DHS Model B Questionnaire, which is designed primarily for use in countries with low contraceptive prevalence. Keeping in view the Indian sociocultural milieu and the objectives of the NFHS, additions and modifications were made to the model questionnaire after extensive deliberations at the workshop. In addition to a standard set of questions in all the states of the NFHS, it was decided at the workshop that individual states could recommend a number of state-specific questions which would be formulated after considering the issues of importance in each state. Based on the recommendations of this workshop, the questionnaires were finalized at IIPS, Bombay. The questionnaires are largely precoded, with fixed response categories.

A pretest of the questionnaires was carried out by IIPS with the help of the PRC, Bhopal, in October, 1991. A I0-day training session for the interviewers and supervisors was conducted at the PRC. For the pretesting of the questionnaire, a total of 150 pretest interviews were completed in two villages near Bhopal and a few urban blocks within Bhopal city. After the pretest, appropriate changes were made in the questionnaires, based on the experience of the pretest. Questionnaires used in each state were bilingual, consisting of questions in both the State language and English. In each state, the entire content of the questionnaires was translated to the state language and then independently translated back to English. Appropriate changes were made in the translation of questions for which the back-translated version did not compare well with the original English version. The PRCs in these states undertook the responsibility of translating the questionnaires into the state language and pretesting the translated version of the questionnaries.

The Household Questionnaire was used to list all usual residents of each sample ousehold, plus all visitors who slept in the household the night before the interview. Some basic information was collected on the characteristics of each person listed, including age, sex, marital status, education, occupation, and relationship to the head of the household, as well as health status. The main purpose of this section of the Household Questionnaire was to identify women who were eligible to respond to the Woman's Questionnaire (ever-married women age 13-49 years). In addition, the Household Questionnaire collected information on household conditions, such as the source of water, type of toilet facilities, materials used in the construction of the house, source of lighting, cooking fuel, ownership of agricultural land and livestock, ownership of various consumer durable goods and characteristics of the head of the household such as religion, caste or tribe. The Household Questionnaire also included household birth and death records wherein all the live births and deaths that took place within the last two years in the household were recorded.

The Woman's Questionnaire Was used to collect information from eligible women—that is, all ever-married women, usual residents as well as visitors, age 13-49 years. The Woman's Questionnaire consisted of seven sections:

Section 1. Respondent's Background

Questions on age, marital status, age at marriage, and education of the eligible woman are included. if the respondent is a visitor, information about her own household is also collected.

Section 2. Reproduction

In this section, information is collected about the births that a woman had during her life. The information collected includes the total number of sons and daughters that a woman has given birth to, information about stillbirths and abortions, a complete birth history (including month and year of birth, current age, sex, survival status, and if dead, age at death for each of the live births), and information about current pregnancy and menstruation status.

Section 3. Contraception

This section collects information on the knowledge, ever use and current use of various family planning methods, intentions for future use, attitudes about family planning, exposure to family planning messages, and for current users, the duration of use, source of the method, and problems experienced with use.

Section 4. Health of Children

The questions in this section relate to births in the year of the survey as well as to all the births in the previous four calendar years. The objective of this section is to obtain information related to the health of children. The topics include antenatal care, breastfeeding, vaccinations and recent illnesses of young children. The questions are organized into two subsections: Section 4A containing questions on pregnancy and breastfeeding and Section 4B containing questions on Immunization and health of children.

Section 5. Fertility Preferences

This section gathers information on the desire for additional children, ideal family size and sex composition of children, preferred and ideal birth intervals, and husband' s attitude about family size.

Section 6. Husband's Backeround and Woman's Work

Questions related to age, education and work status of the husband as well as questions on the work status of the woman herself are included.

Section 7. Height and Weight

The nutritional status of children was measured using both weight and height/length of children under age 4 in most of the states. The results were recorded in this section of the Woman's Questionnaire. However, due to the nonavailability of measuring instruments during the first phase of data collection, the height/length of children was not measured in the first phase states. In these states, only the weight of children was taken as a measure of their nutritional status. The NFHS is the first national survey that collected demographic, health and anthropometric data simultaneously. The measurement of height and weight was a separate operation that was conducted after the individual interview was completed. All interviewers, editors and supervisors were trained in taking anthropometric measurements. For the measurement of the weight of the children, standard spring balance weighing machines (Salter scales) were used. The height/length of the child was measured using adjustable boards made of acrylic and other synthetic materials with a metal frame providing strength, suitable for measuring either the length or the height of children.

The Village Questionnaire was used to collect information on all villages covered in the NFHS. The Village Questionnaire included information on various amenities available in the villages such as electricity, water, transportation, and educational and health facilities.

In addition to the above standard questions used in all the states of the NFHS, a set of state-specific guestions was added in most of the states on issues of importance in those states. Accordingly, a set of questions on knowledge of AIDS was added to the NFHS in Arunachal Pradesh, Assam, Delhi, Goa, Gujarat, Maharashtra, Manipur, Meghalaya, Mizoram, Nagaland, Tamil Nadu, Tripura, and West Bengal. The topics covered by state-specific questions in the other states are: dowry in Bihar, age at marriage in Rajasthan, sex preference for children in Uttar Pradesh, international migration in Kerala, Green Cards in Madhya Pradesh, benefits received from antipoverty programmes in Karnataka, and sex preselection and international migration in Punjab.

2.3 Sample Design

The sample design for the NFHS was discussed during a Sample Design Workshop held in Madurai in October, 1991. The workshop was attended by representatives from the PRCs; the COs; the Office of the Registrar General, India; IIPS and the East-West Center/Macro International. A uniform sample design was adopted in all the NFHS states. The sample design adopted in each state is a systematic, stratified sample of households, with two stages in rural areas and three stages in urban areas. Detailed descriptions of the state sample designs can be found in the state reports.

Sample Size and Allocation

The sample size for each state was specified in terms of a target number of completed interviews with eligible women. The target sample size was set considering the size of the state, the time and resources available for the survey and the need for separate estimates for urban and rural areas of the state. The initial target sample size was 3,000 completed interviews with eligible women for states having a population of 25 million or less in 1991; 4,000 completed interviews for large states with more than 25 million population; 8,000 for Uttar Pradesh, the largest state; and 1,000 each for the six small northeastern states (Arunachal Pradesh, Manipur, Meghalaya, Mizoram, Nagaland and Tripura). In states with a substantial number of backward districts[2] (Bihar, Madhya Pradesh, Rajasthan and Uttar Pradesh), the initial target samples were increased so as to allow separate estimates to be made for groups of backward districts.

The urban and rural samples within states were drawn separately and, to the extent possible, sample allocation was proportional to the size of the urban-rural populations (to facilitate the selection of a self-weighting sample for each state). In states where the urban population was not sufficiently large to provide a sample of at least 1,000 completed interviews with eligible women, the urban areas were appropriately oversampled (except in the six small northeastern states).

The Rural Sample: The Frame, Stratification and Selection

A two-stage stratified sampling design was adopted for the rural areas: selection of villages followed by selection of households. Because the 1991 Census data were not available at the time of sample selection in most states, the 1981 Census list of villages served as the sampling frame in all the states with the exception of Assam, Delhi and Punjab. In these three states the 1991 Census data were used as the sampling frame.

Villages were stratified prior to selection on the basis of a number of variables. The first level of stratification in all the states was geographic, with districts subdivided into regions according to their geophysical characteristics. Within each of these regions, villages were further stratified using some of the following variables: village size, distance from the nearest town, proportion of nonagricultural workers, proportion of the population belonging to scheduled castes/scheduled tribes, and female literacy. However, not all variables were used in every state. Each state was examined individually and two or three variables were selected for stratification, with the aim of creating not more than 12 strata for small states and not more than 15 strata for large states. Female literacy was often used for implicit stratification (i.e., the villages were ordered prior to selection according to the proportion of females who were literate). Primary Sampling Units (PSUs) were selected systematically, with probability proportional to size (PPS). In some cases, adjacent villages with small population sizes were combined into a single PSU for the purpose of sample selection. On average, 30 households were selected for interviewing in each selected PSU.

In every state, all the households in the selected PSUs were listed about two weeks prior to the survey. This listing provided the necessary frame for selecting households at the second sampling stage. The household listing operation consisted of preparing up-to-date notional and layout sketch maps of each selected PSU, assigning numbers to structures, recording addresses (or locations) of these structures, identifying the residential structures; and listing the names of the heads of all the households in the residential structures in the selected PSU. Each household listing team consisted of a lister and a mapper. The listing operation was supervised by the senior field staff of the concerned CO and the PRC in each state. Special efforts were made not to miss any household in the selected PSU during the listing operation. In PSUs with fewer than 500 households, a complete household listing was done. In PSUs with 500 or more households, segmentation of the PSU was done on the basis of existing wards in the PSU, and two segments were selected using either systematic sampling or PPS sampling[3]. The household listing in such PSUs was carried out in the selected segments. The households to be interviewed were selected from the household lists using systematic sampling with equal probability. Each team supervisor was provided with the original household listing, layout sketch map and the household sample selected for each PSU. All the selected households were approached during the data collection, and no substitution of a household was allowed under any circumstances.

THE URBAN SAMPLE: THE FRAME, STRATIFICATION AND SELECTION

A three-stage sample design was adopted for the urban areas in each state: selection of cities/towns, followed by urban blocks, and finally households. Cities and towns were selected using the 1991 population figures while urban blocks were selected using the 1991 list of census enumeration blocks in all the states with the exception of the first phase states. For the first phase states, the list of urban blocks provided by the National Sample Survey Organization (NSSO) served as the sampling frame.

All cities and towns were subdivided into three strata: (1) self-selecting cities (i.e., cities with a population large enough to be selected with certainty), (2) towns that are district headquarters, and (3) other towns. Within each stratum, the cities/towns were arranged according to the same kind of geographic stratification used in the rural areas. In self-selecting cities, the sample was selected according to a two-stage sample design: selection of the required number of urban blocks, followed by selection of households in each of the selected blocks. For district headquarters and other towns, a three-stage sample design was used: selection of towns with PPS, followed by selection of two census blocks per selected town, followed by selection of households from each selected block. As in rural areas, a household listing was carried out in the selected blocks, and an average of 20 households per block was selected systematically.

SAMPLE WEIGHTS

At the national level, the overall sample weight for each household or woman is the product of the design weight for each state (after adjustment for nonresponse) and the state weight. The calculation of the design weights at the state level is described in each state report. The state weights are defined below.

Let P_i be the projected population of the ith state[4]. Let P be the projected population for all India. Then the state weight is calculated as follows:

$$w_i = \frac{\frac{P_i}{P}}{\sum_i \left(\frac{P_i}{P}\right)}, \; i = 1, 2, \ldots, 25$$

Let N_{Hi} be the number of households with completed interviews in the ith state. Then ΣN_{Hi} is the total number of households with completed interviews in the NFHS. The normalized state weight for the households is calculated as follows:

$$W_{Hi} = \frac{N'_{Hi}}{N_{Hi}} = \frac{w_i \times \sum_i N_{Hi}}{N_{Hi}}$$

Similarly, the normalized state weight for women is calculated as follows:

$$W_{wi} = \frac{N'_{wi}}{N_{wi}} = \frac{w_i \times \sum_i N_{wi}}{N_{wi}}$$

where N_{wi} is the number of women with completed interviews in the i_{Hi} state.

2.4 Recruitment, Training and Fieldwork

In order to maintain uniform survey procedures across the states, four manuals dealing with different aspects of the survey were prepared at IIPS. The *Interviewer's Manual* consists of instructions to the interviewers regarding interviewing techniques, field procedures, and instructions on the method of asking each question and recording answers. The *Manual for Field Editors and Supervisors* contains a detailed description of the role of field editors and supervisors in the survey. A list of checks to be made by the field editor in the filled-in questionnaires is also provided in this manual. The *Household Listing Manual* was meant for household listing teams, and contains procedures to be adopted for household listing. The guidelines for the training of the field staff are described in the manual entitled *Training Guidelines.*

The representatives of each of the COs and the PRCs were trained in a series of Training of the Trainers Workshops organized by IIPS at the beginning of each phase of data collection. The purpose of these workshops was to ensure uniformity in data collection procedures in different states. Persons who were trained in each workshop subsequently trained the field staff in each state according to the standard procedures discussed in the Training of Trainers Workshops. In these workshops, detailed discussions were held on the objectives of the NFHS, different aspects of the survey, roles of various organizations participating in the survey, details of each of the three questionnaires used in the survey, methods of data collection and field supervision, and guidelines for the training of the field staff.

The fieldwork in each state was carried out by a number of interviewing teams, each team consisting of one field supervisor, one field editor and four interviewers The number of interviewing teams in each state varied according to the sample size. In each state, interviewers were hired specially for the NFHS, taking into consideration their educational background, experience and other relevant qualifications. All interviewers were females, a stipulation that was necessary to ensure that women who were survey respondents would feel comfortable talking about topics which they may find somewhat sensitive.

Training of the entire field staff lasted for a minimum of 20 days in each state. The training course consisted of instruction in interviewing techniques and field procedures for the survey, a detailed review of each item in the questionnaire, instruction and practice in weighing and measuring children, mock interviews between participants in the classroom and practice interviews in the field. In addition two special lectures were arranged in each state: one on the topic of family planning at the beginning of training on the section on contraception in the Woman's Questionnaire, and one on maternal and child health practices, including immunizations, at the beginning of training on the section on the health of children. In addition to the main training, two days' training was arranged for field editors and supervisors, which focused on the organization of fieldwork as well as methods of detecting errors in field procedures and in the filled-in questionnaires.

Assignment of Primary Sampling Units (PSUs) to the teams and various logistical decisions were made by the staff of each CO, who were designated as co-ordinators. In most cases, each team was allowed a fixed period of time to complete fieldwork in a PSU before moving to the next PSU. Each interviewer was instructed not to conduct more than three individual interviews a day and was required to make a minimum of three callbacks if no suitable informant was available for the household interview or if the eligible woman identified in the selected household was not present at the time of the household interview.

The main duty of the field editor was to examine the completed questionnaires in the field for completeness, consistency and legibility of the information collected, and to ensure that all necessary corrections were made. Special attention was paid to missing information, skip instructions, filter questions, age information, and completeness of the birth history and the health section. If the problems were major, such as discrepancies between the birth history and the health section, the interviewers were required to revisit the respondent to correct the errors. If a return visit was not possible, the editor tried to establish, with the interviewer's assistance, the correct response. If either of these options was not possible, the editor designated the response as either "missing" or "inconsistent". An additional duty of the field editor was to observe ongoing interviews and verify the accuracy of the method of asking questions, recording answers, and following skip instructions correctly.

The field supervisor collected information on the village using the Village Questionnaire. In addition, the field supervisor conducted spot-checks to verify the accuracy of information collected on the eligibility of respondents. During the period of data collection, IIPS assigned one Research Offtcer to the survey in most states for ensuring the use of correct survey procedures and maintaining the quality of the data. Throughout the survey, the staff from the CO, the PRC, and IIPS maintained close contact with all the teams through direct communication and spot-checking. The objective was to provide support and advice to staff in the field and to enhance data quality and the efficiency of interviewers. This objective was accomplished by communicating data problems and possible solutions to the interviewing teams, reminding interviewers about proper probing techniques, and examining the work of the supervisors. In addition, data from the field were simultaneously entered into microcomputers, and field check tables were produced during the fieldwork to assess the quality of the data and to identify problem areas. These tables were discussed with the interviewing teams and supervisors during the fieldwork so that they could improve their performance if needed.

2.5 Field Problems

Every survey is subject to a variety of field problems that cannot be fully anticipated. Especially a survey like the NFHS, which was conducted in 25 different states of India with the co-ordination of more than 30 different organizations, can not be free of problems during the data collection. In some states the NFHS data collection went on smoothly without any significant problems. The major problems encountered in the NFHS in other states are highlighted below.

Transportation

All the data collection teams in most of the states were provided with vehicles in the field to visit the selected PSUs. However, teams in certain states, including Uttar Pradesh, Himachal Pradesh, Jammu, Assam, and other Northeastern states, experienced difficulty in reaching

PSUs located in hilly regions due to the absence of proper approachable roads. These PSUs were covered by foot or by the use of local means of transportation.

Security of Teams

In many of the states covered during the second phase of data collection, fieldwork had to be suspended for about 15 days during the communal riots in December, 1992. In Uttar Pradesh, some selected PSUs had to be replaced because of the presence of dacoits (bandits) in a village within that PSU. In Madhya Pradesh, the good offices of some local saints popular in dacoit-infested areas in Chambal were utilized to complete the data collection in PSUs situated in this area.

Household Identification

In hilly regions and in Goa, houses are not as densely packed as in other parts of India, but are scattered throughout the village. Consequently good village maps were required to identify the sample households. Perhaps because of inadequate training, maps drawn during household listing in some states were not very satisfactory. Field teams were sometimes forced to abandon the map and take the help of knowledgeable local people to trace the sample households.

Drop-out of Members of Interviewing Teams

The drop-out of *ad hoc* staff recruited for the fieldwork is common to all surveys. In some states the NFHS experienced problems with the drop-out of members of interviewing teams in the middle of fieldwork for various reasons. To maintain the quality of data, field staff who dropped out were usually not replaced at any stage, because new recruits would require extensive training which would be difficult to provide; particularly at the later stages of data collection .

Temporary Absenteeism of Households

In a few states, noncontact with some households and eligible women for individual interviews was high in certain PSUs because of temporary absenteeism. These absent households and eligible women had to be revisited at a later date so as to keep the nonresponse to a minimum.

Unseasonal Rains

Due to unseasonal heavy rains, data collection was interrupted in a few states including Karnataka, Kerala, and the Northeastern states.

FUNDS

Fieldwork in isome states was delayed because of delays in the receipt of funds by the interviewing teams.

2.6 DATA PROCESSING

All completed questionnaires for the NFHS were sent for data processing to the office of the concerned CO. This process consisted of office editing, coding, data entry, and machine editing. Although-field editors examined the completed questionnaires in the field, the questionnaires were re-edited at the CO by specially trained office editors. The office editors checked all skip sequences, all circled response codes, and information recorded in the filter questions. Special attention was paid to the consistency of responses to age questions and the accurate completion.of the birth history. In the second stage of office editing, appropriate codes were assigned for the information on occupation, caste, and cause of death, and commonly mentioned "other" responses were added to the coding scheme. One supervisor and four data entry operators were typically responsible for data entry and computer editing operations. For each state, the data were processed with four microcomputers using the data entry and editing software known as the Integrated System for Survey Analysis (ISSA). The data were entered directly from the preceded questionnaires, starting within one week of the receipt of the first set of completed questionnaires. All data entry and editing operations were completed a few days after the end of fieldwork in each state. Computer-based checks were used to clean the data and remove inconsistencies. Age imputation was also completed at this stage. Age variables such as current age, age at first marriage, age of the woman when she started living with her husband, and the ages of all children were imputed for those cases in which information was missing or incorrect entries were detected.

Preliminary reports with selected results were prepared for each state by the end of 1993 and presented to policymakers and programme administrators responsible for Improving family welfare programmes. The NFHS report for each state was prepared by IIPS in collaboration with the concerned PRCs and the East-West Center/Macro International, on the basis of the tabulation plan discussed at a workshop held at Vadodara in December, 1992. Each state-level report contains detailed information pertaining to that state on the survey design and implementation, household and respondent background characteristics, marriage patterns, fertility, family planning, fertility preferences, mortality, maternal and child health, infant feeding and child nutrition, village profile, and detailed findings on the state-specific questions if any.

The preliminary findings of the NFHS relating to the country as a whole were published in October, 1994. The contents and tabulation plan for the detailed national report were decided in a workshop held at Bombay in September, 1994. Based on this tabulation plan, tables for this national report were prepared at IIPS.

2.7 Presentation of Survey Results

In this volume, survey results are reported separately for urban areas, rural areas and total India. A comparison across the 25 States covered in the survey is also presented. For a better understanding of the state differentials, the states are grouped into six regions of the country (north, central, east, northeast, west, and south), but aggregate estimates are not shown for these regions. In the text, reference is sometimes made to "major states". In this report, the major States refer to the 17 states with a 1991 population of more than 5 million[5]. Although both usual residents and visitors were eligible for the individual interviews, the standard tables for women and children are based only on *de facto* women (those who slept in the household the night before the interview) to avoid double counting. All tables in the report are weighted according to the sample design except for Tables 2.1 and 2.2, which summarize the basic characteristics of sample households and eligible women .

2.8 Sample Implementation

Tables 2.1 and 2.2 show the month and year of fieldwork, the number of households and eligible women interviewed and the household and individual response rates. As noted earlier, the data collection for the NFHS was carried out in three phases. The first phase started in Andhra Pradesh in April, 1992 and the third phase was completed in all states except Punjab by June, 1993. The fieldwork in Punjab was completed in September, 1993. Because most of the data collection for the NFHS was done within the span of about one year, adjustments for the different timing of data cellection in different states are not necessary for the all-India estimates of demographic and health parameters.

A total of 88,562 households were interviewed, two-thirds of which were rural. The overall household response rate the number of households interviewed per 100 occupied households — is 96 per cent. The household response rate is slightly lower in urban areas (94 per cent) than in rural areas (96 per cent). The household response rate ranged between 92 and 98 per cent in every state except Arunachal Pradesh, where the household response rate was 88 per cent. In all, interviews were cômpleted with 89,777 eligible women who slept in the household the night before the household interview. The individual response rate — the number of completed interviews per 100 identified eligible women in the household - was 96 per cent in both urban and rural areas. The individual response rate ranged from 91 per cent in Arunachal Pradesh to nearly 100 per cent in Nagaland. Most of the larger states had an individual response rate of more than 95 per cent.

Table 2.1: Nunber of Households and Women Interview

Month end year of fieldwork, and number of households end women interviewed, by residence and state (unweighted), India, 1992-93

State	Month and year of fieldwork		Number of households interviewed			Number of women Interviewed		
	From	To	Urban	Rural	Total	Urban	Rural	Total
India	4/92	9/93	28822	59740	88562	27534	62243	89777
North								
Delhi	2/93	5/93	3377	300	*3677*	3189268		3457
Haryana	1/93	4/93	1033	1702	2735	1002	1844	2846
Himachal Pradesh	6/92	10/92	1036	2083	3119	9302032		2962
Jammu Region of J & K	5/93	7/93	988	1851	2839	945	1821	2766
Punjab	7/93	9/93	937	2276	3213	836	2159	2995
Rajasthan	12/92	5/93	1103	3911	5014	1019	4192	5211
Central								
Madhya Pradesh	4/92	8/92	1459	4398	5857	1476	4778	6254
Utter Pradesh	10/92	2/93	2315	7795	10110	2337	9101	11438
East								
Blhar	3/93	6/93	1088	M60	4748	1267	4682	5949
Orissa	3/93	6/93	1296	3306	4602	1143	3114	4257
West Bengal	4/92	7/92	1086	3152	4238	898	3424	4322
Northeast								
Arunachal Pradesh	5/93	6/93	144	817	961	130	752	882
Assam	12/92	3/93	1230	2025	3255	1107	1899	3006
Manipur	3/93	5/93	346	740	1086	307	646	953
Meghalaya	4/93	6/93	202	790	992	221	916	1137
Mizoram	5/93	6/93	561	526	1087	517	528	1045
Nagaland	5/93	6/93	228	832	1060	240	909	1149
Tripura	2/93	4/93	231	908	1139	221	879	1100
West								
Goa	12/92	2/93	1834	1907	3741	1559	1582	3141
Gujarat	2/93	6/93	1360	2515	3875	1344	2488	3832

{Cont.}.....

Maharashtra	11/92	3/93	1754	2309	4063	1699	2407	4106
South								
Andhra Predesh	4/92	7/92	1096	3112	4208	1116	3160	4276
Karnataka	11/92	2/93	1449	2820	4269	1442	2971	4413
Kerala	10/92	2/93	1220	3167	4387	1218	3114	4332
Tamil Nadu	4/92	7/92	1449	2838	4287	1371	2577	3948

Note: The table is based on the number of households with completed interviews and the nunber of *de facto* women with completed interviews.

Table 2.2: Household and Individual Response Rates

Household and individual response rates, by residence and state (unweighted), India, 1992-93

State	Household response rate			Individual response rate		
	Urban	Rural	Total	Urban	Rural	Total
1	2	3	4	5	6	7
India	94.4	96.1	95.6	96.2	96.0	96.1
North						
Delhi	96.7	98.0	96.8	98.1	98.2	98.1
Haryana	94.2	95.4	94.9	94.2	92.5	93.1
Himachal Pradesh	91.7	96.8	95.0	96.6	94.8	95.3
Jamnu Region of J & K	96.2	97.0	96.7	93.1	93.2	93.2
Punjab	93.9	96.1	95.4	91.1	93.0	92.5
Rajasthan	94.8	95.0	95.0	97.2	94.3	94.8
Central						
Madhya Pradesh	91.5	94.7	93.9	95.4	95.8	95.7
Uttar Pradesh	95.7	97.8	97.3	97.1	97.5	97.4
East						
Bihar	93.9	96.0	95.5	96.6	98.3	97.9
Orissa	93.6	96.9	95.9	94.6	96.1	96.7
West Bengal	92.6	97.3	96.0	93.2	97.0	96.2
Northeast						
Arunachal Pradesh	88.3	88.2	88.2	97.7	89.7	90.8
Assam	94.1	94.4	95.5	98.0	97.3	97.5
Manipur	97.7	95.4	96.1	95.0	94.9	94.9
Meghalaya	96.7	93.6	94.2	98.7	99.2	99.1
Mi zoram	92.6	93.6	93.1	94.5	98.5	96.5
Nagaland	100.0	96.9	97.5	100.0	99.9	99.9
Tripura	96.3	91.0	92.0	97.8	94.5	95.2

(Cont....)

1	2	3	4	5	6	7
West						
Goa	97.5	96.6	97.0	97.9	95.6	96.7
Gujarat	92.5	95.8	94.7	97.5	96.7	97.0
Maharashtra	89.9	96.4	93.5	94.5	94.5	94.5
South						
Andhra Pradesh	93.4	95.6	95.0	97.5	96.0	96.3
Karnataka	94.0	96.5	95.6	94.6	95.5	95.2
Kerala	97.1	97.5	97.4	96.7	96.1	96.3
Tamil Nadu	95.6	96.4	96.1	97.2	97.9	97.7

Note: The household response rate is defined as the member of households interviewed per 100 occupied households. The individual response rate is defined as the number of eligible women interviewed per 100 eligible women identified in the selected households.

NOTES

1 The Demographic and Health Surveys (DHS) programme is an international project designed to collect comparable survey data across countries on fertility, family planning, and maternal and child health.

2 The Ministry of Health and Family Welfare, Government of India, has defined backward districts as those having a crude birth rate of 39 per 1,000 population or higher, estimated on the basis of data from the 1981 Population Census.

3 In some states, an alternative cut-off point of 300 or 600 households was used.

4 The population was projected to November 1992, the midpoint of the fieldwork dates for all the states except Punjab.

5 The major, states are Andhra Pradesh Assam, Bihar, Delhi, Gujarat, Haryana, Himachal Pradesh, Karnataka, Kerala, Madhya Pradesh, Maharashtra, Orissa, Punjab, Rajasthan, Tamil Nadu, Uttar Pradesh and West Bengal.

3

Household and Respondent Background Characteristics

A profile of the demographic and socioeconomic characteristics of households and individual respondents in the NFHS for all India as well as for the 25 states covered in the survey presented in this chapter, After examining the age-sex distribution, marital status, literacy and educational attainment of the household population, the household composition and housing characteristics, the chapter discusses the characteristics of the primary respondents in the survey (ever-married women age 13-49). Information on the household population, household composition, and housing characteristics was collected in the NFHS Household Questionnaire, and information on eligible women was collected in the NFHS Woman's Questionnaire. The chapter also includes some comparisons of the NFHS results with the results of the 1991 Census and the Sample Registration System (SRS).

All usual residents of each sample household, plus all visitors who slept in that household the night before the interview, were listed in the Household Questionnaire. Some basic information was collected on each person listed including age, sex, marital status, and education. In addition, information was collected for each person on whether the person is a usual resident of the household or a visitor, and whether the person slept in the household the night prior to the survey interview. Based on this information, the NFHS household population can be defined in two ways: *de facto* or *de jure*. The *de facto* population refers to all usual residents and visitors who slept in the sample household the night prior to the survey interview, and the *de jure* population refers to all usual residents of the sample household including those who did not sleep in the household the night prior to the survey interview. The *de facto* and *de jure* populations may differ because of temporary population movements. Tables in this and the following chapters are based on the *de facto* sample, unless otherwise specified. It is expected that the *de facto* sample is more representative of women in the country as a whole because it includes all women wherever they were staying the hight before the survey. A *de jure* sample, on the other hand, would miss usual residents who were temporarily staying elsewhere at the time of the survey.

Table 3.1 presents the percentage distributions of the *de facto* and de jure populations, according to their residence status in the household. The information is provided separately for males and females by age and place of residence. In the sample households, fewer males are visitors (3 per cent) than usual residents temporarily absent (5 per cent). Some of this difference may reflect the prevalence of temporary labour migration outside of India, as well as the tendency of men to stay temporarily in group living quarters within India (such as military barracks, hostels and hotels, which are not included in the survey). Almost the same proportion (6 per cent) of females are visitors or usual residents temporarily absent. Visiting (in both the *de facto* and *de jure* populations) is more common among women in the prime childbearing ages (15-29) and among young children. This pattern is likely to result from the common practice of women returning to their parents' house to give birth (particularly for the first delivery), where they typically remain throughout the postpartum period. Thus, the survey estimates would be biased if they were based on only the usual residents of the sample households who were present at the time of the survey, because they would not fully represent the underlying population. Fertility would be particularly affected because visiting is more common among children and women in the prime reproductive ages.

3.1 Age-Sex Distribution of the Household Population

Table 3.2 shows the *de facto* population in the NFHS household sample, classified by age, sex and residence. The total *de facto* sample population is 494,939 and the sample is 26 per cent urban. The proportion urban in the NFHS sample is the same as that observed for all India in the 1991 Census (see Table 1.1).

The age distribution is typical of populations with moderately high fertility, with a high proportion of the population in the younger age groups. Thirty-eight per cent of the population is below 15 years of age and 8 per cent is age 60 or more. The NFHS child population (below

Table 3.1: Usual residents and visitors

Per cent distribution of the *de facro* and *de jure* household populations by resident status in the household according to age, residence end sex, India, 1992-93

	De facto household population				*De jure* household population			
Characteristic Age	Usual resident	visitor	Total percent	Number	Usual resident present	Usual resident absent	Total persent	Number
1	2	3	4	5	6	7	8	9
				MALE				
< 1	87.8	12.2	100.0	6645	90.2	9.8	100.0	6467
1 - 4	92.7	7.3	100.0	25021	92.9	7.1	100.0	24966
5 -14	97.3	2.7	100.0	65780	96.6	3.4	100.0	66222
15-19	97.6	2.4	100.0	24954	95.5	4.5	100.0	25515
20-24	96.7	3.3	100.0	21414	93.1	6.9	100.0	22234
25-29	96.2	3.8	100.0	19838	93.3	6.7	100.0	20439
30-34	96.8	3.2	100.0	16204	94.0	6.0	100.0	16680
35-39	97.4	2.6	100.0	15542	94.8	5.2	100.0	15969
40-44	97.8	2.2	100.0	11910	95.1	4.9	100.0	12248
45-49	98.1	1.9	100.0	10206	95.3	4.7	100.0	10509
50+	98.5	1.5	100.0	35313	96.1	3.9	100.0	36188
Residence								
Urban	96.7	3.3	100.0	67822	95.6	4.4	100.0	68595
Rural	96.7	3.3	100.0	185005	94.7	5.3	100.0	188842
Total	96.7	3.3	100.0	252827	94.9	5.1	100.0	257437

FEMAIL

1	2	3	4	5	6	7	8	9
Age								
<1	87.3	12.7	100.0	6541	90.8	9.2	100.0	6285
1 - 4	92.0	8.0	100.0	23497	92.2	7.8	100.0	23453
5 -14	96.6	3.4	100.0	60726	96.0	4.0	100.0	61035
15-19	90.0	10.0	100.0	25891	91.9	8.1	100.0	24316
20-24	87.8	12.2	100.0	23780	88.7	11.3	100.0	23182
25-29	91.8	8.2	100.0	19724	91.1	8.9	100.0	20500
30-34	95.7	4.3	100.0	15930	93.8	6.2	100.0	16214
35-39	97.2	2.8	100.0	13467	95.5	4.5	100.0	14144
40-44	97.6	2.4	100.0	10575	95.4	4.6	100.0	10718
45-49	97.9	2.1	100.0	8735	94.8	5.2	100.0	9554
50+	97.0	3.0	100.0	33105	95.4	4.6	100.0	33654
Residence								
Urban	94.4	5.6	100.0	63225	94.0	6.0	100.0	63456
Rural	94.0	6.0	100.0	178745	93.5	6.5	100.0	179599
Total	94.1	5.9	100.0	241970	93.6	6.4	100.0	243055
				TOTAL				
Age								
<1	87.6	12.4	100.0	13186	90.5	9.5	100.0	12752
1-4	92.6	7.6	100.0	48518	92.5	7.5	100.0	48419
5 -4	97.0	3.0	100.0	126506	96.3	3.7	100.0	127257
15-19	93.8	6.2	100.0	50845	93.7	6.3	100.0	49830

1	2	3	4	5	6	7	8	9
20-24	92.0	8.0	100.0	45194	90.8	9.2	100.0	45415
25-29	94.0	6.0	100.0	39562	92.2	7.8	100.0	40939
30-34	96.3	3.7	100.0	32135	93.9	6.1	100.0	32894
35-39	97.3	2.7	100.0	29008	95.1	4.9	100.0	30113
40-44	97.7	2.3	100.0	22485	95.2	4.8	100.0	22966
45-49	98.0	2.0	100.0	18941	95.0	5.0	100.0	20063
50+	97.8	2.2	100.0	68418	95.8	4.2	100.0	69843
Residence								
Urban	95.6	4.4	100.0	131047	94.9	5.1	100.0	132051
Rural	95.3	4.7	100.0	363750	94.1	5.9	100.0	368441
Total	95.4	4.6	100.0	494797	94.3	5.7	100.0	500492

Note: Table excludes persons with missing information on sex.

Table 3.2: Household population by ase and sex
Per cent distribution of the de facto household population by age, according to sex and residence, India, 1992-93

	Urban			Rural			Total		
Age	Male	female	total	Male	female	total	Male	female	total
<1	2.2	2.4	2.3	2.8	2.8	2.8	2.6	2.7	2.7
1-4	8.4	8.5	8.5	10.4	10.1	10.3	9.9	9.7	9.8
5 - 9	12.1	11.7	11.9	14.3	13.7	14.0	13.7	13.2	13.4
10-14	11.9	11.8	11.8	12.5	11.9	12.2	12.3	11.9	12.1
15-19	10.1	10.9	10.5	9.8	10.6	10.2	9.9	10.7	10.3
20-24	9·6	10.4	10.0	8.1	9.6	8.8	8.5	9.8	9.1
25-29	8·6	8.7	8.6	7.6	8.0	7.8	7.8	8.1	8.0
30-34	7.3	7.3	7.3	6.1	6.3	6.2	6.4	6.6	6.5
35-39	6·8	6.3	6.6	5.9	5.3	5.6	6.1	5.6	5.9
40-44	5·5	5:0	5.2	4.4	4.2	4.3	4.7	4.4	4.5
45-49	4·6	3.7	4.2	3.8	3.6	3.7	4.0	3.6	3.8
50-54	3·6	3.0	3.3	3.1	2.8	3.0	3.3	2.9	3.1
55-59	2·8	3.2	3.0	2.7	3.5	3.1	2.7	3.4	3.1
60-64	2.4	2.8	2.6	3.1	3.0	3.1	2.9	3.0	2.9
65-69	1·7	1.7	1.7	2.1	1.8	2.0	2.0	1.8	1.9
70-74	1.3	1.2	1.3	1.7	1.4	1.6	1.6	1.3	1.5
75-79	0·5	0.5	0.5	0.6	0.6	0.6	0.6	0.6	0.6
80+	0.7	0.7	0.7	0.9	0.8	0.8	0.8	0.8	0.8
Total per cent	100.0	100.0	100.0	100.0	100.0	100.0	100.0	100.0	100.0
Number	67833	63251	131083	185052	178804	363856	252885	242055	494939
Sex ratio[1]	NA	NA	932	NA	NA	966	NA	NA	957

NA: Not applicable
[1]Sex ratio is the number of females per 1,000 males.

age 15) is proportionately larger in rural areas (39 per cent) than in urban areas (35 per cent), which is consistent with the higher levels of fertility in rural areas.

Age reporting in developing countries is typically prone to errors due to age misstatements and preferences for ages ending in particular digits. An examination of the single- year_age_distributions from the NFHS (see Figure 3.1) indicates distortions of the data due to misreporting of age and preference far particular digits. One of the most commonly used measures of digit preference in age reporting is the Myers' Index (United Nations, 1955). This index provides an overall summary measure of preferences for, or avoidance of, each of the ten digits, from 0 to 9. Myers' Indices computed from the survey population are 48.4 and 20.2 for males and females, respectively. The corresponding indices for males and females from the 1981 Census are 64.5 and 68.0, respec-

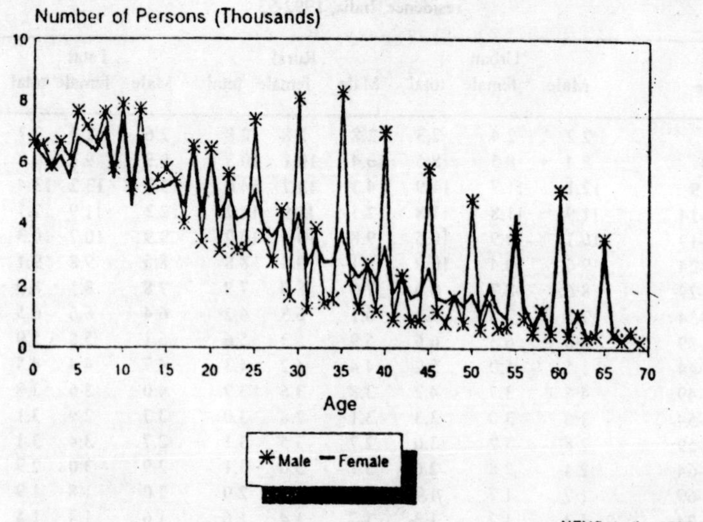

Figure 3.1: Number of Persons Reported at Each Age by Sex

tively (Office of the Registrar General and Census Commissioner, 1984c). Although the method of collecting information on the age of household members was almost the same in the Census and the NFHS. Age reporting in the NFHS seems to be considerably better, particularly for females. In the NFHS, as in the Census, the interviewer collected information on the age of household members from the head of the household or any responsible adult household member. Myers' Indices for males and females in the NFHS indicate that age reporting is much better for females than for males. Figure 3.1 also indicates that the age distribution is smoother for women in the age group 13-49 than for other females.

The better age reporting for females in the age group 13-49 in the NFHS is mainly due to the difference in the method of collecting age information for males and females in the roductive ages. In the Household Questionnaire, the ages of all males and females are reported by the head of the household or another household respondent No extensive probin techniques were adopted for obtaining age information in the household listing. For eligibly women, who were interviewed using the Woman's Questionnaire the age reported by the women herself replaces the age reported in the Household Questionnaire if there is a discrepancy Her age in the Woman's Questionnaire is based on month and year of her birth, if known, or on her reported age otherwise. A variety of probing techniques were used to elicit accurate age information from the respondent to the Woman's Questionnaire.

The age of the woman is one of the most important items of information collected in any demographic survey, because many demographic statistics, and especially fertility estimates, depend on accurate reporting of women's ages. Recognizing the difficulties of obtaining accurate age data in India, the NFHS made special efforts to minimize age reporting errors. The training of interviewers placed great emphasis on procedures for obtaining as accurate information as possible on women's ages. For women who did not know their age or date of birth (74 per cent of ever-married women age 13-49 in the NFHS sample did not know either the month or the year of their birth, several procedures for probing age were used. One method was based on the age of the woman at different significant events in her life, such as the birth of her first child, her age at marriage, her age at menarche, and on the time gap between these events. Reference calendars were also used to try to locate the woman's birth in relation to the dates of major national or local events. Although age errors cannot be totally eliminated, the comparisons with the Census suggest that probing and other elaborate measures used for arriving at the age of the eligible women have helped in reducing the biases in age reporting due to digit preference.

The distribution by five-year age groups is shown in the population pyramid in Figure 3.2. The irregular dip in the proportion of women at age 50-54 is indicative of a possible shifting of women's ages from the 50-54 age group to the 45-49 and 55-59 age groups. This is unusual, because in Demographic and Health Surveys there is usually a slight tendency to increase the age of women from age group 45-49 to 50-54, presumably to move women out of the eligible age range and reduce the workload of the interviewer (Rutstein and Bicego, 1990). Perhaps interviewers in the NFHS were overcompensating because of warnings that questionnaires would be carefully scrutinized for this kind of bias. However, the impact of the apparent shifting on the quality of data on fertility and contraception is minimal because of the small number of older women involved.

Table 3.3 compares the age distributions by sex and residence from the NFHS de jure sample with the 1992 Sample Registration System. By and large, the age distributions by sex are quite similar for the 1992 SRS and the NFHS. Only 5 per cent of males and 4 per cent of females would have to be placed in a different age group for the two age distributions to be identical. Table 3.3 also provides information on sex

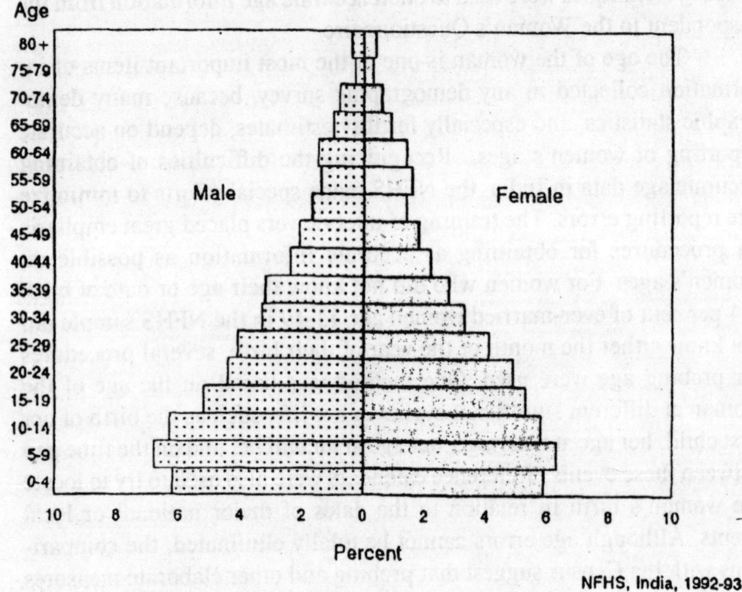

Figure 3.2 Population Pyramid of India

ratios by age for the NFHS. No sex ratios by age can be computed from the SRS published results because only per cent age distributions for the sample registration areas are given and information is not available on absolute numbers of population.

The sex ratio (number of females per 1,000 males) is an important measure that indicates the balance of the sexes in the population. The *de facto* popdation sex ratio, as shown in Table 3.2, is 932 in urban areas, 966 in rural areas and 957 for the country as a whole. Roughly comparable figures from the 1991 Census are 894 for urban areas, 939 for rural areas and 927 for the country as a whole (Office of the Registrar General and Census Commissioner, 1992). The sex ratios are consistently higher in the NFHS. The discrepancy between the two sources is 4 percentage points (38 pe' 1,000) in urban areas and 3 percentage points (27 per 1,000) in rural areas. The population sex ratio is 944 in the NFHS *de jure* sample, 925 in urban areas and 951 in rural areas (Table 3.3). The NFHS *de jure* sex ratio is higher than the Census value by 2 percentage points (17 per 1,000) and the NFHS defacco sex ratio is higher than the Census value by 3 percentage points (30 per 1,000). Since the 1991 Census and the NFHS were conducted only about a year apart, the sex ratios from the two sources should be about the same. Possible reasons for the differences observed are discussed below.

Table 3.4 compares the sex ratios of the de jure population computed from the NFHS and the 1991 Census population for India as well as the states covered in the survey. The states vary considerably with regard to the sex ratio. Tamil Nadu has a balanced sex ratio of 1,000, and the sex ratio is more favourable to females only in Himachal Pradesh (1,070), Kerala (1,068) and Goa (1,019). The sex ratio is lowest in Delhi (824), followed by Rajasthan (880) and Haryana (888).

The overall sex ratio from the NFHS is the same as the 1991 Census value for Meghalaya, 1-3 percentage points lower than the 1991 Census value for Orissa, Rajasthan, and Madhya Pradesh, and higher than the Census value for the remaining states (by less than one percentage point in Andhra Pradesh to more than 11 percentage points in Arunachal Pradesh). It should be noted that in both the NFHS and the 1991 Census, Kerala and Himachal Pradesh have the highest sex ratio and Delhi has the lowest sex ratio. These extreme values are probably due to the selective out-migration of males from Kerala and Himachal Pradesh and the selective in-migration of males to Delhi. Sampling error in the NFHS does not account for the observed difference in sex ratios between the two sources, because the NFHS sample is fairly large. In fact, the sampling error for the *de facto* sex ,tie from the NFHS is only 3.1, yielding a confidence interval of 951-963. Even the lowest value in this range is considerably higher than the Census values. Moreover, both urban and rural sex ratios are higher in the NFHS than in the 1991 Census, suggesting a systematic rather than a random pattern of differences.

The observed differences in the sex ratios between the census and the NFHS in most states can be partly attributed to differences in the two data sources. One difference between the two sources of data is the population coverage. The census includes institutional and homeless persons, who are overwhelmingly male, whereas the NFHS excludes such persons. Aside from the difference in the coverage, the discrepancies in population sex ratios between the NFHS and the 1991 Census could have occurred if the NFHS missed males more than females, or if the census missed females more than males, or if both occurred. It seems highly unlikely that the NFHS missed more males than females because the underenumeration of females is typically more common in India. Moreover, training and supervision of interviewers was much more thorough in the NFHS than in the census. Therefore, the most likely source of the discrepancy in the estimated sex ratio is relative underenumeration of females in the 1991 Census, a possibility that has been mentioned by

Premi (1991), among others. According to post-enumeration checks, Indian censuses have consistently underenumerated females more than males, although the gap has been closing with each successive census. Because of the possible relative underenumeration of females in the 1991 Census, the difference in sex ratio estimates should not be taken as evidence that the NFHS is unrepresentative of the underlying population, especially since other comparisons generally indicate reasonable agreement between the 1992-93 NFHS and other sources of data.

Table 3.3
population by age and.sex from the NFHS and SRS

Per cent distribution of the de jure population by age end sex from NFHS and Sample Registration System (SRS), India, 1992-93

	NFHS (1992-93)			SRS (1992)	
Age	*Male*	*Female*	*Sex ratio*	*Mail*	*Female*
			URBAN		
0-4	10.4	10.7	952	11.1	11.3
5-9	11.9	11.8	914	11.2	11.2
10-14	11.8	11.7	917	10.6	10.6
15-19	10.1	10.5	960	10.3	10.2
20-24	9.6	10.1	975	9.9	10.7
25-29	8.5	8.9	967	9.1	9.2
30-34	7.3	7.3	931	8.2	7.9
35-39	6.9	6.6	886	6.9	6.5
40-44	5.6	4.9	815	5.7	5.4
45-49	4.7	4.0	802	4.7	4.4
50-54	3.6	3.1	793	3.9	3.5
55-59	2.9	3.2	1040	2.9	2.9
60-64	2.4	2.8	1058	2.1	2.2
65-69	1.7	1.7	937	1.4	1.7
70+	2.5	2.5	914	1.8	2.3
Total	100.0	100.0	925	100.0	100.0
Medium age	22.7	22.3	NA	U	U
			RURAL		
0-4	12.9	12.8	944	13.8	13.5
5-9	14.0	13.7	930	12.1	11.9
10-14	12.4	12.0	917	11.4	11.1
15-19	9.8	9.8	950	11.0	10.2
20-24	8.3	9.3	1071	9.6	9.7
25-29	7.7	8.3	1017	7.7	7.8
30-34	6.2	6.4	990	6.7	6.8
35-39	6.0	5.5	886	5.8	5.9

{Cont}.........

40-44	4.5	4.2	902	4.9	5.0
45-49	3.9	3.9	956	4.3	4.5
50-54	3.2	2.9	864	3.6	3.7
55-59	2.7	3.5	1253	3.2	3.2
60-66	3.1	3.0	922	2.3	2.4
65-69	2.1	1.8	826	1.8	2.0
70+	3.3	2.7	791	2.0	2.3
Total	100.0	100.0	951	100.0	100.0
			TOTAL		
Indian age	20.3	20.6	NA	U	U
0-4	12.2	12.2	946	13.2	13.0
5-9	13.5	13.2	926	11.9	11.8
10-14	12.2	11.9	917	11.2	11.0
15-19	9.9	10.0	953	10.9	10.2
20-24	8.6	9.5	1043	9.7	9.9
25-29	7.9	8.4	1003	8.1	8.1
30-34	6.5	6.7	972	7.0	7.1
35-39	6.2	5.8	886	6.0	6.1
40-44	4.8	4.4	875	5.0	5.0
45-49	4.1	3.9	909	4.4	4.5
50-54	3.3	2.9	844	3.7	3.7
55-59	2.7	3.5	1193	3.1	3.1
60-64	2.9	3.0	952	2.2	2.3
65-69	2.0	1.8	851	1.7	1.9
70+	3.1	2.7	818	1.9	2.3
Total	100.0	100.0	944	100.0	100.0
Medium age	20.8	20.9	NA	U	U

NA: Not applicable.
U: Not available.
Source for SRS: Office of the Registrar General (1994).

3.2 Marital Status

The NFHS gathered information on the marital status of all household members age 6 years and over. Table 3.5 shows the marital status distribution of the *de facto* household population by age and sex according to residence. Among females age 6 or more years, 54 per cent are currently married and 37 per cent have never been married. The percentage never married is higher for males (48 per cent) than for females. The percentage of females never married is lower in rural areas (35 per cent) than in urban areas (39 per cent). Percentages currently divorced and separated are small, regardless of age, sex, or type of place of residence.

Table 3.4: Sex Ratio
Sex ratio of the *dr jure* NFHS household population and the 1991 Census population, by residence end state, India, 1991-93

	NFHS (1992-93)			Census (1991)		
State	*Urban*	*Rural*	*Total*	*Urban*	*Rural*	*Total*
India	925	951	944	894	939	927
North						
Delhi	828	763	824	830	807	808
Haryana	895	886	888	868	864	865
Himachal Pradesh	945	1084	1070	831	990	976
Jamnu Region of J & K	965	983	980	U	U	U
Punjab	927	906	912	868	888	882
Rajasthan	885	879	880	879	919	910
Central						
Madhya Pradesh	923	901	906	893	941	911
Uttar Pradesh	903	921	917	860	884	879
East						
Bihar	893	968	956	844	921	911
Orissa	907	974	963	866	988	971
West Bengal	876	969	940	858	940	917
Northeast						
Arunachal Pradesh	920	980	973	728	880	859
Assam	899	953	947	838	934	923
Manipur	999	981	987	975	951	958
Meghalaya	976	949	955	910	966	955
Mizoram	983	989	986	932	912	921
Nagaland	1007	987	991	749	917	886
Tripura	997	988	989	958	942	945
West						
Goa	1000	1035	1019	930	993	967
Gujarat	912	962	944	907	949	934
Maharashtra	937	988	966	875	972	934
South						
Andhra Pradesh	969	983	979	959	977	972
Karnataka	968	971	970	930	973	960
Kerala	1070	1067	1068	1034	1037	1036
Tamil Nadu	996	1001	1000	960	981	974

Note: Sex ratio is the number of females per 1,000 males.
U: Not available
Source for Census: Office of the Registrar General and Census Commissioner (1992)

The percentage widowed is also quite small except in the older ages. Forty-seven per cent of women age 60-64, one-half of women age 65-69, and three-quarters of women age 70 or over are widows. The corresponding percentages among males are 12, 13 and 25, respectively. The higher percentage of older women than men who are widowed reflects sex differentials in age at marriage, longevity, and remarriage rates.

Of interest from the point of view of fertility trends is the proportion of persons (especially females) who marry young. Marriage is rare for either males or females under age 15. At age 15-19, 7 per cent of males and 39 per cent of females have married. By age 25-29, marriage is nearly universal for females and the proportion of males ever married reaches 76 per cent. Overall, women marry at much younger ages than men, and both men and women marry at much younger ages in rural areas than in urban areas. Nearly one-quarter of women in their child-bearing years (age 15-49) are not currently married. This is one of the major factors that has depressed the level of fertility in India. A more detailed discussion of marriage patterns is contained in the next chapter, which is devoted entirely to the topic of nuptiality.

3.3 Household Composition

Table 3.6 shows the per cent distribution of households by various characteristics of the household head (sex, age, marital status, religion and caste/tribe), as well as the number of usual household members. Ninety-one per cent of household heads are male, and proportionately slightly more female headed households are found in urban than in rural areas. The median age of household heads is one year younger in urban areas (44 years) than in rural areas (45 years). There is a greater concentration of household heads in the age group 30-49 in urban areas (54 per cent) than in rural areas (48 per cent). On the other hand, the proportion of household heads age 60 and above is higher in rural areas (22 per cent) than in urban areas (17 per cent). This pattern may reflect underlying differences in household composition, for example, whether the oldest generation is present in the household. As shown earlier, rural areas have a slightly higher proportion of old age population than urban areas, especially for males (Table 3.2).

Table 3.5: Marital status of the household population
Per cent distribution of the *de facto* household population age, 6 and above by marital status, according to age, sex and residence, India, 1992-93

Age	Marital Status						
	Never married	*Currently married*	*Widowed*	*Divorced*	*Separated*	*DK/ missing*	*Total per cent*
	1	*2*	*3*	*4*	*5*	*6*	*7*
				URBAN			
				Mail			
6-9	99.1	0.3	0.2	--	0.1	0.3	100.0
10-12	99.5	0.2	0.1	--	0.1	0.1	100.0
13-14	99.6	0.2	0.1	--	0.1	--	100.0
15-19	97.3	2.5	0.1	--	0.1	--	100.0
20-24	75.1	24.1	0.3	0.2	0.4	--	100.0
25-29	35.0	63.9	0.4	0.2	0.5	--	100.0
30-34	10.4	88.2	0.6	0.2	0.5	--	100.0
35-39	4.5	94.3	0.8	0.1	0.4	--	100.0
40-44	2.5	96.0	0.9	0.2	0.4	--	100.0
45-49	1.8	96.1	1.6	0.2	0.4	--	100.0
50-54	1.2	93.5	4.8	0.1	0.3	--	100.0
55-59	1.2	92.3	6.3	0.1	0.1	--	100.0
60-64	1.8	87.9	9.3	0.3	0.7	--	100.0
65-69	1.8	85.9	11.4	0.1	0.8	--	100.0
70+	2.6	73.6	23.1	0.2	0.4	--	100.0
6+	49.3	48.3	1.9	0.1	0.3	--	100.0
15-59	4.7	58.3	0.6	0.1	0.4	--	100.0
				Female			
6-9	99.1	0.4	0.1	--	0.1	0.3	100.0
10~2	99.4	0.3	0.1	--	--	0.1	100.0
13-14	97.9	2.1	--	--	--	--	100.0
15-19	78.3	21.1	0.1	0.2	0.3	--	100.0
20-24	31.8	66.3	0.5	0.2	1.2	--	100.0
25-29	9.1	87.9	1.4	0.4	1.3	--	100.0
30-34	3.2	91.7	2.8	0.6	1.7	--	100.0
35-39	1.8	92.4	4.7	0.2	1.0	--	100.0
40-44	1.9	88.4	8.2	0.3	1.3	--	100.0
45-49	1.4	83.6	13.7	0.3	1.1	--	100.0
50-54	0.9	75.1	22.7	0.3	1.0	--	100.0
55-59	0.7	65.8	32.0	0.4	1.1	--	100.0
60-64	0.9	47.6	50.1	0.3	1.0	0.1	100.0
65-69	1.3	43.8	54.3	0.3	0.3	--	100.0
70+	1.3	19.7	77.6	0.5	0.7	0.1	100.0
6+	39.4	50.8	8.8	0.2	0.8	0.1	100.0
15-59	25.1	70.5	3.1	0.3	1.1	--	100.0
6-9	99.1	0.3	0.1	--	0.1	0.4	100.0

{Cont.}

	1	2	3	4	5	6	7
			RURAL **Male**				
10-12	99.2	0.5	0.1	--	0.1	0.1	100.0
13-14	98.7	1.1	--	--	0.1	--	100.0
15-19	91.8	7.8	0.1	0.1	0.1	0.1	100.0
20-24	56.2	42.6	0.5	0.2	0.5	--	100.0
25-29	19.7	78.8	0.7	0.1	0.6	--	100.0
30-34	6.1	92.0	1.0	0.2	0.6	0.1	100.0
35-39	2.6	94.8	1.7	0.2	0.6	0.1	100.0
40-44	1.9	95.0	2.4	0.1	0.6	--	100.0
45-49	1.4	94.5	3.4	0.1	0.6	--	100.0
50-54	1.5	91.7	6.1	0.1	0.6	--	100.0
55-59	1.7	89.4	8.2	0.2	0.5	--	100.0
60-64	1.8	85.3	12.2	0.1	0.5	0.1	100.0
65-69	1.8	83.4	14.0	0.2	0.6	--	100.0
70+	1.6	71.9	25.9	0.2	0.4	--	100.0
6+	47.0	49.5	2.9	0.1	0.4	0.1	100.0
15-49	34.3	63.9	1.1	0.1	0.5	--	100.0
			RURAL **Female**				
6-9	98.8	0.4	03	--	0.1	0.3	100.0
10-12	98.8	0.9	0.1	--	0.1	0.1	100.0
13-14	93.8	6.1	--	--	0.1	--	100.0
15-19	54.6	44.4	0.2	0.1	0.7.	--	100.0
20-24	13.2	84.5	0.8	0.2	1.2	--	100.0
25-29	2.9	93.5	1.6	0.3	1.6	--	100.0
30-34	1.3	93.5	3.2	0.5	1.6	--	100.0
35-39	0.7	92.2	5.3	0.3	1.6	--	100.0
40-44	0.6	88.9	8.6	0.2	1.7	--	100.0
45-49	0.5	86.4	11.6	0.3	1.2	--	100.0
50-54	0.5	76.8	21.4	0.2	1.0	0.1	100.0
55-59	0.3	72.1	26.4	0.2	1.0	0.1	100.0
60-64	0.6	52.5	45.9	0.2	0.5	0.2	100.0
65-69	0.6	47.6	50.8	0.2	0.6	0.2	100.0
70+	0.6	22.6	75.9	0.4	0.5	--	100.0
6+	35.4	54.6	8.8	0.2	0.9	0.1	100.0
15-49	15.7	79.6	3.1	0.3	1.3	--	100.0
			TOTAL **Male**				
6-9	99.1	0.3	0.1	—	0.1	0.3	100.0

{Cont}.....

	1	2	3	4	5	6	7
10-12	99.3	0.4	0.1	—	0.1	0.1	100.0
13-14	99.0	0.8	—	—	0.1	--	100.0
15-19	93.3	6.3	0.1	0.1	0.1	0.1	100.0
20-24	61.9	37.0	0.4	0.2	0.4	--	100.0
25-29	24.2	74.4	0.6	0.1	0.6	--	100.0
30-34	7.4	90.9	0.9	0.2	0.6	0.1	100.0
35-39	3.1	94.6	1.4	0.2	0.6	--	100.0
40-44	2.0	95.3	1.P	0.1	0.5	--	100.0
45-49	1.5	95.0	2.9	0.1	0.5	--	100.0
50-54	1.4	92.2	5.7	0.1	0.5	0.1	100.0
55-59	1.6	90.2	7.7	0.2	0.4	--	100.0
60-64	1.8	85.9	11.6	0.2	0.5	--	100.0
65-69	1.8	84.0	13.4	0.1	0.6	0.1	100.0
70+	1.8	72.3	25.3	0.1	0.4	--	100.0
6+	35.4	54.6	8.8	0.2	0.9	0.1	100.0
15-49	36.2	62.2	0.9	0.1	0.4	--	100.0
				Female			
6-9	98.9	0.4	0.2	--	0.1	0.3	100.0
10-12	99.0	0.7	0.1	--	--	0.1	100.0
13-14	94.9	5.0	--	--	--	--	100.0
15-19	60.9	38.2	0.2	0.1	0.6	--	100.0
20-24	18.3	79.5	0.7	0.2	1.2	--	100.0
25-29	4.6	91.9	1.6	0.3	1.5	--	100.0
30-34	1.8	93.0	3.1	0.5	1.6	--	100.0
35-39	1.0	92.2	5.1	0.3	1.4	--	100.0
40-44	0.9	88.8	8.5	0.2	1.6	--	100.0
45-49	0.8	85.6	12.2	0.3	1.2	--	100.0
50-54	0.6	76.3	21.8	0.3	1.0	--	100.0
55-59	0.4	70.5	27.8	0.3	1.0	0.1	100.0
60-64	0.7	51.3	46.9	0.2	0.6	0.2	100.0
65-69	0.8	46.6	51.7	0.2	0.5	0.2	100.0
70+	0.7	21.9	76.3	0.4	0.6	0.1	100.0
6+	36.553.6	8.8	0.2	0.9	0.1	100.0	
15-49	18.377.1	3.1	0.3	1.2	--	100.0	

DK: Don't know.

-- Less than 0.05 per cent.

Table 3.6 Household Composition

Per cent distribution of households by selected characteristics of household head and household size according to residence, India, 1992-93

Characteristic	Residence		
	Urban	Rural	Total
1	2	3	4
Sex of household head			
Male	90.4	90.9	90.8
Female	9.6	9.1	9.2
Age of household head			
< 20	0.3	0.7	0.6
20-24	2.6	3.1	2.9
25-29	7.5	8.5	8.3
30-34	11.8	11.2	11.4
35-39	14.9	13.9	14.2
40-44	14.1	12.0	12.5
45-49	12.7	11.1	11.6
50-54	10.4	9.3	9.6
55-59	8.4	7.9	8.0
60+	17.2	22.3	20.9
Median age	44.2	45.1	45.0
Marital status of household head			
Never married	2.6	2.1	23
Currently married	86.9	86.5	86.6
Widowed	9.6	1.4	10.1
Divorced	0.2	0.2	0.2
Separated	0.7	0.8	0.8
Religion of household head			
Hindu	76.7	84.5	82.3
Muslim	15.4	9.9	11.4
Christian	3.2	2.5	2.7
Sikh	1.8	1.9	1.8
Jain	1.3	0.2	0.5
Buddhist	1.3	0.7	0.8
Other	0.3	0.5	0.4
Caste/tribe of household head			
Scheduled caste	9.1	13.9	12.6
Scheduled tribe	3.3	11.3	12.6
Other	87.6	74.8	78.3
Number of usual memebrs			
1	3.3	2.6	2.8

{Cont.....}

1	2	3	4
2	7.1	7.3	7.2
3	11.3	10.3	10.5
4	18.6	15.5	16.1
5	18.7	17.9	18.2
6	14.7	15.1	15.3
7	9.8	11.1	10.7
8	6.1	7.0	6.8
9+	10.4	13.2	12.4
Mean size	5.4	5.7	5.7
Total per cent	100.0	100.0	100.1
Number of households	24424	64138	88562

Eighty-seven per cent of household heads are currently married, regardless of place of residence. Only 2 per cent of the household heads have never been married and 11 per cent of the household heads are widowed, divorced or separated.

Table 3.6 also shows that 82 per cent of household heads are Hindus, 11 per cent are Muslims, and another 3 percent are Christians. Sikhs constitute 2 per cent of household heads and Jains, Buddhists and others constitute less than 1 per cent each. The religious composition of the household heads in the NFHS is similar to that of the population observed in the 1991 Census (see Table 1.1). The percentage Muslim is higher in urban areas (15 per cent of household heads) than in rural areas (10 per cent). Households with Christian, Jain and Buddhist heads are also more concentrated in urban areas. Thirteen per cent of household heads are classified as belonging to scheduled castes and 9 per cent are members of scheduled tribes. Both groups (especially the scheduled tribes) are disproportionately concentrated in rural areas. According to the 1991 Census, the percentages of the population belonging to scheduled castes and scheduled tribes in India are 17 and 8 per cent, respectively (see Table 1.1). The mean NFHS household size is 5.7 persons per household. The average household size is slightly higher in rural areas than in urban areas.

States differ greatly in terms of the religion and caste/tribe of household heads (Table 3.7). A large majority of household heads are Hindus in 20 of the 25 states. More than one- fourth of the household heads in Assam and 21 per cent in West Bengal are Muslims. The percentage of Muslim household heads is 19 per cent in Kerala, 17 per cent in Jammu, 16 per cent each in Uttar Pradesh and Bihar, and 11 per cent each in Maharashtra and Karnataka. No other state has more than 10 per cent of Muslim households. Christians head more than 93 per cent of households in Mizoram and Nagaland, 76 per cent in Meghalaya, 31 per cent in Goa, 29 per cent in Manipur, 22 per cent in Kerala and 15 per cent in Arunachal Pradesh. In the other states, the proportion of Christian household heads is 6 per cent or less. Sikhs are concentrated primarily in Punjab, where they constitute 58 per cent of household heads. Interestingly, 38 per cent of the household heads in Arunachal Pradesh and 12 per cent in Meghalaya profess "other" religions. The 1991 Census also found a high proportion of the population in the "other" religious group in Arunachal Pradesh and Meghalaya — 36 and 17 per cent, respectively (Office of the Registrar General and Census Commissioner, 1995).

Between 21 and 30 per cent of the households in Jammu, Haryana, Punjab, Himachal Pradesh and Rajasthan belong to scheduled castes. Scheduled castes are also concentrated in Tamil Nadu, Uttar Pradesh, Andhra Pradesh and Karnataka where they constitute 12-20 per cent of household heads. No scheduled caste households were identified in Arunachal Pradesh, Manipur, Mizoram and Nagaland. Similarly, Haryana and Punjab do not have scheduled tribes. Scheduled tribes are more concentrated in the northeastern states, particularly in Mizoram, Nagaland, Meghalaya, and Arunachal Pradesh (where more than three-fourths of household heads belong to scheduled tribes). Scheduled tribes constitute 29 per cent of the households in Manipur, 28 per cent in Madhya Pradesh and 24 per cent in Orissa.

3.4 Educational Attainment

The educational level of household members is an important characteristic because educational attainment can affect reproductive behaviour, the use of contraceptives, the health of children, proper hygienic practices and the status of women. Table 3.8 shows the extent of literacy and the level of educational attainment among the male and female household population age 6 and above by age and residence 57 per cent of females age 6 and above and 31 per cent of males are illiterate. The 1992-93 levels of illiteracy in the NFHS for the population age 6 and above are somewhat lower than the 1991 Census figures of 61 per cent for females and 36 per cent for males for the population age 7 and above (see Table 1.1). In the NFHS, a higher per centage of males than females have completed each level of schooling. While only 9 per cent of females have at least a high school education, 20 per cent of males have completed at least high school. The median number of years of school-

Table 3.7 Religion and caste/tribe of household head
Per cent distribution of households by religion and caste/tribe of the household head, according to state, India, 1992-93

	Religion of household								Caste/tribe of household head			
State	Hindu	Muslim	Cristian	Sikh	Jain	Buddhist	other	Total percent	Scheduled caste	scheduled tribe	Total Other	per cent
India	82.3	11.4	2.7	1.8	0.5	0.8	0.4	100.0	12.6	9.1	78.3	100.0
North												
Delhi	82.4	9.7	1.0	5.3	1.3	0.1	0.1	100.0	5.0	0.9	94.1	100.0
Haryana	88.4	4.3	0.1	6.9	0.3	0.1	0.1	100.0	28.3	–	71.6	100.0
Himachal Pradesh	96.8	1.3	0.1	0.8	–	0.2	0.8	100.0	23.4	5.7	70.8	100.0
Jammu Region of J&K	77.2	17.0	0.2	5.7	–	–	–	100.0	30.2	0.9	68.9	100.0
Punjab	39.7	1.2	1.5	57.5	0.1	–	0.1	100.0	28.0	–	72.0	100.0
Rajasthan	92.3	5.5	0.3	1.0	0.7	–	0.2	100.0	20.7	17.3	62.0	100.0
Central												
Madhya Pradesh	93.0	4.9	0.7	0.2	0.7	0.2	0.2	100.0	7.2	27.5	65.3	100.0
Uttar Ptadesh	82.9	15.8	0.1	0.6	0.3	0.1	0.2	100.0	18.0	1.1	80.9	100.0
East												
Bihar	82.1	15.7	0.9	0.2	0.1	0.2	0.8	100.0	9.8	8.6	81.6	100.0
Orissa	96.7	1 5	1.5	0.1	–	–	0.2	100.0	9.5	23.9	66.6	100.0
West Bengal	77.2	20.7	0.6	–	0.1	0.5	0.9	100.0	8.7	4.8	86.5	100.0
Northeast												
Arunachal Pradesh	36.7	0.8	15.0	0.3	–	9.3	37.9	100.0	–	76.1	23.9	100.0

Assam	69.3	26.1	4.2	0.3	0.1	–	–	100.0	4.1	16.0	79.9	100.0
Manipur	60.2	5.4	28.5	0.1	0.1	–	5.6	100.0	–	28.7	71.3	100.0
Meghalaya	9.4	2.4	76.0	–	–	0.3	11.9	100.0	0.2	88.9	10.9	100.0
Mizoram	2.3	0.7	95.5	–	0.1	1.4	–	100.0	–	97.1	2.9	100.0
Nagaland	4.8	0.8	93.2	–	0.4	–	0.8	100.0	–	95.8	4.2	100.0
Tripura	86.4	8.4	2.7	–	0.1	2.4	–	100.0	0.6	16.5	82.9	100.0
West												
Goa	64.0	4.7	30.9	0.1	0.1	0.1	0.1	100.0	2.2	1.8	96.0	100.0
Gujarat	89.5	8.5	0.5	0.1	1.2	0.2	0.1	100.0	5.8	14.9	79.3	100.0
Maharashtra	77.3	11.1	1.0	0.2	1.8	7.7	1.0	100.0	6.6	10.0	83.4	100.0
South												
Andhra Pradesh	87.7	8.4	3.7	0.1	–	–	–	100.0	14..9	6.0	79.1	100.0
Karnataka	86.3	10.6	2.2	–	0.7	–	0.2	100.0	11.9	5.7	82.4	100.0
Kerala	58.3	19.1	22.3	0.1	–	–	0.2	100.0	3.6	3.6	92.8	100.0
Tamil Nadu	88.1	5.4	6.3	–	0.1	–	0.1	100.0	19.8	0.3	79.9	100.0

– Less than 0.05 per cent.

Table 3.8 Educational level of the household population

Percent distribution of the de facto household population age 6 and baove by literacy and level of education, and median number of completed years of schooling, according to age, sex and residence, India, 1992-93

	Educational level									
Age	Literare	Litrate, primary complete	Primary school complete	Middle school complete	High school complete	Above high School	missing	total percent	Number	Median number of years of schooling
					URBAN Male					
6-9	22.5	75.4	1.8	—	—	—	0.3	100.0	6455	1.8
10-14	9.5	29.2	45.2	15.3	0.7	—	0.1	100.0	8049	5.7
15-19	10.3	5.4	15.4	30.0	34.5	4.4	—	100.0	6876	9.4
20-24	11.9	5.9	12.9	17.6	30.1	21.5	0.1	100.0	6497	10.1
25-29	13.6	6.3	14.2	15.5	26.4	23.9	0.1	100.0	5832	10.0
30-34	14.0	6.9	13.4	14.7	27.1	23.8	0.2	100.0	4947	10.1
35-39	16.2	7.4	13.6	12.9	25.6	24.3	0.1	100.0	4632	10.0
40-44	15.9	8.4	12.4	12.7	25.7	24.8	0.1	100.0	3718	10.0
45-49	18.3	9.3	14.2	11.7	25.2	21.0	0.2	100.0	3100	9.4
50+	25.9	13.4	15.4	9.5	21.9	13.5	0.3	100.0	8788	7.0
Total	15.9	18.3	17.0	14.2	20.6	13.9	0.1	100.0	58894	7.7
					Femal e					
6 - 9	25.1	72.5	2.1	—	—	—	0.3	100.0	5911	1.8
10-14	15.7	26.0	42.2	14.9	1.0	—	0.1	100.0	7433	5.5
15-19	19.2	5.3	15.5	23.3	32.0	4.7	—	100.0	6904	9.1
20-24	26.3	5.5	13.7	13.6	23.1	17.7	—	100.0	6581	8.6

1	2	3	4	5	6	7	8	9	10	11
25-29	31.2	5.5	13.4	12.8	20.0	17.1	—	100.0	5492	7.8
30-34	33.9	7.1	13.9	11.3	18.7	15.0	—	100.0	4627	7.1
35-39	34.4	8.6	15.3	10.0	20.1	11.6	—	100.0	3988	5.9
40-44	40.8	9.0	15.1	10.1	15.8	9.2	—	100.0	3141	5.1
45-49	43.9	10.7	17.1	8.5	13.2	6.7	—	100.0	2361	4.2
50+	61.6	11.7	12.3	5.7	5.9	2.4	0.4	100.0	8383	0.0
Total	32.5	17.2	16.7	11.4	14.4	7.7	0.1	100.0	54821	5.0
					Total					
6-9	23.8	74.0	1.9	—	—	—	0.2	100.0	12366	1.8
10-14	12.5	27.7	43.8	15.1	0.9	—	0.1	100.0	15481	5.6
15-19	14.8	5.3	15.5	26.6	33.2	4.6	—	100.0	13780	9.2
20-24	19.2	5.7	13.3	15.6	26.6	19.6	—	100.0	13079	9.5
25-29	22.1	5.9	13.8	14.2	23.3	20.6	0.1	100.0	11324	9.1
30-34	23.6	7.0	13.6	13.0	23.0	19.6	0.1	100.0	9574	8.8
35-39	24.6	8.0	14.4	11.6	23.0	18.4	—	100.0	8619	8.4
40-44	27.3	8.7	13.7	11.5	21.1	17.7	—	100.0	6859	8.0
45-49	29.4	9.9	15.4	10.3	20.0	14.8	0.1	100.0	5461	7.0
50+	43.4	12.6	13.9	7.7	14.1	8.1	0.3	100.0	17171	3.9
Total	23.9	17.8	16.9	12.8	17.6	10.9	0.1	100.0	113715	6.3
					RURAL					
					Male					
6 - 9	40.2	58.1	1.2	—	—	—	0.5	100.0	20569	1.2
10-14	20.9	35.2	35.0	8.5	0.4	—	0.1	100.0	23123	4.5
15-19	23.0	8.6	19.9	27.3	19.8	1.4	0.1	100.0	18078	7.8

1	2	3	4	5	6	7	8	9	10	11
20-24	27.1	7.8	15.2	17.3	25.0	7.5	0.1	100.0	14916	7.9
25-29	35.2	9.0	15.7	14.1	18.4	7.6	—	100.0	14006	5.9
30-34	39.5	10.4	16.0	12.6	15.3	6.0	0.1	100.0	11257	5.0
35-39	40.7	11.3	15.8	12.0	14.4	5.8	—	100.0	10910	4.6
40-44	43.0	11.9	16.2	10.7	13.1	5.0	0.1	100.0	8192	4.1
45-49	44.5	13.6	16.4	9.2	12.7	3.4	0.2	100.0	7106	3.4
50+	58.5	15.2	13.3	5.2	6.2	1.4	0.2	100.0	26525	0.0
Total	37.1	21.0	16.8	11.0	10.9	3.1	0.2	100.0	154683	3.6
					Female					
6 - 9	52.9	45.9	0.8	—	—	—	0.4	100.0	19296	0.0
10-14	42.9	26.4	24.6	5.6	0.3	—	0.1	100.0	21350	2.7
15-19	52.8	6.7	15.0	14.5	10.4	0.6	—	100.0	18986	0.0
20-24	62.2	6.2	11.8	8.6	8.8	2.4	—	100.0	17199	0.0
25-29	69.3	6.5	10.5	6.0	6.0	1.7	—	100.0	14232	0.0
30-34	71.7	6.9	10.4	5.2	~.6	1.2	—	100.0	11304	0.0
35-39	74.1	7.1	10.4	4.6	3.2	0.6	—	100.0	9479	0.0
40-44	78.0	7.2	8.3	3.3	2.6	0.5	—	100.0	7434	0.0
45-49	82.2	7.5	6.7	1.P	1.4	0.3	—	100.0	6374	0.0
50+	90.5	5.0	3.0	0.6	0.4	0.1	0.3	100.0	24722	0.0
Total	65.5	14.3	10.5	5.2	3.7	0.7	0.1	100.0	150376	0.0
					Total					
6-9	46.3	52.2	1.0	—	—	—	0.4	100.0	39866	1.0
10-14	31.5	31.0	30.0	7.1	0.3	—	0.1	100.0	44472	3.9
15-19	38.2	7.6	17.4	20.7	15.0	1.0	0.1	100.0	37064	5.7

20-24	45.9	6.9	13.3	12.7	16.3	4.8	0.1	100.0	32116	4.2
25-29	52.4	7.7	13.1	10.0	12.2	4.6	—	100.0	28238	0.0
30-34	55.7	8.7	13.2	8.9	9.9	3.6	0.1	100.0	22561	0.0
35-39	56.2	9.3	13.3	8.6	9.2	3.4	—	100.0	20389	0.0
40-44	59.7	9.7	12.4	7.2	8.1	2.9	—	100.0	15626	0.0
45-49	62.4	10.7	11.8	5.8	7.4	1.P	0.1	100.0	13480	0.0
50+	73.5	10.3	8.3	3.0	3.4	0.8	0.2	100.0	51247	0.0
Total	51.1	17.7	13.7	8.2	7.4	1.9	0.1	100.0	305059	0.0
					Total					
					Male					
6 - 9	36.0	62.2	1.3	—	—	—	0.4	100.0	27024	1.4
10-14	17.9	33.6	37.6	10.2	0.5	—	0.1	100.0	31171	4.9
15-19	19.5	7.7	18.7	28.0	23.8	2.3	0.1	100.0	24954	8.3
20-24	22.5	7.2	14.5	17.4	26.6	11.7	0.1	100.0	21414	8.7
25-29	28.8	8.2	15.2	14.5	20.8	12.4	0.1	100.0	19838	7.6
30-34	31.7	9.4	15.2	13.3	18.9	11.4	0.1	100.0	16204	6.6
35-39	33.4	10.1	15.2	12.3	17.7	11.3	—	100.0	15542	5.9
40-44	34.6	10.8	15.0	11.3	17.0	11.2	0.1	100.0	11910	5.6
45-49	36.6	12.3	15.7	10.0	16.5	8.8	0.2	100.0	10206	5.1
50+	50.4	14.8	13.8	6.3	10.1	4.4	0.2	100.0	35313	0.0
Total	31.2	20.2	16.8	11.9	13.6	6.1	0.1	100.0	213577	4.8
					Female					
6 - 9	46.4	52.1	1.1	—	—	—	0.4	100.0	25208	1.0
10-14	35.9	26.3	29.2	8.0	0.5	—	0.1	100.0	28782	3.8

1	2	3	4	5	6	7	8	9	10	11
15-19	43.8	6.3	15.1	16.8	16.2	1.7	—	100.0	25891	5.0
20-24	52.3	6.0	12.3	10.0	12.8	6.6	—	100.0	23780	0.0
25-29	58.7	6.2	11.3	7.9	9.9	6.0	—	100.0	19724	0.0
30-34	60.7	7.0	11.4	6.9	8.7	5.2	—	100.0	15930	0.0
35-39	62.3	7.5	11.8	6.2	8.2	3.9	—	100.0	13467	0.0
40-44	67.0	7.8	10.3	5.3	6.5	3.1	—	100.0	10575	0.0
45-49	71.9	8.4	9.5	3.7	4.6	2.0	—	100.0	8735	0.0
50~	83.2	6.7	5.4	1.9	1.8	0.7	0.3	100.0	33105	0.0
Total	56.7	15.1	12.1	6.9	6.6	2.6	0.1	100.0	205197	0.0
					Total					
6 - 9	41.0	57.3	1.2	—	—	—	0.4	100.0	52232	1.2
10-14	26.6	30.1	33.6	9.2	0.5	—	0.1	100.0	59953	4.5
15-19	31.9	7.0	16.9	22.3	19.9	2.0	—	100.0	50845	7.1
20-24	38.2	6.6	13.3	13.5	19.3	9.1	0.1	100.0	45194	5.9
25-29	43.7	7.2	13.3	11.2	15.4	9.2	0.1	100.0	39562	4.8
30-34	46.1	8.2	13.3	10.1	13.8	8.3	0.1	100.0	32135	3.8
35-39	46.8	8.9	13.6	9.5	13.3	7.8	—	100.0	29008	3.5
40-44	49.8	9.4	12.8	8.5	12.1	7.4	—	100.0	22485	1.2
45-49	52.8	10.5	12.9	7.1	11.0	5.6	0.1	100.0	18941	0.0
50+	66.2	10.9	9.7	4.2	6.1	2.6	0.3	100.0	68418	0.0
Total	43.7	17.7	14.5	9.4	10.1	4.4	0.1	100.0	418773	2.5

Note: This table and all subsequent tables are based on the *de facro* population unless otherwise indicated. Table excludes cases uith missing information on sex.

— Less than 0.05 percent.

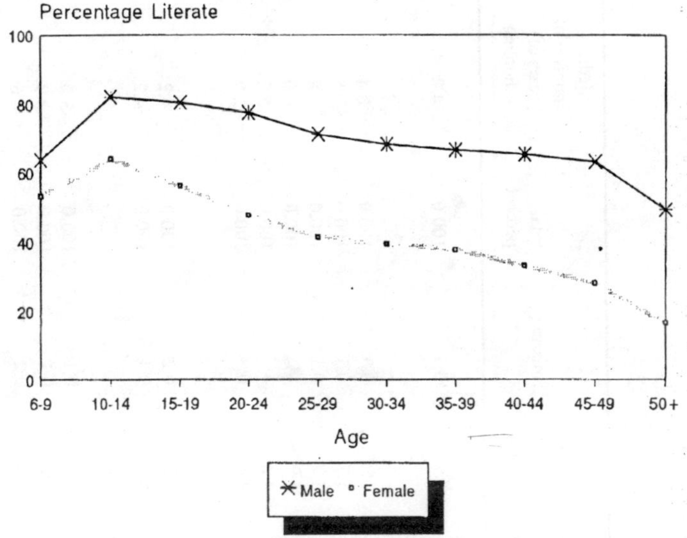

Figure 3.3 Percentage Literate by Age and Sex

ing is 4.8 for males and 0.0 for females, the latter indicating that the majority of females have never been to school.

Despite the low overall level of literacy, cohort differences in literacy suggest that there has been progress over time (Table 3.8 and Figure 3.3). For example, while only 17 per cent of women age 50 and over are literate, the literacy rate for females almost doubles to 33 per cent for those age 40-44, and steadily increases to 48 per cent for those age 20-24, and 64 per cent for those age 10-14. The literacy gap between males and females has narrowed over time, but even at age 10-14, a much higher percentage of males than females is literate (82 versus 64 per cent).

Urban areas have a wide lead over rural areas in both iiteracy and the level of education attained. The percentage of females who are illiterate is twice as high in rural areas (66 per cent) as in urban areas (33 per cent). The corresponding percentages for males are 37 and 16. Differences between urban and rural areas in the proportion of the population that has attended or completed primary school are, however, minimal, with 31-35 per cent of both the urban and rural groups attending or completing this level of school. Among those who are literate, however, 77 per cent in urban areas and 64 per cent in rural areas completed at

Table 3.9: Educational level of the household population by State

Percent distribution of the *de focro* household population age 6 and above by Literacy end Level of education and median number of completed years of schooling, according to sex end state, India, 1992-93

	Educational level								
Age	Illiterare	Literacy, <primary complete	Primary school complete	Middle school complete	High school complete	Above high School	missing	total percent	Median number of years of schooling
					MALE				
India	31.2	20.2	16.8	11.9	13.6	6.1	0.1	100.0	4.8
North									
Delhi	14.3	16.1	15.9	14.4	23.3	15.7	0.3	100.0	8.4
Haryana	27.7	18.4	18.6	12.0	17.6	5.7	0.1	100.0	5.5
Himachal Pradesh	20.7	22.0	21.7	13.7	16.9	4.9	0.1	100.0	5.8
Jammu Region of J & K	25.8	17.1	16.7	18.7	15.8	5.9	--	100.0	6.0
Punjab	34.1	14.1	17.5	12.1	18.0	4.2	--	100.0	5.2
Rajasthan	39.7	18.9	15.5	11.4	10.2	4.0	0.3	100.0	2.9
Central									
Madhya Pradesh	36.2	19.0	18.4	10.3	11.0	5.0	0.2	100.0	4.2
Utter Pradesh	36.4	16.8	15.2	12.5	13.8	5.3	0.1	100.0	4.2
East									
Pihar	39.5	17.4	13.5	8.9	13.9	6.7	0.1	100.0	3.0
Orissa	31.2	26.3	18.3	8.9	10.2	5.0	0.1	100.0	3.9
West Bengal	24.6	28.3	15.8	12.8	10.7	7.6	0.2	100.0	4.6

1	2	3	4	5	6	7	8	9	10
Northeast									
Arunachal Pradesh	38.1	25.2	14.3	9.2	9.0	4.1	--	100.0	2.8
Assam	30.1	28.6	14.1	13.3	9.4	4.4	0.1	100.0	4.0
Manipur	14.9	25.9	14.8	16.6	17.8	10.1	--	100.0	6.7
Meghalaya	33.2	29.3	14.5	11.2	9.1	2.6	--	100.0	3.1
Mizoram	6.6	32.7	25.2	16.5	14.6	4.4	--	100.0	6.2
Nagaland	20.1	26.5	18.9	14.2	16.5	3.8	--	100.0	5.7
Tripura	18.7	32.0	18.1	17.3	8.7	5.1	--	100.0	4.9
West									
Goa	11.7	23.6	17.7	14.9	22.1	9.9	0.1	100.0	7.6
Gujarat	24.6	22.0	20.2	10.9	15.5	6.7	0.1	100.0	5.5
Maharashtra	20.5	24.3	18.9	13.2	15.5	7.4	0.2	100.0	5.9
South									
Andhra Pradesh	39.7	15.4	12.3	12.0	13.8	6.4	0.4	100.0	3.8
Karnataka	31.9	21.3	17.6	8.0	14.6	6.6	0.1	100.0	4.6
Kerala	10.0	24.1	24.2	20.9	15.1	5.3	0.2	100.0	7.0
Tami Nadu	23.0	16.3	23.3	14.3	14.8	6.2	0.1	100.0	5.8
					FEMALE				
India	56.7	15.1	12.1	6.9	6.6	2.6	0.1	100.0	0.0
North									
Delhi	29.2	15.8	15.1	11.1	16.0	12.5	0.2	100.0	5.6
Haryana	54.1	15.1	14.5	6.2	7.6	2.5	--	100.0	0.0
Himachal Pradesh	42.6	17.8	20.3	8.8	8.6	1.9	--	100.0	2.4

1	2	3	4	5	6	7	8	9	10
Jammu Region									
of J & K	48.2	13.3	14.4	11.2	9.3	3.6	--	100.0	1.7
Punjab	48.0	11.1	16.9	8.8	12.2	3.0	--	100.0	2.0
Rajasthan	74.6	9.8	7.3	3.5	3.1	1.4	0.4	100.0	0.0
Central									
Madhya Pradesh	65.7	13.2	10.6	4.5	3.8	2.0	0.2	100.0	0.0
Uttar Pradesh	68.5	10.2	8.9	5.2	5.0	2.2	0.1	100.0	0.0
East									
Bihar	71.4	11.0	7.3	3.6	4.8	1.8	0.1	100.0	0.0
Orissa	58.6	18.2	12.4	4.8	4.4	1.6	--	100.0	0.0
West Bengal	44.8	25.9	12.5	8.9	4.9	2.8	--	100.0	1.0
Northeast									
Arunachal Pradesh	57.9	19.2	10.9	6.5	4.7	0.8	--	100.0	0.0
Assam	49.3	22.2	11.3	10.3	5.1	1.8	--	100.0	1.0
Manipur	37.0	21.8	11.9	10.9	11.4	7.0	--	100.0	2.0
Meghalaya	39.8	27.9	14.9	9.0	6.7	1.6	--	100.0	2.0
Mizoram	*11.1*	*35.6*	*23.1*	*17.0*	*11.6*	*1.5*	--	*100.0*	*5.4*
Naga Land	28.2	24.5	19.2	12.9	13.7	1.5	--	100.0	4.6
Tripura	35.6	28.6	16.4	12.4	4.4	2.6	--	100.0	2.8
West									
Goa	26.9	21.8	16.3	12.4	16.1	6.4	0.1	100.0	5.2
Gujarat	48.7	17.2	15.0	6.6	9.1	3.2	0.1	100.0	1.7

Maharashtra	44.1	19.7	16.2	7.7	8.4	3.7	0.2	100.0	0.0
South									
Andhra Pradesh	61.5	11.8	9.2	7.9	6.8	2.4	0.3	100.0	0.0
Karnataka	53.5	15.9	14.1	5.7	8.2	2.5	0.1	100.0	0.0
Kerala	17.6	21.7	23.0	19.1	14.1	4.4	0.1	100.0	6.4
Tamil Nadu	43.9	14.9	18.9	10.1	9.4	2.7	--	100.0	3.6
					TOTAL				
India	43.7	17.7	14.5	9.4	10.1	4.4	0.1	100.0	2.5
North									
Delhi	21.0	15.9	15.5	12.9	20.0	14.3	0.3	100.0	73
Haryana	40.1	16.9	16.7	9.3	12.9	4.2	--	100.0	3.4
Himachal Pradesh	32.1	19.8	21.0	11.2	12.6	3.3	0.1	100.0	4.6
Jammu Region of J & K	36.9	15.2	15.6	15.0	12.6	4.8	--	100.0	4.5
Punjab	40.8	12.7	17.2	10.5	15.2	3.7	--	100.0	4.1
Rajasthan	56.1	14.6	11.6	7.6	6.9	2.8	0.3	100.0	0.0
Central									
Madhya Pradesh	50.2	16.3	14.7	7.5	7.6	3.6	0.2	100.0	0.0
Utter Pradesh	52.0	13.5	12.1	8.9	9.5	3.8	0.1	100.0	0.0
East									
Bihar	55.4	14.2	10.4	6.3	9.3	4.3	0.1	100.0	0.0
Orissa	44.8	22.3	15.4	6.9	7.4	3.3	--	100.0	1.8
West Bengal	34.4	27.1	14.2	11.0	7.9	5.3	0.1	100.0	3.3

1	2	3	4	5	6	7	8	9	10
Northeast									
Arunachal Pradesh	47.9	22.3	12.7	7.8	6.9	2.4	—	100.0	1.2
Assam	39.5	25.5	12.8	11.8	7.3	3.1	—	100.0	2.6
Manipur	26.0	23.8	13.4	13.7	14.6	8.5	—	100.0	5.1
Meghalaya	36.4	28.6	14.7	10.2	7.9	2.1	—	100.0	2.5
Mizoram	8.9	34.2	24.1	16.7	13.1	3.0	--	100.0	5.9
Nagaland	24.2	25.5	19.0	13.6	15.1	2.7	--	100.0	5.1
Tripura	27.2	30.3	17.3	14.8	6.5	3.8	--	100.0	3.9
West									
Goa	19.4	22.7	17.0	13.6	19.0	8.2	0.1	100.0	6.5
Gujarat	36.3	19.7	17.7	8.8	12.4	5.0	0.1	100.0	4.1
Maharashtra	32.1	22.0	17.6	10.5	12.0	5.6	0.2	100.0	4.5
South									
Andhra Pradesh	50.6	13.6	10.8	9.9	10.3	4.4	0.4	100.0	0.0
Karnataka	42.6	18.6	15.8	6.9	11.4	4.6	0.1	100.0	2.9
Kerala	14.0	22.9	23.6	20.0	14.6	4.8	0.2	100.0	6.7
Tamil Nadu	33.6	16.6	21.1	12.1	12.1	4.4	0.1	100.0	5.0

— Less then 0.05 per cent.

least primary school. Attending high school or above is also more common in the urban than the rural sample, both for those who are literate and for the whole population. The literacy gap between males and females is greater in rural than in urban areas. Whereas the percentage of rural females who are illiterate (66 per cent) exceeds the percentage of rural males who are illiterate (37 per cent) by 29 percentage points, the difference is only 17 percentage points in urban areas (33 per cent versus 16 per cent).

There are large interstate variations in the level of female and male literacy and education (Table 3.9). More than 80 per cent of females age 6 and above are literate in Mizoram (89 per cent) and Kerala (82 per cent). Between 71 and 73 per cent of women in Delhi, Nagaland and Goa are literate. At the other extreme, nearly three-fourths of females age 6 and over are illiterate in Rajasthan (75 per cent) and Bihar (72 per cent). The percentage of females who have at least a high school education is highest in Delhi (29 per cent), followed by Goa (23 per cent), Kerala (19 per cent), Manipur (18 per cent), and Punjab and Nagaland (15 per cent each). Less than 10 per cent of females have at least a high school education in nearly half of the states. In every state, the percentage literate is higher for males than for females and (with a couple of minor exceptions) a higher percentage of males have completed each level of schooling than females. The literacy gap between males and females is particularly large in Rajasthan, Uttar Pradesh and Bihar, where the male literacy rate is more than twice as high as the female literacy rate. The male-female ratio in literacy is also very high in Madhya Pradesh (1.86), Orissa (1.66), Haryana (1.58) and Andhra Pradesh (1.57). The male-female gap in literacy is very small in Mizoram, Meghalaya, Nagaland and Kerala.

Among males who are literate more than one-quater (29 per cent) have at least a high school education. There are interesting statewise variations in the tendency of literate men to continue with their education through the high school level. Although Kerala has the second highest male literacy rate in the country, a lower promotion of literate males finish at least high School in Kerala (23 per cent) than in any other major state except Orissa and Assam. On the other hand, in the low literacy states of Bihar and Andhra Pradesh, more than one-third of literate men have completed at least high school. In Delhi, which is predominantly urban, almost half of literate males (46 per cent) have completed at least high school.

In the case of females, Delhi again has the highest proportion of high school graduates among the literate population (40 per cent), but

Table 3.10 School Attendance
Percentage of the *de jacro* household population age 6-14 years attending school by sex, residence end state, India, 1992-93

	Male			Female			Total		
State	Urban	Rural	Total	Urban	Rural	Total	Urban	Rural	Total
India									
Age 6 -14 years	85.3	72.2	75.5	79.2	52.2	58.9	82.4	62.6	67.5
6 -10 years	86.2	71.4	75.0	81.8	55.0	61.3	84.1	63.5	68.4
11-14 years	84.2	73.4	76.3	75.7	47.9	55.3	80.1	61.2	66.2
North									
Delhi	87.3	89.9	87.5	86.6	82·8	86.3	87.0	86.9	86.9
Haryana	90.8	85.9	87.2	88.8	69.5	74.7	89.8	78.2	81.3
Himachal Pradesh	96.4	93.6	93.8	93.8	87.1	87.6	95.1	90.4	90.8
Jammu Region of J & K	95.2	90.7	91.3	96.3	77.0	79.6	95.7	84.1	85.7
Punjab	88.9	81.1	83.4	89.0	73.1	77.8	88.9	77.4	80.8
Rajasthan	86.2	72.0	74.2	71.9	33.5	40.6	78.6	54.4	58.8
Central									
Madhya Predesh	84.7	64.3	69.0	81.6	46.3	54.8	83.2	55.9	62.3
Utter Pradesh	77.1	71.7	72.8	69.5	42.6	48.2	73.5	58.1	61.3
East									
Bihar	84.3	59.8	63.6	67.8	33.6	38.3	76.7	46.9	51.3
Orissa	88.2	74.7	76.8	78.6	58.9	62.0	83.5	67.0	69.6
West Bengal	83.3	68.6	72.5	71.8	60.1	62.9	77.9	64.2	67.7

Northeast									
Arunachal Pradesh	82.4	76.1	76.8	71.1	64.6	65.3	76.7	70.3	71.0
Assam	79.4	73.4	74.0	72.6	65.2	66.0	76.1	69.5	70.1
Manipur	96.2	92.1	93.6	93.5	83.9	86.8	94.9	88.1	90.2
Meghalaya	93.8	69.9	74.3	92.5	71.6	75.7	93.1	70.6	75.0
Mizoram	96.5	89.5	92.8	93.0	84.2	88.5	94.7	86.9	90.7
Nagaland	96.7	88.0	90.1	97.3	86.8	89.0	97.0	87.4	89.6
Tripura	86.2	81.0	81.9	89.9	74.0	76.7	88.0	77.6	79.4
West									
Goa	95.0	94.3	94.7	91.8	93.0	92.5	93.4	93.7	93.5
Gujarat	89.2	78.8	82.4	81.8	61.7	68.4	85.7	70.5	75.7
Maharashtra	90.7	83.3	86.2	87.8	69.2	76.6	89.3	76.4	81.5
South									
Andhra Pradesh	85.0	66.8	71.8	76.3	46.6	54.8	80.6	56.8	63.3
Karnataka	84.6	72.8	76.4	80.1	57.3	64.4	82.4	65.3	70.5
Kerala	94.5	94.8	94.7	96.3	94.3	94.8	95.4	94.6	94.8
Temil Nadu	87.3	85.3	86.0	86.4	74.8	78.7	86.8	80.1	82.4

Kerala also slightly exceeds the national average. For India as a whole, literate males are more likely to have completed at least high school (29 per cent) than literate females (21 per cent). The earlier age at marriage for females may be one important factor that prevents them from acquiring higher education.

Table 3.10 shows school attendance rates for the school-age population, by sex, residence, and state. The results are presented for children age 6-14, because the Indian Constitution established a goal of providing free and compulsory education for children below age 15. In the country as a whole, only 68 per cent of children age 6-14 are attending school. As expected, the proportion attending is higher for males than for females: 76 per cent for males compared with 59 per cent for females (Figure 3.4). Urban attendance is also higher than rural attendance (82 per cent compared with 63 per cent). The gap between girls and boys in school attendance is more pronounced in rural than in urban areas, especially at age 11-14, where only 48 per cent of rural girls as opposed to 73 per cent of rural boys are in school. In spite of the substantial educational advances that have been made over time, 41 per cent of school-age girls in India are still not attending school.

As interesting feature of Table 3.10 is that attending rates for males do not differ much by age group (6-10 and 11-14), that is, as male children get older they tend to stay in school. In comparison, the attendance rates for females decline from age 6-10 to age 11-14 years. Urban females experience a 7 per cent decline in attendance and rural females, whose level of education is much lower to begin with experience a 13 per cent decline in attendance from age 6-10 to age 11-14. These differences in attendance rates by age reflect the drop out of children from school at higher ages as well as the improvement in school attendance in recent years.

School attendance is almost universal in Kerala, Goa, Himachal Pradesh, Mizoram and Manipur where more than 90 per cent of School-age children are in school. In every state except Kerala and Meghalaya, proportionately more boys than girls age 6-14 attend school. The attendance rate for both boys and girls is higher in u'ban than in rural areas in every state except Goa, More than 50 per cent of school-age girls in Bihar (62 per cent), Rajasthan (59 per cent), and Uttar Pradesh (52 per cent) are not attending School. The gap between male and female attendance rates is also substantial in these states. The attendance rates for school-age boys in these states are 64 per cent in Bihar, 74 per cent in Rajasthan, and 73 per cent in Uttar Pradesh.

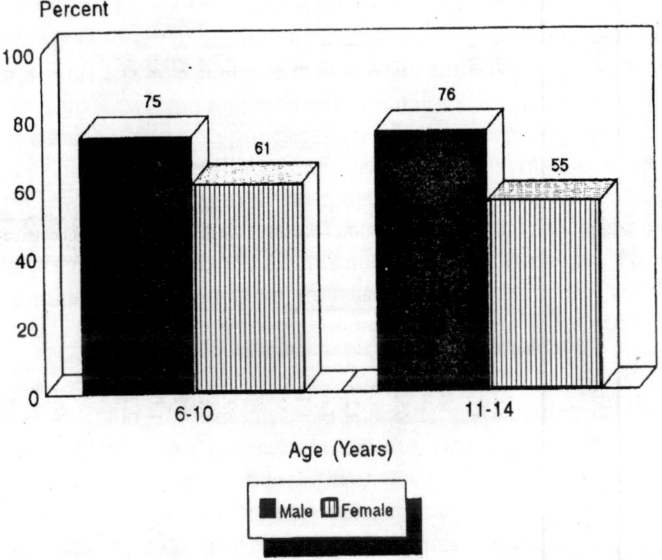

Figure 3.4 School Attendance by Age and Sex

3.5 HOUSING CHARACTERISTICS

The NFHS gathered information on the foliowing housing characteristics: electricity, source of bathing/washing water and drinking water, sanitation facility, type of cooking fuel, place where livestock is kept, number of rooms in the house and the housing materials used for construction of the walls roof and floor. The data on housing are summarized by residence in Table 3.11. Overall, only 51 per cent of households have electricity. A large majority of households in urban areas have electricity (83 per cent), whereas only 39 per cent of the households in rural areas have electricity.

The source of water and availability of sanitary facilities are important determinants of the health status of household members, particularly of children. Thirty-three per cent of households get piped water for drinking, another 35 per cent get water from a handpump, and 26 per cent from wells. There are large urban-rural differences in the source of drinking water. More than two-thirds of households in urban areas get piped water, whereas only about one-fifth of rural households use piped water for drinking. The sources of water used for bathing/washing and drinking are similar in urban and rural areas, except that surface water is less likely to be used for drinking.

Table 3.11 Housing Characteristics

Per cent distribution of households by housing characteristics, according to residence, India, 1992-93

	Residence		
Housing Characteristic	Urban	Rural	Total
Electricity			
Yes	82.8	38.7	50.9
No	17.2	61.3	49.1
Source of bathing/washing water			
Piped	65.3	18.3	31.3
Handpump	17.6	35.6	30.6
Well water	12.3	30.2	25.3
Surface water	3.6	14.3	11.4
Other	1.1	1.5	1.4
Source of drinking water			
Piped	69.5	19.3	33.1
Handpump	18.1	41.6	35.1
Well water	9.2	32.1	25.8
Surface water	1.0	5.1	3.9
Other	2.2	2.0	2.0
Sanitation facility			
Flush toilet	60.1	6.9	21.6
Pit toilet/latrine	15.5	5.9	8.6
Other	0.3	0.1	0.1

No facility	24.1	87.1	69.7
Type of fuel for cooking			
Wood	29.6	77.0	63.9
Cow dung cates	3.0	12.2	9.7
Coal/coke/Lignite/chercoel	8.6	2.3	4.1
Kerosene	22.5	1.9	7.6
Electricity	1.0	0.1	0.4
Liquid petroleun gas	33.4	1.9	10.6
Other	1.9	4.5	3.8
Type of house			
Kachcha	17.2	60.4	48.5
Semi -pucca	26.2	28.4	27.8
Pucca	56.6	11.2	23.7
Placewhere livestoct is Irept			
Inside the house	4.8	19.5	15.4
Outside the house	9.5	47.5	37.0
Ho livestock	85.7	33.0	47.6
Persons per room			
< 3.0	63.4	58.6	59.9
3.0-4.9	21.8	25.4	24.4
5.0-6.9	21.8	25.4	24.4
7.0+	9.9	5.0	5.0
Don't know/missing	--	0.1	0.1

1	2	3	4
Mean	2.7	2.8	2.8
Total percent	100.0	100.0	100.0
Number of households	24424	64138	88562

- - Less than 0.05 per cent.

The lack of availability of sanitary facilities poses a serious health problem. Only 22 per cent of the households have a flush toilet (using either piped water or bucket water for flushing), 9 per cent have a pit toilet or latrine and a substantial majority (70 per cent) have no facility at all. There are large urban-rural differences as well; three-fifths of households in urban areas but only 7 per cent in rural areas have a flush toilet, whereas 24 per cent of households in urban areas and an overwhelming majority (87 per cent) in rural areas have no toilet facility.

Several types of fuel are used for cooking, but wood is the most common fuel. Overall, 64 per cent of households rely on wood, 11 per cent use liquid petroleum gas, 10 per cent use cow dung cakes, 8 per cent use kerosene, 4 per cent use coal/coke/charcoal and the rest (4 per cent) depend on other fuels. Again,there are large urban-rural differences. Almost 6 in 10 urban households use liquid petroleum gas or kerosene and only 3 in 10 urban households use wood, whereas a substantial majority of rural households (77 per cent) rely on wood for cooking.

Based on the materials used for the construction of the walls, roof and floor, houses in the NFHS are classified as either kachch (made from mud, thatch or other low-quality materials), pucca (made from high-quality materials throughout, including the roof, walls and floor), or semi-pucca (made from partly low-quality and partly high-quality materials). Almost one-half (49 per cent) of houses are kachcha, 28 per cent are semi-pucca and slightly less than one-quarter (24 per cent) are pucca. Sixty per cent of the houses in rural areas can be classified as kachcha. The quality of housing is better in urban areas: 57 per cent of houses in urban areas are pucca, and another 26 per cent of houses are semi-pucca.

The NFHS also collected information on whether households own any livestock. A follow-up question was asked on where the livestock are usually kept at night, because keeping them inside the house may adversely affect the health of the residents. Overall, 52 per cent of households own livestock, 67 per cent in rural areas and 14 per cent in urban areas. Only 15 per cent of all households and 20 per cent of rural households have livestock that are kept inside the house at night.

Crowded conditions may affect health as well as the quality of life. The number of persons per room in the household is used as a simple measure of crowding. On average, there are 2.8 persons per room in India. A majority of households (60 per cent) have fewer than three persons per room. However, 16 per cent of households have five or more persons per room and 5 per cent of households are very crowded, with seven or more persons per room.

Table 3.12 Housing characteristics by states

Housing characteristics of households, according to state, India, 1992-93

State	Per cent with electricity	Per cent with drinking water from pump/pipe	Percent with andy toilet/ latrine facility	Per cent using wood as fuel for cooking	Per cent with pucca house construction	Mean number of persons per room
India	50.9	68.2	30.3	63.9	23.7	2.8
North						
Delhi	95.5	99.5	84.1	6.4	81.0	2.6
Haryana	85.0	73.0	26.9	55.6	39.6	2.9
Himachal Pradesh	90.2	57.6	12.6	84.8	22.7	2.1
Jammu Region of J & K	86.7	57.3	19.(	M.9	32.5	2.8
Punjab	92.0	98.6	36.7	44.9	52.6	2.7
Rajasthan	51.9	57.3	19.8	81.D	38.1	3.0
Central						
Madhya Pradesh	62.4	55.8	21.3	68.2	13.8	2.8
Uttar Pradesh	31.9	74.3	22.9	68.3	20.1	3.0
East						
Bihar	16.6	63.6	16.5	51.1	15.5	2.8
Orissa	27.8	50.9	12.2	68.7	9.5	2.4
West Bengal	32.9	84.9	40.4	31.6	22.5	2.8
North east						
Arunachal Pradesh	63.1	75.8	73.6	87.7	2.2	2.9

Assam	20.4	43.2	49.6	87.8	2.2	2.4
Manipur	62.1	47.0	83.1	80.5	4.9	2.1
Meghalaya	42.6	47.6	54.3	82.0	3.9	2.0
Mizoram	76.0	40.1	98.3	66.2	6.0	2.4
Nagaland	76.9	72.1	79.3	97.4	8.4	1.9
Tripura	45.1	44.1	79.4	91.1	3.1	2.4
West						
Goa	91.7	56.5	48.0	51.3	54.0	1.8
Gujarat	76.6	75.1	35.8	55.9	33.2	3.3
Maharashtra	73.6	78.5	40.8	55.2	30.6	3.2
South						
Andhra Pradesh	62.2	63.4	24.4	77.0	31.3	2.8
Karnataka	64.0	75.6	31.2	75.4	16.5	2.7
Kerala	60.3	21.0	70.9	87.4	19.9	1.4
Tamil Nadu	63.8	74.6	29.4	77.7	22.7	2.5

An interstate comparison of housiog conditions is presented in Table 3.12. percentage of households with electricity is lowest in Bihar (17 per cent), closely followed by Assam (20 percent), Orissa (28 per-cent), and Uttar Pradesh (32 per cent). Apart From Delhi, which is mostly urban, more than 70 per cent of households have electricity in Punjab and Goa (92 per cent each), Himachal Pradesh (90 per cent), Jammu (87 per cent), Haryana (85 per cent), Gujarat and Nagaland (77 per cent each), Mizoram (76 per cent), and Maharashtra (74 per cent)· Piped water or water from a handpump is used for drinking in a majority, of households in all State rates except Assam, Manipur, Meghalaya, Miroram, Tripura (40-48 per cent), and Kerala. In Kerala, more than 60 per cent of households obtain their drinking water from wells, which in many cases are within the house. Toilet facilities are inadequate in almost all states. Delhi (which is mostly urban), Arunachal Pradesh, Manipur, Mizoram, Nagaland, Tripura, and Kerala are the only states where more than 70 per cent of the households have some form of toilet facility. Again with the exception of Delhi, as well as Punjab and West Bengal, the majority of households in every state use wood as cooking fuel. Less than 10 per cent of households in the northeastern states and in Orissa are classified as pucca. Delhi (81 per cent), Goa (54 per cent) and Punjab (53 per cent) are the only states where a majority of households live in pucca houses. Households in Kerala are least crowded (with an average of only 1.4 persons per room) and households in Gujarat, Maharashtra, Rajasthan and Uttar Pradesh are most crowded (with an average of 3.0 persons per room or more).

Table 3.13 contains a number of measures related to the socioeconomic status of the household (household ownership of agricultural land, various kinds of livestock, and durable goods). Overall, 48 per cent of households are landless; not surprisingly, urban households are more than twice as likely to be landless as rural households. In rural areas, among those who have land, 37 per cent irrigate all of their land and 21 per cent irrigate some of their land. More than half (52 per cent) of all households have livestock, and rural households are five times as likely to own livestock as urban households. Twenty-nine per cent of rural households have one or more bullocks, 35 per cent have cows, 28 per cent have buffaloes: and 17 per cent have goats.

The possession of durable goods is another indicator of a household's socioeconomic level, although these goods may also have other benefits. For example, having access to a radio or television may expose household members to innovative ideas; a refrigerator prolongs the wholesomeness of food; and a means of transportation allows greater

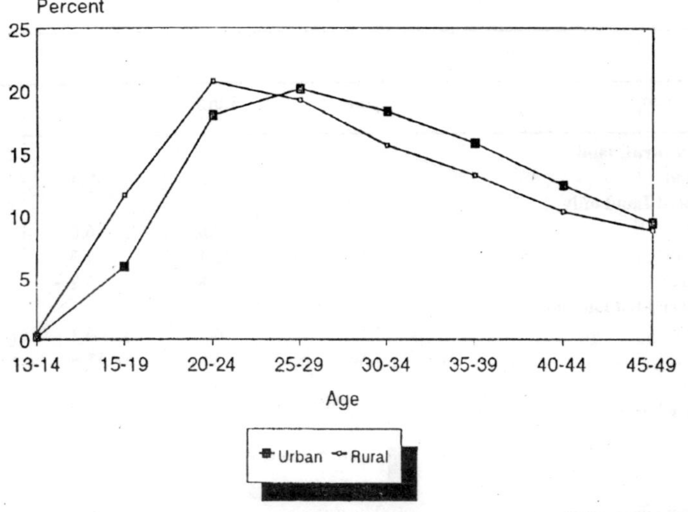

Figure 3.5 Age Distribution of Ever-Married Women by Residence

access to many services outside the local area. Fifty-three per cent of households in India own a clock or a watch, 42 per cent own a bicycle, 39 per cent own a radio, 21 per cent own a television, and 18 per cent own a sewing machine. Other durable goods found in Indian households include: motorcycles or scooters (8 per cent) and refrigerators (7 per cent). Urban households are much more likely to have each of these durable goods.

3.6 Background Characteristics of Respondents

Whereas the previous tables considered characteristics of households, based on results from the NFHS Household Questionnaire, this section examines selected background characteristics of primary respondents (ever-married women age 13-49), based on the NFHS Woman's Questionnaire.

Table 3.14 shows several important background characteristics of respondents: age, marital status, education, religion, caste/tribe, work status, and husband's education. The data shown in the first three columns and in all subsequent tables, are based on the weighted sample of women. The weighted number of cases may not add up to the total of 89,777 women due to rounding.

Table 3.13 : Household ownership of land , Livestock and durable goods
Percentage of households owing agricultural land, livestock and various consumer durable goods according to residence, India, 1992-93

	Residence		
Item owned	Urban	Rural	Total
AgriaulturaL land			
No Land	81.0	36.0	48.4
Irrigated Land only			
<1Acre	1.7	7.6	6.0
1-5 Acres	3.5	12.1	9.7
6+ Acres	1.5	3.8	3.2
Non-irrigated land only			
< 1Acre	2.1	6.3	5.1
1-5 Acre	4.8	15.6	12.6
6+ Acre	2.1	5.1	4.3
Irrigated and non-irrigated land			
<1 Acre	0.5	2.4	1.0
1-5 Acres	1.3	6.4	5.0
6+ Acres	1.5	4.8	3.9
Total per cent	100.0	100.0	100.0
Livestock			
Buttock	3.0	29.1	21.9
Cow	6.7	34.8	27.1
Buffalo	4.4	27.8	21.4
Coat	4.3	17.2	13.7
Sheep	0.2	1.9	1.4
Camel	0.1	0.5	0.3
Other	0.8	2.8	2.3
No livestock	85.7	33.0	47.6
Consumer durable goods			
Sewing machine	35.5	11.3	18.0
Clock/watch	78.7	43.1	52.9
Radio	59.4	31.6	39.3
Television	51.7	8.9	20.7
Refrigerator	20.1	1.7	6.8
Bicycle	47.5	39.7	41.8
Motorcycle/scooter	19.2	3.8	8.1
Car	3.2	0.3	1.1
Number of households	24424	64138	88562

Note: Information on the ownership af bullock carts, threshers, tractors and water pumps is not included under consumer durable goods because information on these items was not collected for all states.

Table 3.14: Background Characteristics of Respondents
Per cent distribution of ever-married Women age 13-49, by selected background characteristics, according to residence; India, 1992-93

	Residence			Number of women	
Background charactaristic	Urban	Rural	Total	Weighted	Unweighted
1	2	3	4	5	6
Age					
13-14	0.2	0.5	0.4	352	275
15-19	5.9	11.6	10.1	9095	7816
20-24	18.0	20.7	20.0	17983	17233
25-29	20.1	19.2	19.4	17442	17734
30-34	18.3	15.6	16.3	14660	15161
35-39	15.8	13.2	13.9	12461	12875
40-44	12.4	10.3	10.9	9748	10195
45-49	9.4	8.8	9.0	8036	8491
Marital status					
Currently married	94.1	94.4	94.3	84678	84558
Widowed	4.0	3.7	3.8	3421	3526
Divorced	0.4	0.3	0.3	274	367
Separated	1.5	1.6	1.6	1404	1326
Education					
Illiterate	36.8	72.4	63.1	56656	52142
Literate, < primary complete	7.4	6.4	6.7	5997	6473
Primary school complete	15.4	10.3	11.7	10478	11169
Middle school complete	12.0	5.6	7.2	6508	7463
High school complete	17.9	4.4	7.9	7128	8675
Above high school	10.6	0.8	3.4	3011	3855
Religion					
Hindu	75.6	84.3	82.0	73648	70129
Muslim	16.6	10.4	12.0	10806	9494
Christian	2.9	2.2	2.4	2142	5923
Sikh	1.8	1.9	1.9	1673	2616
Jain	1.3	0.5	0.5	428	376
Buddhist	1.5	0.6	0.8	734	514
Other	0.3	0.4	0.4	345	725
Caste/tribe					
Scheduled caste	9.1	13.3	12.2	10970	10571
Scheduled tribe	3.2	10.8	8.8	7934	10780
Other	87.6	75.9	78.9	70872	68426
Work status					
Not working	79.5	64.6	68.5	61462	61870
Working in family					

{Cont.}

farm/business	3.6	15.3	12.2	10987	11356
Employed by someone else	12.8	17.4	16.2	14575	13144
Self-employed	4.1	2.7	3.1	2752	3407
Husband's education					
Illiterate	17.0	41.0	34.7	31142	28539
Literate, < primary complete	8.2	10.8	10.1	9073	9028
Primary school complete	14.9	16.1	15.8	14148	13987
Middle school complete	13.1	11.6	12.0	10735	11451
High school complete	25.9	15.7	18.3	16461	17713
Above high school	20.7	4.8	8.9	8025	8881
Don't know/missing	0.2	0.2	0.2	193	178
Total per cent	100.0	100.0	100.0	NA	NA
Number of women					
Weighted	23455	65322	89777	89777	NA
Unweighted	27534	62243	89777	NA	89777

NA: Not applicable

Up to age 20-24, the percentage in each age group increases reflecting the increase in the proportion married in successive age groups. The decline after age 20-24, by which time most women have already married, reflects the normal pyramidal shape of the age distribution. The age pattern of eligible women differs slightly between the urban and rural areas with a modal age of 25-29 in the urban sample and of 20-24 in the rural sample (Figure 3.5). Moreover, the percentages in the yunger age groups are smaller in urban areas, reflecting the somewhat later age at marriage in urban area (see the earlier discussion of Table 3.5).

Overall, 94 per cent of respondents (ever-married women) are currently married, and the proportion currently married is nearly the same in urban and rural areas. Among the remainder, most are widowed (4 per cent), less than 1 per cent are divorced and 2 per cent are separated.

The literacy level of ever-married women age 13-49 in India is quite low. Sixty-three per cent of respondents are illiterate and the percentage illiterate is even higher in rural areas (72 per cent). Only 11 per cent have completed at least high school. Ever-married women in urban areas are substantially better educated than their rural counterparts. For example, 41 per cent of urban respondents, compared with 11 per cent of rural respondents, have completed at least middle school. The distribution of ever-married women by educational level is similar to that of all females in the *de facto* household population age 6 and above, but as a group, the primary respondents are less literate than the female household population in the childbearing ages (Table 3.7). This difference reflects a tendency for illiterate women to marry at younger ages than literate women.

The pattern of distribution of respondents by religion and caste/tribe is similar to the pattern of distribution of household heads by the same characteristics, as discussed in Section 3.3. Table 3.14 also shows the distribution of respondents by the respondent's work status and her husband's education. In the NFHS, work is defined as any kind of job for which the woman is paid in cash or in kind as well as unpaid work on a family farm or business. Overall, 69 per cent of respondents report that they are not working (80 per cent in urban areas and 65 per cent in rural areas). The proportion working on a family farm or in some other family business is 12 per cent overall and 15 per cent in rural areas. Sixteen per cent of respondents report that they are employed by someone other than a family member. The percentage self- employed is almost the same in urban and rural areas (3-4 per cent).

Thirty-five per cent of husbands are illiterate (17 per cent in urban areas and 41 per cent in rural areas). The per centage of husbands with at least a high school education is more than twice as high in urban areas (47 per cent) as in rural areas (21 per cent).

The states vary substantially with respect to literacy and the educational level of ever-married women Table 3.15). The literacy rate among ever-married women is highest in Mizoram (92 per cent), closely followed by Kerala (84 per cent). More than 70 per cent of ever- married women are illiterate in Rajasthan (82 per cent), Bihar (78 per cent), Uttar Pradesh (76 per cent) and Madhya Pradesh (74 per cent). The percentage of interviewed women who have completed at least high school ranges from only 5 per cent in Rajasthan to 37 per cent in Delhi.

Table 3.16 shows interstate variations in the work status of interviewed women. Approximately half of women report that they are working in Manipur, Andhra Pradesh, Maharashtra, Himachal Pradesh, Karnataka and Tamil Nadu. Women are least likely to work in Punjab (8 per cent) and Uttar Pradesh (13 per cent). Delhi follows the national pattern of low levels of urban employment of married women. In most states, the majority of working women work for someone outside the family. The particularly high proportion of females in Tamil Nadu working for someone outside the family (35 per cent) is consistent with various government programmes to promote female employment in the state. However, in Haryana, Himachal Pradesh, Jammu, Rajasthan, Madhya

Table 3.15: Education of respondents

Per cent distribution of ever-married Women age 13-49 by education and state, India, 1992-93

State	Educational						
	Illiterate	Literate, <primary complete	Primary school complete	Middle school complete	High school complete	Above high School	Total per cent
India	63.1	6.7	11.7	7.2	7.9	3.4	100.0
North							
Delhi	37.4	3.5	11.6	10.6	19.8	17.1	100.0
Haryana	63.8	3.1	12.8	6.0	11.0	3.4	100.0
Himachal Pradesh	49.7	7.2	21.0	8.7	10.6	2.8	100.0
Jammu Region of J & K	56.7	1.5	11.8	11.2	13.2	5.6	100.0
Punjab	52.6	2.3	17.8	9.0	14.1	4.2	100.0
Rajasthan	82.2	2.2	6.7	3.5	3.6	1.8	100.0
Central							
Madhya Pradesh	74.4	4.3	9.2	4.7	4.7	2.6	100.0
Uttar Pradesh	75.7	2.0	7.9	5.6	5.6	3.2	100.0
East							
Bihar	78.3	2.9	7.6	3.1	5.6	2.5	100.0
Orissa	67.4	9.1	14.0	3.4	4.6	1.4	100.0
West Bengal	50.6	17.2	12.4	10.3	5.9	3.7	100.0
Northeast							
Arunachal Pradesh	69.5	5.7	9.5	7.9	6.2	1.1	100.0

Assam	59.3	13.8	10.1	9.8	5.0	2.1	100.0
Manipur	47.6	10.3	8.9	10.6	14.5	8.1	100.0
Meghalaya	51.4	15.7	13.7	8.8	8.2	2.2	100.0
Mizoram	8.4	32.1	25.6	19.2	12.8	1.8	100.0
Nagaland	43.0	11.7	16.3	13.3	14.1	1.7	100.0
Tripura	41.3	15.4	19.4	15.5	5.4	3.2	100.0
West							
Goa	33.7	16.3	12.6	10.2	19.8	7.4	100.0
Gujarat	55.3	8.7	13.0	6.9	11.9	4.2	100.0
Maharashtra	50.2	10.5	16.6	8.0	10.4	4.4	100.0
South							
Andhra Pradesh	68.7	4.7	8.7	7.6	7.6	2.8	100.0
Karnataka	61.6	6.5	12.8	5.5	10.5	3.1	100.0
Kerala	16.0	14.5	23.2	25.0	15.5	5.8	100.0
Tamil Nadu	50.1	6.9	17.6	10.3	12.1	3.1	100.0

Table 3.16 Work status of respondents
Per cent distribution of ever-married Women age 13-49 by work status, according to state, India, 1992-93

State	Work Status				
	Not working	Working in family farm/business	Working for someone else	Self-employed	Total percentage
India	68.5	12.2	16.2	3.1	100.0
North					
Delhi	80.7	1.8	10.9	6.7	100.0
Haryana	71.1	18.6	8.6	1.8	100.0
Himachal Pradesh	52.3	40.9	5.9		100.0
Jammu Region of J & K	72.5	20.8	5.3	0.9	100.0
Punjab	92.3	1.8	4.7	1.5	100.0
Rajasthan	68.6	23.0	6.1	2.3	100.0
Central					
Madhya Pradesh	67.6	20.8	6.1	2.3	100.0
Uttar Pradesh	86.6	7.9	3.9	2.3	100.0
East					
Bihar	75.1	6.8	15.5	2.5	100.0
Orissa	75.1	2.5	18.3	4.1	100.0
West Bengal	77.0	6.3	13.1	3.6	100.0

Northeast					
Arunachal Pradesh	55.1	18.6	7.7	18.6	100.0
Assam	81.6	1.0	15.4	2.1	100.0
Manipur	46.5	17.7	11.6	24.1	100.0
Meghalaya	58.2	16.6	18.2	6.9	100.0
Mizoram	66.8	15.3	11.7	6.2	100.0
Nagaland	56.3	15.1	5.1	23.5	100.0
Tripura	74.3	10.3	12.9	2.5	100.0
West					
Goa	70.3	4.9	18.0	6.8	100.0
Gujarat	56.8	18.4	22.1	2.7	100.0
Maharashtra	51.0	20.0	25.6	3.4	100.0
South					
Andhra Pradesh	46.6	18.4	29.4	5.6	100.0
Karnataka	53.0	17.0	27.3	2.7	100.0
Kerala	75.3	1.2	19.6	3.9	100.0
Tamil Nadu	53.3	9.2	35.3	2.2	100.0

Table 3.17 Respondent's Level of education by background charateristics

Per cent distribution of ever-married women age 13-49 by highest level of education attained, according to selected background, characteristics and residence, India, 1992-93

	Respondent's Level of Education							
Background Characteristic	Illiterare	Literate, <primary complete	Primary school complete	Middle school complete	High school complete	Above high School	Total per cent	Number
1	2	3	4	5	6	7	8	9
				URBAN				
Age								
13-14	(60.8)	(18.9)	(15.7)	(4.9)	(--)	(--)	100.0	42
15-19	44.1	6.6	19.1	14.8	14.8	0.7	100.0	1376
20-24	35.1	5.9	16.5	14.9	19.5	8.1	100.0	4229
25-29	33.2	5.5	14.0	13.4	19.4	14.5	100.0	4705
30-34	34.2	7.5	14.1	11.3	18.5	14.4	100.0	4291
35-39	35.2	8.3	15.8	10.0	19.4	11.3	100.0	3715
40-44	41.6	9.0	15.1	10.1	15.2	9.1	100.0	2899
45-49	44.2	10.9	16.5	8.6	13.3	6.4	100.0	2197
Religion								
Hindu	34.7	6.7	15.3	12.6	18.9	11.7	100.0	17730
Muslim	52.1	11.1	16.4	8.5	9.2	2.7	100.0	3902
Christian	17.6	7.3	13.1	15.0	30.2	16.8	100.0	692
Sikh	25.3	1.7	16.8	11.8	28.0	16.6	100.0	419
Jain	7.8	5.1	13.1	9.3	34.2	30.5	100.0	311
Buddhist	50.8	9.8	14.9	12.4	9.1	3.0	100.0	342
Other	37.0	10.9	10.2	11.0	20.2	10.2	100.0	59

Caste/tribe								
Scheduled caste	64.2	5.9	12.1	7.7	7.7	2.2	100.0	2140
Scheduled tribe	53.6	7.3	12.6	9.0	12.3	5.3	100.0	762
Other	33.3	7.6	15.9	12.5	19.1	11.6	100.0	20553
Husband's education								
Illiterate	83.5	6.0	6.7	2.5	1.1	--	100.0	3983
Lit., < primary complete	58.7	18.0	15.4	6.3	1.2	0.3	100.0	1926
Primary school complete	51.4	10.9	22.5	9.4	5.3	0.5	100.0	3501
Middle school complete	32.3	9.5	23.8	22.1	11.3	1.0	100.0	3073
High school complete	18.0	6.0	19.6	18.4	31.2	6.7	100.0	6067
Above high school	5.3	2.3	6.8	9.4	34.7	41.5	100.0	4848
Missing	55.4	5.4	3.4	6.5	15.3	14.0	100.0	57
Total	36.8	7.4	15.4	12.0	17.9	10.6	100.0	23455
				RURAL				
Age								
13-14	74.3	7.9	15.8	2·0	--	--	100.0	311
15-19	71.2	5.4	11.9	7·5	3.9	0·1	100.0	7719
20-24	67.4	5.8	11.7	7·8	6.4	1·0	100.0	13755

Cont.......

1	2	3	4	5	6	7	8	9
25-29	70.3	6·4	10.4	5·9	5.7	1·3	100.0	12735
30-34	71.8	6.7	10.4	5.2	4.7	1.2	100.0	10369
35-39	73.7	7.2	10.6	4·6	3.3	0·6	100.0	8746
40-44	78.6	6·8	8.2	3·5	2.4	0-5	100.0	6850
45-49	82.4	7.3	6·8	1·9	1·4	0.2	100.0	5838
Religion								
Hindu	73.5	5·9	10.0	5·4	4.4	0·8	100.0	55919
Muslim	74.0	9·4	9.9	4·5	1.8	0-4	100.0	6905
Christian	40.5	12.0	15.9	14.4	13.8	3.4	100.0	1450
Sikh	59.0	3.6	19.8	7·0	9.2	1·5	100.0	1254
Jain	16.8	13.0	14.4	18.5	31.4	6·0	100.0	117
Buddhist	67.0	12.7	10.7	6.5	3.1	--	100.0	392
Other	79.0	7.7	8.6	3·4	1.0	0·4	100.0	286
Caste/tribe								
Scheduled caste	85.4	3.8	5·8	3.1	1·8	0.1	100.0	8830
Scheduled tribe	87.6	4·4	3.9	2·5	1'4	0.2	100.0	7172
Other	68.0	7·2	12.1	6·5	5.3	1·0	100.0	50319
Husband's education								
Illiterate	93.8	2.8	2·7	0.6	0.1	--	100.0	27159
Lit., <primary com.	74.4	14.1	8·4	2.6	0·5	--	100.0	7147
Primary school com.	68.4	9·9	15.4	4·7	1.6	--	100.0	10647
Middle school com.	56.8	9.1	18.0	12.1	3.8	0.1	100.0	7662

Above high school	23.4	4.5	16.0	14.9	28.6	12.5	100.0	3177
Missing	71.8	3.8	14.9	4.6	4.8	--	100.0	136
Total	72.4	6.4	10.3	5·6	4.4	0.8	100.0	66322
				TOTAL				
Age								
13-14	72.7	9.2	15.8	2.3	--	--	100.0	352
15-19	67.1	5.6	13.0	8.6	5.6	0.2	100.0	9095
20-24	59.8	5.8	12.8	9.5	9.5	2.6	100.0	17983
25-29	*60.3*	6.1	11.3	7.9	9.4	4.9	100.0	17442
30-34	*60.8*	6.9	11.5	7.0	8.8	5.0	100.0	14660
35-39	*62.2*	7.5	12.1	6.2	8.1	3.8	100.0	12461
40-44	67.6	7.4	10.2	5.5	6.2	3.1	100.0	9748
45-49	72.0	8.3	9.5	3.7	4.7	1.9	100.0	8036
Rel igion								
Hindu	64.1	6.1	11.3	7.2	7.9	3.4	100.0	73648
Muslim	*66.1*	10.0	12.2	5.9	4.5	1.2	100.0	10806
Christian	33.1	10.5	15.0	14.6	19.1	7.8	100.0	2142
Sikh	50.5	3.1	19.0	8.2	13.9	5.3	100.0	1673
Jain	10.3	7.2	13.5	11.8	33.4	23.8	100.0	428

Cont.......

1	2	3	4	5	6	7	8	9
Buddhist	59.4	11.3	12.7	9.3	5.9	1.4	100.0	734
Other	71.7	8.3	8.8	4.7	4.3	2.2	100.0	345
Caste/tribe								
Scheduled caste	81.3	4.2	7·0	4.0	3.0	0.5	100.0	10970
Scheduled tribe	84.3	4.7	4·7	3.1	2.4	0.7	100.0	7934
Other	57.9	7.3	13.2	8.2	9.3	4.1	100.0	70872
Husband's education								
Illiterate	92.5	3.2	3.2	0.8	0.3	—	100.0	31142
Lit., <primary complete	71·1	14.9	9.9	3.4	0.7	0.1	100.0	9073
Primary school complete	64.2	10.1	17.2	5.9	2.5	0.1	100.0	14148
MiddLe school corplete	49.8	9.2	19.7	15.0	5.9	0.4	100.0	10735
High school complete	35.5	5.9	19.3	15.6	20.6	3.1	100.0	1646
Above high school	12.5	3.2	10.4	11.6	32.3	30.0	100.0	8025
Missing	67.0	4.3	11.5	5.2	7.9	4.1	100.0	193
Total	63.1	6.7	11.7	7.2	7.9	3.4	100.0	89777

() Based on 25-49 unweighted cases

-- Less than 0.05 per cent

Table 3.18: Exposure to mass media

Per cent of ever-married women age 13-49 who usually watch television or listen to the radio at least once a week or visit a cinema at least once a month or who are not regularly exposed to any of these media, by selected background characteristics, India, 1992-93

	Exposure to mass media				
Background Characteristic	Watches television at least once a week	Listens to the radio at least once a week	Visits a cinema/theater at least once a week	Not regularly exposed to any media	Number of women
Age					
13-14	17.3	34.1	19.6	54.6	352
15-19	22.6	41.0	18.2	50.5	9095
20-24	30.7	44.6	18.0	46.5	17983
25-29	33.0	44.5	17.1	46.1	17442
30-34	34.3	43.7	14.4	46.8	14660
35-39	35.3	43.6	13.3	46.0	12461
40-44	32.8	43.7	10.9	47.6	9748
45-49	31.2	40.8	9.2	50.8	8036
Residence					
Urban	68.2	63.5	27.6	19.1	23455
Rural	18.9	36.4	10.6	57.3	66322
Education					
Illiterate	15.1	28.9	9.2	64.2	56654
Lit.,<middle comple.	45.0	59.7	20.1	27.7	16475
Middle school comp.	63.5	70.9	26.8	14.5	6508
High school comp.	83.0	80.7	31.9	6.4	10138
Rel igim					
Hindu	31.2	43.3	15.7	47.7	73648
Muslim	21.6	40.4	11.0	51.4	10806
Christian	41.3	57.4	18.9	32.4	2142
Sikh	54.7	41.9	3.1	37.1	1673
Jain	85.0	78.0	28.4	8.6	428
Buddhist	46.6	50.4	15.6	36.4	734
Other	19.0	29.7	11.0	63.1	345
Caste/tribe					
Scheduled caste	22.7	34.8	13.8	56.0	10970
Scheduled tribe	12.0	25.3	6.3	70.2	7934
Other	35.4	46.8	16.2	43.4	70872
Total	31.8	43.5	15.0	47.3	89777

Pradesh and Uttar Pradesh, the majority of working women work on the family farm or in the family business. The percentage of women who are self-employed is highest in Nagaland and Manipur.

Among ever-married women age 13-49, the proportion illiterate generally increases with age, reflecting improvements in levels of education over time (Table 3.17). A notably high proportion of women in the age groups 13-14 and 15-19 (73 and 67 per cent, respectively) are illiterate because women who marry young tend to be drawn selectively from among the less educated.

Almost two-thirds of Hindu and Muslim women are illiterate, as are one-third of Christians and one-half of Sikhs. The percentage of women who have completed at least a high school education is lowest among Muslims (6 per cent), followed by Buddhists (7 per cent), Hindus (11 per cent), Sikhs (19 per cent), and Christians (27 per cent). Jains are the most highly educated group. Fifty-seven per cent of Jain women have completed at least high school and only 10 per cent are illiterate. Between 81 and 84 per cent of women belonging to scheduled castes and scheduled tribes are illiterate compared with 58 per cent of other women. A similar disadvantage of scheduled castes and scheduled tribes is also found at each level of schooling. With respect to the husband's education, 93 per cent of women with illiterate husbands are illiterate themselves. Among husbands who have completed high school (but have not gone on to a higher level of Education), three-fourths have married women with lower levels of education. As expected, urban respondents have lower levels of illiteracy and higher levels of education for all the background characteristics considered.

Tables 3.18 and 3.19 provide information on exposure of respondents to mass media. This type of information can be used as one measure of modernity and it can also help health and family welfare planners design appropriate information, education and communication IEC) programmes. Almost half (47 per cent) of NFHS respondents are not regularly exposed to any kind of mass media (television, radio or cinema). Only 44 per cent of women normally listen to the radio at least once a week; 32 per cent watch television at least once a week; and 15 per cent go to a cinema hall or theatre to see a movie at least once a month. It was noted earlier (Table 3.13) that 39 per cent of households own a radio and only 21 per cent own a television. These facts point out the difficulty of diffusing information on family planning, health and other topics through the mass media.

Exposure to mass media varies sharply according to women's place of residence, education, religion, and caste/tribe, but not as much

Table 3.19: Exposure to mass media by state

Per cent of ever-married women age 13-49 who usually watch television or listen to the radio st least once a week or visit a cinema at least once a month or who are not regularly exposed to any of these media, by state, India, 1992-93

	Exposure to mass media			
State	Watches television at least once a week	Listens to the radio at least once a week	Visits a cinema/theater at least once a week	Not regularly exposed to any media
India	31.8	43.5	15.0	47.3
North				
Delhi	82.8	63.6	5.7	13.3
Haryana	49.0	42.2	2.0	39.9
Himachal Pradesh	47.1	54.6	2.9	33.2
Jammu Region of J & K	50.1	64.2	2.5	27.8
Punjab	57.3	42.0	2.3	34.5
Rajasthan	17.9	27.2	5.2	69.9
Central				
Madhya Pradesh	26.7	32.7	10.0	59.0
Utter Predesh	19.0	29.7	4.1	64.5
East				
Bihar	12.7	25.9	5.2	70.5
Orissa	16.1	34.9	7.4	60.5
West Bengal	33.3	48.3	16.1	38.7
Northeest				
Arunachal Pradesh	28.7	40.7	14.4	53.4
Assam	18.0	32.8	4.2	60.9
Manipur	38.2	63.1	16.5	32.2
Meghalaya	23.8	37.6	5.4	53.6
Mizorarn	25.3	55.1	0.6	38.7
Nagaland	22.5	42.4	1.5	55.4
Tripura	34.3	56.7	6.7	34.5
West				
Goa	70.6	69.3	3.9	14.8
Gujarat	39.4	47.0	9.5	44.6
Maharashtra	46.4	52.3	14.9	37.2
South				
Andhra Pradesh	39.1	62.4	48.8	24.8
Karnataka	39.5	62.9	30.3	29.9
Kerala	42.2	71.3	18.3	20.8
Tamil Nadu	50.4	59.7	42.6	22.0

according to their age. The proportion who watch television at least once a week ranges from 31 to 35 per cent across the different age groups, except among women under age 20 who are less likely to watch television. This lower percentage no doubt occurs because women who marry young are selectively drawn from among the less educated and lower socioeconomic groups, as mentioned earlier. The proportion who listen to the radio at least once a week ranges from 34 to 45 per cent, increasing up to age 20-24, after which it decreases slightly. The number who go to the cinema/theatre at least once a month ranges from 9 to 20 per cent, with younger women more likely to attend than older women .

Media exposure is much greater in urban than in rural areas, regardless of the type of media. Eighty-one per cent of urban women are regularly exposed to any media compared with only 43 per cent of rural women. Differences in media exposure by education are even more pronounced, with greater exposure for the more educated. Only 36 per cent of illiterate women are regularly exposed to any media compared with 94 per cent of women with at least a high school education. Hindus are slightly more exposed to mass media than Muslims (52 per cent compared with 49 per cent). Between 63 and 68 per cent of Christian, Sikh and Buddhist women are regularly exposed to mass media, as are 91 per cent of Jain women. Women from scheduled tribes are least exposed to all kinds of media. Scheduled caste women are also less likely to be exposed to mass media than non-SC/ST women. These differences may partly reflect underlying differences in place of residence or education.

Interstate variations in media exposure are presented in Table 3.19. More than threefourths of women are regularly exposed to television, radio or the cinema in Delhi, Goa, Kerala, Tamil Nadu, and Andhra Pradesh. Less than 40 per cent of women are regularly exposed to mass media in Rajasthan, Bihar, Uttar Pradesh, Assam and Orissa. The states differ most in the exposure of women to television. Only 13-19 per cent of women watch television at least once a week in Bihar, Orissa, Assam, Rajasthan and Uttar Pradesh. On the other hand, more than 70 per cent of women regularly watch television in Delhi and Goa. The penetration of television is also relatively high in Punjab, Tamil Nadu and Jammu, where more than half of women are regularly exposed to television. The southern states have the highest percentage of women who visit a cinema/theatre at least once in month. Among the remaining states, cinema watching is more common in Manipur, West Bengal, Maharashtra, Arunachal Pradesh and Madhya Pradesh.

4

NUPTIALITY

The findings on marriage patterns from the National Family Health Survey are explained in this chapter. Marriage is important in its own right, and also because it influences fertility and population growth, affects the nature of family relationships, and is inextricably linked to the status of women. After examining current marital status distributions, this chapter considers age at first marriage, age at first cohabitation, and marriage between relatives. State differentials in age at marriage and the incidence of consanguineous marriages are also presented in this chapter. Before discussing the findings of the NFHS on marriage patterns in India, it is useful to describe the salient features of the marriage system in India.

4.1 MARRIAGE IN INDIA

Marriage is the basis of social life and is a matter of great importance in India. By that very fact, marriage is subject to strict rules and prohibitions. One of these rules, laid down by Hindu scriptures, is that marriage should take place as soon as the girl reaches puberty, or else the father or guardian commits a grave fault. If he finds a good bridegroom, the father may arrange her marriage even before puberty (Renou, 1959). Child wives are expected to live with their parents until puberty. Traditionally, virginity was highly respected, and was regarded as a sign of the elite and an index to high caste. Consequently, marriages with no possibility of suspicion regarding the virginity of the girl were considered most desirable. This is one of the reasons why even today parents are very concerned and anxious once their daughters attain puberty (Kapadia, 1966). According to Kapadia, a further impetus to prepuberty marriages was given by attaching social prestige to them. To have one's daughter betrothed before puberty was also considered a sign of one's affluence, influence or status. "Under the operation of these various forces early marriages became more popular, and with the passing of time the practice became so compelling that a departure from it was a matter of social disgrace" (Kapadia, 1966).

Various laws have been enacted in India to prevent child marriages. The Child Marriage Restraint Act, which is commonly known as the Sarda Act, was enacted in 1929 and was applicable at that time only to British India. Initially the Act placed restrictions on marriages of girls below age 12 and boys below age 15. However, in its final form, the Act specified the minimum age at marriage for females and males to be 14 and 18 years, respectively. Through an amendment of this Act in 1949, the legal minimum age at marriage for females was raised to 15. According to the Child Marriage Restraint Act of 1978, the minimum legal age at marriage in India is 18 years for women and 21 years for men. Registration of marriages is not compulsory in India.

Traditionally, divorce and separation have not been common in India. Marriage has been considered as a union of souls and not merely of bodies. Writing about Hindu marriage, Dass in his study on Rigvedic Culture observes: "It is more solemn affair in a man or woman's life, upon which depends his or her worldly and spiritual welfare and final emancipation from bonds that tie him or her down to the earth. It is certainly not a thing to be donned or doffed at one's pleasure. It is an eternal bond that binds two souls together for ever and each suffers for other's lapses and derelictions. It is not a contract with them, but a sacrament and there is no breaking away or parting from the union" (as quoted by Goyal, 1988).

However, the proportion of widows has been relatively high in India because of the considerable age gap between husbands and wives, high levels of mortality, and restrictions on remarriage. Traditionally, remarriage is more permissible for men than for women. Remarriages among high caste Hindu women were socially prohibited, but such restrictions did not exist for low caste Hindu women (Agarwala, 1985). The restrictions on remarriages still prevail, particularly in rural areas.

Another facet of marriage in India is the dowry. The custom of dowry in the form of the presentation of gifts to the bridegroom by parents or guardians of brides has prevailed in India since ancient times. According to the Hindu Dharmashastras, among the eight forms of marriages, the most approved form, the Brahma Vivah, is that in which a maiden or virgin girl is decorated with ornaments and is given by her father to a suitable partner. The most emphatically denounced form of marriage is that in which money is paid to the father or kinsman of the bride by the bridegroom, in other words, where the bride is purchased (Prabhu, 1963; Kapadia, 1966). The custom of giving dowry may also be rooted in the desire of parents to show affection for their daughters who are married at a very early age (Hooja, 1969). These days, however the dowry is a matter of status for the bride's family —the bigger the dowry and grander the ceremony, the greater the prestige to the family.

Although the practice is officially outlawed, a dowry is still expected in the majority of cases. For poorer families the marriage can become a huge financial burden. Many families are forced to borrow the money, either for the daughter's dowry or to stage a lavish ceremony and feast (or both), usually at high rates of interest. The system of dowry also perpetuates early marriages in that parents wish to have their daughter marry young, when less dowry is demanded.

4.2 Current Marital Status

Table 4. 1 shows the current marital status of women by residence and age. Information on marital status comes from the Woman's Questionnaire, except for the information on never-married women, which comes from the Household Questionnaire. Table 4.1 contains similar information to Table 3.5, which also includes information for males and covers a wider range of ages. The percentages never married in the two tables differ slightly due to differential nonresponse among eligible women.

Table 4.1 suggests that marriage is virtually universal in India and that marriages in rural areas take place at relatively young ages. At age 15-19, 39 per cent of women in India have ever been married. The proportions ever married at age 15-19 are much lower in urban areas (22 per cent) than in rural areas (46 per cent). Not only do the marriages take place at later ages in urban areas, the proportion of women age 35-49 who remain unmarried is also slightly higher in urban areas (2 per cent) than in rural areas (less than 1 per cent). The per cent of ever-married women increases rapidly with age from 82 per cent of women age 20-24 to 98 per cent of women age 30-34. Only 1 per cent of women age 35-39 remain unmarried. The proportions divorced and separated together account for less than 2 per cent of the total sample of women age 15-49. Only 3 per cent of women age 15-49 are widowed, and the proportion widowed increases with age from less than 1 per cent among women below age 25 to 13 per cent among women age 45- 49. The lower proportion of widows at younger ages may partly be due to lower mortality and partly due to the greater likelihood of widows remarrying in the younger age groups (Agarwala, 1985).

The proportions of women of different ages who are currently married in each state are presented in Table 4.2. Early marriages are common in Madhya Pradesh, Andhra Pradesh and Bihar where more

Table 4.1: Current Marital status
Per cent distribution of Women age 15-49 by current marital status, according to age and residence, India, 1992-93

Age	Never married	Currently married	Widowed	Divorced	Separated	Total percent
			Marital status			
			URBAN			
15-19	78.2	21.3	0.1	0.1	0.3	100.0
20-24	31.8	66.4	0.5	0.2	1.1	100.0
25-29	8.9	88.1	1.Z	0.3	1.4	100.0
30-34	3.1	92.2	2.6	0.5	1.7	100.0
35-39	1.7	92.4	4.5	0.2	1.3	100.0
40-44	1.9	88.1	8.4	0.3	1.3	100.0
45-49	1.6	82.8	13.9	0.3	1.4	100.0
Total	24.6	70.9	3.0	0.3	1.1	100.0
			RURAL			
15-19	54.4	44.7	0.1	0.1	0.6	100.0
20-24	13.2	84.5	0.8	0.2	1.3	100.0
25-29	2.9	93.4	1.6	0.3	1.8	100.0
30-34	1.1	93.7	3.2	0.4	1.7	100.0
35-39	0.6	92.1	5.5	0.3	1.6	100.0
40-44	0.3	89.1	8.8	0.1	1.6	100.0
45-49	0.5	86.0	11.9	0.2	1.3	100.0
Total	15.3	80.0	3.2	0.2	1.3	100.0

TOTAL

15-19	60.7	38.4	0.1	0.1	0.6	100.0
20-24	18.5	79.4	0.7	0.2	1.3	100.0
25-29	4.7	91.9	1.5	0.3	1.7	100.0
30-34	1.7	93.2	3.0	0.4	1.7	100.0
35-39	0.9	92.2	5.2	0.2	1.5	100.0
40-44	1.1	88.5	8.7	0.2	1.5	100.0
45-49	0.6	85.3	12.5	0.2	1.3	100.0
Total	17.9	77.4	3.1	0.3	1.3	100.0

than 50 per cent of women age 15-19 are currently married. Marriages also occur relatively early in Haryana and Uttar Pradesh, where 40-44 per cent of women age 15-19 and 88 per cent of women age 20-24 are currently married. Women tend to marry late in Kerala, Punjab and in the smaller states of Goa, Manipur, Mizoram and Nagaland, with less than 15 per cent of women age 15-19 in these states being currently married. In almost every state, the percentage currently married increases with an increase in the age of women up to age 25-29, levels off at age 30-39 and thereafter gradually declines, mainly because of the increase in widowhood at later ages.

Table 4.2 also provides information on the percentage of ever-married women who have been married more than once. Overall, 2 per cent of ever-married women in India have been married more than once. The proportion is low in all states, varying from 0.3 per cent in Goa to around 3 per cent in Mizoram.

4.3 Age at First Marriage

The description of marriage patterns can be sharpened by examining values of the Singulate Mean Age at Marriage (SMAM), which is calculated from the age-specific proportions never married for age groups 15-19 through 45-49 (Hajnal, 1953; Shryock and Siegel, 1980). Table 4.3 presents female and male SMAMs computed from the 1961, 1971, and 1981 Census, and from the NFHS, for India and the states. For India as a whole, female values of SMAM from the NFHS are 21.5 years in urban areas, 19.3 in rural areas, and 20.0 overall. On average, males marry 5 years later than females. Marriage ages are consistently higher in urban areas, with urban men marrying about two years later than rural men, and urban women also marrying two years later than their rural counterparts. Together, the Census and NFHS SMAMs in Table 4.3 also indicate how age at marriage has been changing in the country. Between 1961 and 1992-93, the SMAM for females rose by 4. 1 years, from 15.9 years of age to 20.0. Over the same period, the SMAM for males rose by 3.1 years, from 21.9 to 25.0.

There are large interstate variations in SMAM. In almost every state, men marry later than women, and men and women marry earlier in rural areas than in urban areas. The female SMAM is lowest in Madhya Pradesh (17.4 years) and highest in Goa (25.1 years). Among the major states (states with a population of more than 5 million in 1991), the female SMAM is higher than 20 years in Kerala, Assam, Punjab, Delhi, Orissa, Tamil Nadu, Himachal Pradesh and Gujarat. On the other hand, the mean age at marriage for females is less than 19 years in Madhya

Pradesh, Bihar, Andhra Pradesh, Rajasthan, Haryana and Uttar Pradesh. The female age at marriage is relatively high in the northeastern states, particularly in Manipur. Similar differences across the states are also observed for the SMAM for males. The difference between the male and female SMAMs is relatively large (6-7 years) in West Bengal, Assam, Tripura, Karnataka and Kerala.

More detailed information from the NFHS on female age at first marriage is shown in Table 4.4, which shows the percentage of all women who were ever married by specified exact ages. The table shows a clear trend toward rising age at marriage, with especially large declines in marriage at very young ages. The proportion marrying before age 13 declines from 27 per cent in the 45-49 age cohort to less than 7 per cent in the 15-19 age cohort, and the proportion marrying before age 15 declines from 45 per cent in the 45-49 age cohort to 17 per cent in the 15-19 age cohort. Although marriages before age 15 have declined considerably, marriages before the legal minimum age at marriage of 18 years are still quite common. For instance, 54 per cent of women currently age 20-24 married before age 18, and this percentage is much higher in rural (63 per cent) than in urban areas (33 per cent). Declines in age at marriage are less pronounced, but, still large, at higher exact age cut-offs.

Table 4.5 shows the median age at first marriage[1] for females by age group and selected background characteristics. The median age at first marriage is used instead of the mean age at marriage (where both are calculated directly from reported ages at marriage) because the median, unlike the mean, is not biased by age truncation. (The survey interview marks the point of age truncation.) For example, in the 20-24 age cohort in Table 4.5, the mean age at first marriage will ultimately be influenced by marriages that occur in this cohort after the survey. But the median age at first marriage for the cohort will not be so affected, because more than 50 per cent of the women in the cohort married before age 20, implying that the median is determined before the survey occurred. It follows that the variation in median age at first marriage by age cohort, from oldest to youngest, reflects a trend over time that is not biased by age truncation.

Table 4.2 Percentage currently married by age

Percentage of women age 15-49 who are currently married and percentage of ever-married women married more than once, by age and state, India, 1992-93

State	Current age								Percent married more than once'
	15-19	20-24	25-29	30-34	35-39	40-44	45-49	Total	
India	38.4	7P.4	91.9	93.2	92.2	88.5	85.3	77.4	1.6
North									
Delhi	18.6	69.5	92.4	95.3	94.4	91.8	84.1	74.3	0.6
Haryana	44.1	88.4	97.0	97.2	95.3	91.2	88.4	82.5	1.1
Himachal Pradesh	19.3	74.9	94.3	92.6	95.3	89.5	86.7	73.9	1.8
Jammu Region of J&K	18.0	62.9	91.9	94.6	94.2	90.7	88.4	68.7	0.9
Punjab	14.4	66.9	93.3	96.0	94.9	92.2	87.8	70.8	0.7
Rajasthan	38.3	87.5	97.9	97.2	96.0	93.1	90.4	81.3	0.9
Central									
Madhya Pradesh	61.9	88.7	94.1	94.2	95.0	95.0	89.0	86.9	2.5
Uttar Pradesh	39.6	88.0	96.8	96.3	95.3	92.0	88.6	80.8	1.6
East									
Bihar	50.3	88.6	95.2	96.1	93.1	90.6	86.0	82.9	1.8
Orissa	27.5	70.9	90.7	93.5	89.7	90.9	83.6	71.8	1.5
West Bengal	40.0	77.5	88.6	88.7	88.9	85.1	83.1	74.8	1.8
Northeast									
Arunachal Pradesh	28.6	75.8	88.8	91.3	90.2	87.8	82.7	72.0	2.1

Assam	31. 0	60.9	80.5	87.2	86.8	78.3	77.5	65.5	2.0
Manipur	6.0	41.0	67,4	81.7	88.5	86.0	86.1	55.5	1.2
Meghalaya	18.3	61 .0	84.4	88.1	85.6	83.9	77.0	64.8	2.0
Mizoram	9.2	40.8	70.0	80.2	92.8	85.6	81.7	56.6	2.8
Nagaland	11.3	50.6	75.1	81.3	90.5	81. Z	88.9	61.0	0.4
Tripura	25.8	61.5	82.1	85.8	91.9	85.5	80.3	67.2	1.2
West									
Goa	3.1	28.8	68.3	86.2	90.9	85.6	81.2	55.7	0.3
Gujarat	22.0	74.5	92.3	95.2	94.4	89.1	86.6	73.9	2.1
Maharashtra	36.2	78.3	89.0	92.3	91.1	87.6	86.2	75.8	1.7
South									
Andhra Pradesn	52.2	85.7	92.3	91.9	89.1	84.3	81.4	80.1	1.6
Karnataka	37.0	72.8	89.7	90.0	89.6	81.9	79.0	72.8	0.4
Kerala	13.4	52.8	82.8	87.3	88.6	83.6	78.4	64.6	2.1
Tamil Nadu	24.4	71.4	88.2	88.8	89.2	87.1	82.2	71.5	0.9

Ever-married women age 13-49.

Table 4.3: Singulate mean age at marriage

Singulate mean age at marriage from selected sources, by sex and state, India, 1961-1993

	1961 Census		1971 Census		1981 Census		NFHS 1992-93 Urban		NFHS 1992-93 Rural		NFHS 1992-93 Total	
State	Male	Female	Male	Female	Male	Female	Male	Female	Male	Female	Male	Female
India	21.9	15.9	22.6	17.2	23.5	18.4	26.3	21.5	24.4	19.3	25.0	20.0
North												
Delhi	23.3	18.7	24.0	20.0	24.3	20.5	24.4	21.0	24.1	19.0	24.3	20.9
Haryana	U	U	20.9	17.7	25.1	17.9	24.4	19.9	22.69	17.9	231	18.4
Himachal Pradesh	22.2	15.6	23.5	17.8	24.2	19.1	26.1	22.3	24.9	20.2	25.0	20.4
Jammu Region of J & K	U	U	U	U	U	U	27.5	23.1	26.0	20.9	26.3	21.2
Punjab	22.6	17.5	24.1	20.1	25.0	21.1	25.5	21.7	24.6	20.9	24.8	
Rajasthan	19.6	14.2	19.9	15.1	20.6	16.1	24.9	20.5	22.2	17.9	22.7	18.4
Central												
Madhya Pradesh	18.7	13.9	19.5	15.0	20.8	16.6	24.9	19.7	21.0	16.7	22.0	11.4
Uttar Pradesh	19.4	14.5	19.8	15.5	21.3	16.7	25.2	20.9	22.4	17.9	23.0	18.6
East												
Bihar	18.9	14.3	20.0	15.3	21.6	16.6	25.3	20.3	22.7	17.6	23.2	18.0
Orissa	21.9	16.4	22.7	17.3	24.3	19.1	27.2	21.8	25.3	20.4	25.6	20.7
West Bengal	24.3	15.9	24.6	18.0	26.0	19.3	27.6	21.8	25.0	18.1	25.9	19.2
Northeast												
Arunachal Pradesh	U	U	25.6	19.6	U	U	25.6	19.8	24.8	20.0	24.9	20.0

Assam	25.9	18.6	25.8	18.7	U	U	29.2	23.0	t1.7	21.4	27.9	21.6
Manipur	24.8	19.9	26.4	22.2	27.3	23.4	29.0	26.5	28.0	24.2	28.3	25.0
Meghalaya	U	U	25.5	20.2	26.0	21.0	27.1	23.3	24.6	20.6	25.1	21.2
Mizoram	U	U	U	U	U	U	28.5	24.0	26.9	21.4	27.8	22.9
Nagaland	26.2	22.2	27.8	24.0	29.0	24.8	26.3	19.0	25.7	22.8	25.8	22.7
Tripura	24.1	16.3	25.3	18.4	26.8	20.3	28.6	22.4	27.1	20.9	27.3	21.2
West												
Goa	27.1	20.9	U	U	28.5	23.0	30.7	25.0	30.5	25.2	30.6	25.1
Gujarat	21.7	17.1	22.4	18.5	23.3	19.6	24.8	20.6	23.5	20.0	23.9	20.2
Maharashtra	22.6	15.8	23.8	11.6	24.4	18.8	25.8	21.0	24.1	17.9	24.9	19.3
South												
Andhra Pradesh	22.3	15.2	22.8	16.3	23.1	17.3	25.6	20.3	22.8	17.3	23.6	18.1
Karnataka	24.7	16.4	25.2	17.9	26.0	19.3	26.9	20.8	25.6	19.0	26.1	19.6
Kerala	26.6	20.2	27.0	21.3	27.5	22.1	28.7	23.2	27.9	21.7	28.1	22.1
Tamil Nadu	25.3	18.4	26.1	19.6	26.1	20.3	27.3	21.3	25.9	20.0	26.4	20.5

U: Not available.

Table 4.4: Age at first marriage
Percentage of women married by specific exact ages, by current age and residence, India, 1992-93

Current age	13	15	18	20	22	25	Per cent never married
		Percentage ever married before age:					
URBAN							
15-19	1.8	5.5	NA	NA	NA	NA	78.2
20-24	3·9	10.9	32.6	52.5	NA	NA	31.8
25-29	5.9	16.1	40.9	59.9	73.5	86.5	8.9
30-34	6·8	16.9	46.2	65.1	78.1	89.3	3.1
35-39	8·9	20.8	51.9	69.8	81.5	91.4	1.7
40-44	11.9	25.6	56.1	73.6	85.0	92.9	1.9
45-49	13.6	27.9	59.2	77.2	87.4	94.4	1.6
20-9	7.4	17.9	44.9	63.7	75.8	84.6	11.0
25-9	8.6	20.2	49.0	67.4	79.7	90.1	4.1
RURAL							
15-19	8.6	21.3	NA	NA	NA	NA	54.4
20-24	14.9	32.0	62.8	78.8	NA	NA	13.2
25-29	18.1	38.0	71.2	84.7	91.8	95.8	2.9
30-34	22.2	41.5	74.6	87.4	93.8	97.2	1.1
35-39	24.7	44.9	77.8	88.8	94.8	97.6	0.6
40-44	27.0	47.6	79.8	90.8	96.5	98.5	0.3
45-49	31.6	51.6	80.8	91.0	96.3	98.5	0.5
20-49	21.2	40.4	72.4	85.5	91.8	94.5	4.4
25-49	23.4	43.4	75.8	87.9	94.2	97.2	1.3
TOTAL							
15-19	6.8	17.0	NA	NA	NA	NA	60.7
20-24	11.8	26.1	54.2	71.4	NA	NA	18.5
25-29	14.7	31.8	62.6	77.7	86.6	93.1	4.7
30-34	17.6	34.2	66.2	80.7	89.1	94.9	1.7
35-39	19.9	37.6	70.0	83.1	90.8	95.7	0.9
40-44	22.4	40.8	72.4	85.3	92.7	96.5	1.1
45-49	26.7	45.1	75.0	87.3	94.0	97.5	0.6
20-49	17.2	33.9	64.5	79.2	87.1	91.6	6.4
25-49	19.1	36.6	68.0	81.9	89.9	95.1	2.2

NA: Not applicable

[1] The current age groups include both never-married and ever-married women.

The median age at first marriage increases steadily from 15.5 years for women in the 40- 49 age cohort to 17.4 years in the 20-24 age cohort, a rise of 2.0 years. The median age at marriage is higher among women who are currently living in urban areas than among those women currently living in rural areas, but both groups show a similar decline across cohorts. Indeed, the decline has been slightly greater in urban than in rural areas. Urban women marry about three years later than rural women.

Table 4.5 Median age at first marriage by background characteristics
Median age at first marriage among women age 20-49 years, by current age and selected background characteristics, India, 1992-93

Background characteristic	Current age						
	20-24	25-29	30-34	35-39	40-49	20-49	25-49
Residence							
Urban	19.7	18.8	18.3	17.8	17.1	18.4	18.1
Rural	16.5	15.9	15.6	15.3	15.0	15.7	15.5
Education							
Illiterate	15.5	15.3	15.2	14.9	14.7	15.1	15.0
Lit., < midde complete	18.0	17.1	16.9	16.7	16.6	17.1	16.8
Middle school complete	19.1	18.7	18.3	18.4	18.1	18.6	18.4
High school and above	NC	21.7	21.4	21.0	20.8	NC	21.3
Religion							
Hindu	17.2	16.4	16.1	15.8	15.4	16.1	15.9
Muslim	17.2	16.4	16.0	15.8	15.5	16.2	15.9
Christian	NC	20.4	20.5	19.9	19.4	NC	20.0
Sikh	NC	20.4	19.6	18.9	18.8	NC	19.5
Other	18.8	17.7	18.1	16.7	16.1	17.7	17.1
Caste/tribe							
Scheduled caste	15.9	15.3	15.2	14.8	14.5	15.2	15.0
Scheduled tribe	16.4	16.1	15.8	15.b	15.6	15.9	15.8
Other	17.8	16.8	16.5	16.2	15.7	16.6	16.3
Total	17.4	16.6	16.3	15.9	15.5	16.4	16.1

NC: Not calculated because less than 50 percent of the women have married for the first time by age 20

The median age at first marriage is higher the more educated the woman is, with the median among women who have completed high school exceeding the median among illiterate women by six years. There are also differences by religion, with Christians and Sikhs marrying four

Tabte 4.6 Median age at first marriage by state
Median age at first marriage among women age 20-49 years, by current age and state, India, 1992-93

	Current age						
State	20-24	25-29	30-34	35-39	40-49	20-49	25-49
India	17.4	16.6	16.3	15.9	15.5	16.4	16.1
North							
Delhi	19.7	18.7	18.5	18.5	17.2	18.6	18.3
Haryana	17.1	16.4	16.2	15.9	15.8	16.3	16.0
Himachat Pradesh	19.7	18.6	17.9	17.2	16.6	18.Z	17.7
Jammu Region of J & K	NC	19.1	18.3	16.7	16.4	18.6	17.8
Punjab	NC	19.8	19.1	18.8	18.7	19.5	19.0
Rajasthan	15.9	15.2	14.9	15.1	15.0	IS.2	15.0
Central							
Madhya Pradesh	15.4	14.9	14.5	14.3	14.0	14.7	14.5
Uttar Pradesh	16.4	15.6	15.2	15.0	14.5	15.4	15.1
East							
Bihar	15.8	15.4	14.9	14.6	13.9	15.0	14.7
Orissa	18.5	17.4	17.0	16.2	15.9	17.0	16.6
West Bengat	17.3	16.6	16.4	15.8	15.1	16.3	16.0
Northeast							
Arunachat Pradesh	18.5	17.9	18.Z	18.2	18.9	18.3	18.2
Assam	18.7	17.6	17.2	16.8	16.2	17.4	16.9
Manipur	NC	22.1	21.S	20.5	19.8	NC	20.8
Meghalaya	SC	19.1	18.4	19.0	19.4	19.3	19.0
Mizoram	NC	21.9	20.4	20.9	21.1	NC	21.0
Nagaland	NC	21.0	19.3	20.0	20.1	NC	20.1
Tripura	18.9	17.8	18.1	16.9	16.3	17.6	17.2
West							
Goa	SC	Z4.1	ZZ.S	Z1.0	Z0.0	NC	Z1.7
Gujarat	19.1	18.3	18.Z	17.6	17.4	18.Z	17.9
Maharashtra	17.5	16.6	16.4	16.1	15.3	16.4	16.1
South							
Andhra Pradesh	15.9	15.4	IS.2	15.0	14.6	15.3	15.1
Karnataka	17.9	16.9	16.6	16.6	16.2	16.8	16.6
Kerala	NC	20.6	20.3	19.6	19.0	NC	19.8
Tamil Nadu	19.3	18.7	18.6	18.0	17.1	18.3	18.1

NC: Not calculated because less than 50 per cent of the women have married for the first time by age 20 years later than Hindus. There is no difference in the median age at first marriage between Hindus and Muslims in any of the age groups. The differences in the median age at marriage by caste/tribe are moderate. The median age at marriage for women age 25-49 is lowest among scheduled caste women (15.0 years), and highet among non-SC/ST women (16.3 years), with scheduled tribe women marrying, on average, about half a year earlier than non-SC/ST women.

States differ considerably in the median age at first marriage (Table 4.6). At least half of women age 20-49 married at or below age 15 in Madhya Pradesh, Bihar, Rajasthan, Uttar Pradesh, and Andhra Pradesh. Only in a few smaller states (Manipur, Mizoram, Nagaland and Goa and Kerala is the median age at marriage 20 years or higher.

The median age at marriage exhibits a consistent gradual rise from the oldest to the youngest cohorts in all states except Rajasthan and the smaller states of Arunachal Pradesh, Meghalaya, Mizoram and Nagaland. However, even these five states have exhibited a rise in the median age at marriage among the younger cohorts. The increase in the age at marriage has been the greatest in Goa, where the median increased from 20.0 years for the women age 40-49 to 24.1 years for the 25-29 age cohort, a rise of more than four years. The difference in the median age at marriage between the youngest and oldest cohorts is also more than two years in Himachal Pradesh, Jammu, Orissa, Tripura, Delhi, Assam, Manipur, West Bengal, Maharashtra and Tamil Nadu.

In the NFHS, respondents were asked about their knowledge of the legal minimum age at marriage for males and females in India. Table 4.7 presents the percentage of women who reported correctly the minimum legal age at marriage in India, according to selected background characteristics. Perhaps because of its weak enforcement, the legal minimum age at marriage is not widely known among women in India. Overall, only one-third of respondents can correctly identify 18 as the legal minimum age at marriage for females, and only one-fifth can correctly identify 21 as the legal minimum age at marriage for males. The provisions of the law are better known in urban areas, where 57 per cent of the respondents can correctly identify the legal minimum age at marriage for females, than in rural areas, where only 25 per cent know the legally mandated minimum age for females. Knowledge of legal minimum age requirements also varies by literacy and educational attainment. Sixty-three per cent of women with a high school education or above know the legal minimum age at marriage for males, and 79 per cent know it for females. In contrast, only 7 and 16 per cent of illiterate women correctly specify the legal minimum age at marriage for males and females, respectively. Jain women are most likely to know the minimum legal age at marriage for males and females, with Hindu and Muslim women least likely to know about the legal age requirements for marriage. Knowledge about the legal minimum age at marriage is also relatively high among non-SC/ST women than among scheduled caste and scheduled tribe women. For every group of women shown in Table 4.7, the legal minimum age at marriage for males is less well known than is the legal minimum age at marriage for females.

Table 4.7 Knowledge of minimum legal age at marriage
Per cent distribution of ever-married women age 13-49 who correctly know the minimum legal age at marriage for males and females, by selected background characteristics, India, 1992-93

Background characteristic	Per centage who correctly know Legal minimum age at marriage: For males	For females	Number of women
Age			
13-19	15.8	27.5	9447
20-29	21.2	34.2	35424
30-39	20.9	35.2	27122
40-49	17.3	31.2	17784
Residence			
Urban	38.9	57.3	23455
Rural	13.0	24.7	66322
Education			
Illiterate	7.4	16.2	56656
Lit., < middle complete	26.7	50.1	16475
Middle school complete	42.8	67.1	6508
High school and above	63.0	79.3	10138
Religion			
Hindu	19.6	32.5	73648
Muslim	14.8	31.4	10806
Christian	30.9	49.6	2142
Sikh	33.3	41.3	1673
Jain	59.8	78.3	428
Buddhist	29.9	48.9	734
Other	9.5	21.3	345
Caste/tribe			
Scheduled caste	12.5	22.8	10970
Scheduled tribe	7.5	15.5	7934
Other	22.3	36.8	70872
Total	19.8	33.2	89777

Table 4.8 Knowledge of minimum legal age at marriage by state
Percentage of ever-married women age 13-49 who correctly know the minimum Legal age at marriage for males end females, by state. India, 1992-93

State	Percentage who correctly know legal minimum age at marriage: For males	For females
India	19.8	33.2
North		
Delhi	50.5	65.4
Haryana	27.5	40.9
Himachal Pradesh	28.9	56.3
Jammu Region of J & K	21.0	33.9
Punjab	33.0	41.1
Rajasthan	18.0	26.9
Central		
Madhya Pradesh	15.9	24.6
Uttar Pradesh	17.7	26.9
East		
Bihar	12.8	18.9
Orissa	6.5	19.1
West Bengal	10.7	31.6
Northeast		
Arunachal Predesh	3.7	19.0
Assam	3.8	18.8
Manipur	5.1	20.9
Meghalaya	13.7	27.7
Mizoram	28.4	54.7
Nagaland	16.9	23.2
Tripura	5.6	28.2
West		
Goa	24.7	35.9
Gujarat	23.6	33.7
Maharashtre	31.4	49.1
South		
Andhra Pradesh	27.0	38.0
Karnataka	23.7	40.9
Kerala	27.6	65.3
Tamil Nadu	19.6	38.9

Legal minimum age requirements for marriage are best known in the high literacy states of Kerala, Delhi, Himachal Pradesh, and Mizoram, where behveen 55 and 65 per cent of women can correctly identify age 18 as the legal minimum age at marriage for females (Table 4.8). Less than one quarter of women know the minimum legal age at marriage for females in Assam, Bihar, Arunachal Pradesh, Orissa, Manipur, Nagaland and Madhya Pradesh. Interestingly, knowledge of the minimum legal age requirements is not widespread in Manipur and Goa, the two states with the highest mean age at marriage for females (25 years, see Table 4.3). Thus the fact that a large majority of women in Manipur and Goa are married after attaining the legal minimum age at marriage apparently reflects social norms and economic conditions more than knowledge of the legal minimum age at marriage. In every state, the legal minimum age at marriage is better known for males than females.

4.4 Age at First Cohabitation

Table 4.9 shows median ages at which the respondents stated living with their husbands. The age at first marriage (Table 4.5) and the age at first cohabitation given, hble 4.9 may differ because formal marriage is not always immediately followed by living with the husband, which generally does not occur until after the gauna ceremony[2]. In the country as a whole, the median age at first marriage is about 8 months earlier than the median age at first cohabitation with the husband. As the median age at marriage has risen and early marriages have become less popular, the difference between the age at marriage and the age at first cohabitation has been reduced. Tn urban areas, the difference is negligible.

4.5 Marriage Between Relatives

Table 4.10 provides information on marriage between relatives. For both social and biological reasons, marriage between relatives has implications for fertility as well as mortality and morbidity of the couple's children. For example, Bittles *et al.*, (1992) found a positive association between consan guinity and fertility in 19 out of 22 populations. They also found that mortality was significantly higher among children of marriages between blood relatives than among other children. In analyzing the relationship between inbreeding and demographic rates, it is important to control for socioeconomic variables because of a tendency for marriages between relatives to be more common in lower socioeconomic groups whose fertility and mortality are higher primarily for socioeconomic reasons. Such a refined analysis is infeasible in this report, however, and will have to await further studies.

Table 4.10 indicates that overall 10 per cent of ever-married women in India married a first cousin (on either their father's side or their mother's side). In addition, 4 per cent married, second cousin, uncle, or other blood relative, and 2 per cent married a brother-in-law or other non-blood relative. Thus, consanguineous marriages are not very common in the country, accounting for 14 per cent of the marriages of ever-married women age 13-49. The percentages marrying a close relative vary only slightly by age, being somewhat more common in the younger cohorts, particularly among women age 13-14. This may reflect a tendency for these marriages to occur at a young age, that is, the age difference may reflect selectivity rather than, a trend over time. Interestingly, however, urban women are somewhat more likely than rural women to have married a close relative, contrary to the general pattern observed elsewhere (Rao *et al.*, 1972; Rao and 'nbaraj, 1977; Khlat and Khoury, 1991). The relatively high prevalence of consanguineous mairiages in urban areas may be due to the urban concentration of Muslim women, who are particularly prone to marry relatives.

Consanguinity does not vary much with literacy and education, although women with at least a high school education are less likely to have married a close relative. As mentioned earlier, Muslim women are more likely to have entered into a consanguineous marriage than are non-Muslim women. Twenty-seven per cent of Muslim women married a blood relative. Consanguineous marriages are also relatively high among Buddhists, and such marriages are particularly low among Sikhs and Jains. Consanguineous marriages are less common among scheduled tribes (10 per cent) than among nontribal groups (around 15 per cent).

Marriage between close relatives is more common in the southern states (with the exception of Kerala) and in Maharashtra (Table 4.11). By far the largest proportion of ever- married women age 13-49 who have married a blood relative are in Tamil Nadu (47 per cent), followed by Andhra Pradesh and Karnataka (35 per cent each) and Maharashtra (25 per cent). The incidence of consanguineous marriages is less than 10 per cent in all other states except Goa. Previous studies have alsq observed considerably higher levels of consanguinity in South India than in North India (Kapadia, 1958; Sanghvi, 1966; Roychoudhury, 1976; Bittles *et al.*, 1991). In every state, consanguineous marriages are mainly between first cousins, either on the father's side or on the mother's side. Uncle-niece marriages are rare everywhere except in Tamil Nadu and Andhra Pradesh.

Table 4.9: Age at first cohabitation with husband

Percentage of women who started living with husband by specific exect ages, and median age at first cohabitation with husband, by current age and residence, India, 1992-93

Current Age	Percentage who started living with husband before age: 13	15	18	20	22	25	Per cent never cohabited	Media age at first cohabitation with husband
					URBAN			
15-19	0.8	4.5	NA	NA	NA	NA	78.2	NC
20-24	1.8	8.3	31.3	52.0	NA	NA	31.8	19.8
25-29	2.3	12.4	39.3	59.3	73.3	86.4	8.9	18.9
30-34	2.7	12.7	44.1	64.2	77.8	89.2	3.1	18.4
35-39	3.8	15.1	19.5	69.1	81.2	91.3	1.7	18.0
40-44	5.1	19.8	53.1	72.5	86.6	92.8	1.9	17.6
45-49	5.2	20.8	55.8	75.6	87.1	94.1	1.6	17.4
20-49	3.1	13.5	42.8	62.9	75.5	84.5	11.0	18.6
25-49	3.5	15.3	6.7	66.5	79.4	90.0	4.1	18.3
					RURAL			
15-19	2.7	14.6	NA	NA	NA	NA	54.4	NC
20.24	4.8	21.9	58.1	77.1	NA	NA	13.2	17.2
25-29	5.P	26.1	65.8	82.4	91.0	95.5	2.9	16.6
30-34	6.5	27.2	68.6	85.2	93.0	96.8	1.1	16.4
35-39	8.0	29.1	71.2	86.7	94.1	97.3	0.6	16.2
40-44	8.6	31.8	73.0	88.4	95.6	98.2	0.3	16.1
49-49	9.9	34.3	73.5	87.9	95.1	98.0	0.5	16.0

20-49	6.7	27.1	66.6	83.5	91.0	94.2	4.4	16.5
25-49	7.4	8.0	69.6	85.5	93.3	96.9	1.3	16.3
				TOTAL				
15-19	2.2	11.9	NA	NA	NA	NA	60.7	NC
20-24	3.9	18.0	50.6	70.0	NA	NA	18.5	17.9
25-29	4.9	22.2	58.3	75.9	86.0	92.9	4.7	17.1
30-34	5.4	22.9	61.3	79.0	88.5	94.5	1.7	16.9
35-39	6.8	25.4	64.7	81.4	90.2	95.5	0.9	16.7
40-44	7.5	28.1	66.8	83.3	92.0	96.2	1.1	16.5
45-49	8.6	30.7	68.7	84.6	93.0	97.1	0.6	16.3
20-49	5.6	23.2	59.7	77.4	86.5	91.3	6.4	17.0
25-49	6.2	25.0	62.9	79.9	89.2	94.8	2.2	16.8

NA: Not applicable.
NC: Not calculated because less than 50 per cent of women in the age group 15-19 started living with their husbands by age 15.
1 The current age groups include both never-married and ever-married women.

Table 4.10 Marriage between relatives

Per cent distribution of ever-married uomen by relationship to current (Last) husband, according to selected background characteristics, India, 1992-93

Background characteristic	First cousin		Second cousin	Uncle	Other blood relation	Brother-in-law	Other non-blood relation	Not related	Missing	Total per-cent	Number of Women
	Father's side	Mother's side									
Age											
13-14	10.1	5.4	0.3	2.0	2.6	0.6	0.4	78.6	—	100.0	352
15-19	6.1	5.7	1.1	0.8	2.8	0.4	1.9	81.2	0.1	100.0	9095
20-24	5.8	4.9	0.9	1.0	2.5	0.5	1.6	82.9	0.1	100.0	17983
25-29	5.3	4.3	1.0	0.9	2.3	0.5	1.4	84.2	0.1	100.0	17442
30-34	4.9	4.2	0.9	0.8	2.2	0.5	1.4	85.0	0.1	100.0	14660
35-39	5.9	4.6	1.0	1.0	2.4	0.4	1.6	82.9	0.1	100.0	12461
40-44	5.4	4.4	1.1	1.0	2.5	0.3	1.2	84.0	0.1	100.0	9748
45-49	5.3	4.5	0.8	1.0	2.0	0.4	1.1	84.8	0.1	100.0	8036
Residence											
Urban	5.7	5.0	1.1	0.9	2.9	0.3	1.8	82.2	0.1	100.0	23455
Rural	5.4	4.5	0.9	0.9	2.2	0.5	1.3	84.1	0.1	100.0	66322
Education											
Illiterate	5.8	5.0	0.9	1.0	2.3	0.5	1.2	83.3	0.1	100.0	56656
Lit.,< middle complete	6.3	4.5	1.1	1.0	2.7	0.4	1.9	82.1	0.1	100.0	16475
Middle school complete	4.6	4.8	1.0	0.9	2.5	0.4	2.1	83.7	0.1	100.0	6508
High school and above	3.5	2.7	0.8	0.7	2.3	0.2	1.8	87.9	0.1	100.0	10138
Religion											
Hindu	4.8	3.9	0.9	1.0	2.3	0.4	1.4	85.2	0.1	100.0	73648

Muslim	11.3	10.1	1.5	0.4	3.5	0.6	1.4	71.1	0.1	100.0	10806
Christian	4.8	3.7	0.7	1.1	2.6	0.2	1.1	85.9	—	100.0	2142
Sikh	0.6	0.6	0.2	0.1	0.9	0.8	3.0	93.8	0.1	100.0	1673
Jain	1.0	2.6	0.7	—	1.2	—	1.9	92.5	—	100.0	428
Buddhist	11.2	5.7	0.1	0.1	2.3	0.9	2.9	76.9	—	100.0	734
Other	4.9	3.6	—	0.2	2.4	0.3	1.6	86.5	0.6	100.0	345
Caste/tribe											
Scheduled caste	5.5	5.0	1.0	1.6	2.4	0.6	1.3	82.5	0.1	100.0	10970
Scheduled tribe	3.8	3.7	0.3	0.4	1.5	0.3	0.9	88.9	0.1	100.0	7934
Other	5.7	4.6	1.0	0.9	2.5	0.4	1.5	83.2	0.1	100.0	70872
Total	5.5	4.6	0.9	0.9	2.4	0.4	1.5	83.6	0.1	100.0	89777

— Less than 0.05 per cent.

Table 4.11 Marriage Between Relatives by State

Per cent distribution of ever-married women by relationship to current (lest) husband, according to state, India, 1992-93

State	First cousin: Father's side	First cousin: Mother's side	Second cousin	Uncle	Other blood relation	Brother-in-leu	Other non-blood relation	Not related	Miss-ing	Total per-cent
India	5.5	4.6	0.9	0.9	2.4	0.4	1.5	83.6	0.1	100.0
North										
Delhi	1.9	1.6	0.8	—	1.9	0.4	3.4	90.0	0.1	100.0
Haryana	0.4	0.3	0.3	—	0.8	1.4	6.0	90.8	—	100.0
Himachal Pradesh	0.2	0.3	0.3	—	0.5	0.6	1.0	97.0	—	100.0
Jammu Region of J & K	3.4	3.5	6.7	0.4	1.8	0.3	6.4	83.5	—	100.0
Punjab	0.4	0.5	—	—	0.7	0.9	2.4	95.0	—	100.0
Rajasthan	0.5	0.5	0.3	—	0.6	0.3	0.8	96.6	0.3	100.0
Central										
Madhya Pradesh	2.0	2.0	0.1	—	0.8	0.3	0.7	94.0	0.2	100.0
Utter Pradesh	3.9	3.2	0.4	—	1.3	0.9	1.1	89.2	0.1	100.0
East										
Bihar	2.2	2.2	0.3	0.3	1.2	0.5	0.5	92.7	0.1	100.0
Orissa	2.8	2.1	0.6	0.2	1.3	0.5	1.5	91.0	0.1	100.0
West Bengal	2.6	1.8	0.5	0.1	1.2	0.2	2.9	90.7	—	100.0
Northeast										
Arunachal Pradesh	0.6	2.3	0.1	0.9	5.0	0.5	4.5	86.2	--	100.0

Assam	0.6	1.0	0.1	--	0.4	0.5	0.7	96.7	--	100.0
Manipur	1.5	0.6	--	--	2.6	0.2	0.2	94.9	--	100.0
Meghalaya	1.9	0.4	0.1	0.3	0.8	0.3	0.8	95.4	--	100.0
Mizoram	0.1	0.2	0.2	--	0.4	--	0.3	98.6	--	100.0
Nagaland	0.7	0.8	--	--	1.1	0.8	1.0	95.6	--	100.0
Tripura	0.6	0.8	0.5	--	0.9	0.2	4.0	92.9	--	100.0
West										
Goa	6.3	3.5	0.5	0.3	3.8	0.1	0.7	84.8	--	100.0
Gujarat	2.3	2.1	0.4	0.1	0.8	0.1	0.8	93.3	0.1	100.0
Maharashtra	12.9	7.6	0.3	0.2	4.4	0.3	2.4	71.7	0.1	100.0
South										
Andhra Pradesh	14.5	10.5	1.6	4.2	4.2	0.2	1.2	63.5	0.1	100.0
Karnataka	10.6	16.5	2.0	0.6	6.0	0.5	1.0	62.8	--	100.0
Kerala	3.7	2.7	1.1	--	1.8	0.2	1.4	89.0	--	100.0
Tamil Nadu	13.6	10.8	6.4	7.4	8.3	0.4	1.3	51.8	--	100.0

-- Less than 0.05 percent

NOTES

1 Median age at first marriage is not calculated for age cohorts in which fewer than 50 per cent of the women were married by the age that defines the lower boundary of the age group.

2 After marriage the bride often returns to her parental home until the gauna ceremony, which usually occurs when the bride is considered to be mature enough to begin cohabitating with her husband. The difference in the age at formal marriage and the age at first cohabitation with the husband is often large for women who marry before menarche.

5

FERTILITY

A major objective of the National Family Health Survey is to estimate fertility levels, differentials and trends in India and in individual states. This chapter presents a description of current and past fertility levels, cumulative fertility and family size, fertility levels by sociodemographic characteristics, pregnancy outcomes, birth intervals and durations of postpartum amenorrhoea, abstinence and nonsusceptibility. Age at first birth and age at last birth, teenage childbearing and age at menopause are also discussed.

Most of the fertility measures presented in this chapter are based on the complete birth histories of ever-married women age 15-49. Several procedures were established to facilitate the complete and accurate reporting of births. First, women were asked separately about the number of their sons and daughters presently living at home, those living elsewhere and those who had died. Then, more complete details were collected for each live birth, including information on the sex, year and month of birth, age and survival status of the child. Interviewers received extensive training in probing techniques to help respondents recall the details of all births. In addition, interviewers were instructed to check any documents (such as horoscopes, school certificates or vaccination cards) that might provide information on the child's date of birth. Finally, for any interval of four or more years between births, interviewers were required to record the reason for the long interval to help in identifying any live births that might have been omitted during the time period. This additional probe also helped to obtain more accurate information on stillbirths and abortions.

Despite all the measures taken to improve data quality, the NFHS is subject, to some degree, to the same kinds of errors that are inherent in all retrospective sample surveys—namely, the omission of some births (especially births of children who died at a very young age) and the displacement of births due to the difficulty of determining dates of birth accurately. These problems may be particularly common in states where the level of female literacy is relatively low.

5.1 Current Fertility Levels, Differentials and Trends

The discussion of fertility levels, differentials and trends is based on both summary and age-specific measures of fertility. Summary measures include the crude birth rate (CBR), the general fertility rate (GFR), and the total fertility rate TFR). Alternative measures of the crude birth rate are calculated from births recorded in the Household Questionnaire and from births recorded in the birth history in the Woman's Questionnaire. The crude birth rate calculated from births recorded in the Household Questionnaire pertains to the two-year period immediately preceding the survey. All other measures are calculated for the three-year period preceding the survey. Because the fieldwork for the NFHS was conducted at different times in each state, the three-year fertility rates do not correspond exactly to any particular calendar years, but they are centred roughly on 1990-1992. A three-year period was chosen for the NFHS rates as a compromise among three objectives: to obtain the most current information, to reduce the effects of sampling variation, and to minimize problems with the displacement of births from recent years to earlier years.

The NFHS fertility estimates can be compared with estimates from the Sample Registration System (SRS) for 1990-92 (Office of the Registrar General, 1994). Estimates of various fertility measures from the NFHS and SRS are shown by place of residence in Table 5.1 and discussed in the following sections.

Crude Birth Rate

The two sets of crude birth rates discussed above are shown in Table 5.1. The CBR from the household birth record is Calculated as the annual number of births in the two-year period before the date of interview per 1,000) usual residents. The denominator for this CBR estimate is adjusted by projecting the population at the time of the survey backward to the midpoint of the time period using the intercensal population growth rate in India, for urban and rural areas separately. The CBR estimate based on the birth history in the Woman's Questionnaire is calculated as a sum of products, where each product is an age-specific fertility rate multiplied by the proportion of women in the specified age group, out of the total *de facto* population, both male and female. Although the NFHS estimates of the CBR are based on information from two different parts of the interview (often with different respondents), the two estimates agree quite closely. The three-year CBR of 28.7 is slightly higher than the two-year household-based) rate of 28.0, as would be expected when fertility is declining. The SRS national crude birth rate for 1990-92 excluding Jammu and Kashmir (29.6) is very close to the NFHS crude birth rate for 1990-92 (28.7). The urban CBR is 21 per cent lower than the rural CBR in the NFHS and 25 per cent lower in the SRS.

Table 5.1:
Age-specific and cumulative fertility rates and crude birth rates from the NFHS and the SRS, by residence, India, 1990-92

	NFHS (1990-92)'			SRS (1990-92)		
Age	Urban	Rural	Total	Urban	Rural	Total
15-14	0.075	0.131	0.116	0.046	0.087	0.078
20-24	0.203	0.243	0.231	0.196	0.248	0.235
25-29	0.154	0.177	0.170	0.160	0.204	0.193
30-34	0.071	0.108	0.097	0.080	0.130	0.117
35-39	0.027	0.051	0.044	0.038	0.078	0.068
40-44	0.006	0.019	0.015	0.016	0.036	0.031
45-49	0.004	0.006	0.005	0.006	0.014	0.012
TFR 15-44	2.68	3.64	3.36	2.68	3.92	3.61
TFR 15-49	2.70	3.67	3.39	2.71	3.99	3.67
GFR	98	133	123	93	129	121
NFHS CBR based on						
Household birth record	23.6	29.6	28.0	NA	NA	NA
Woman's birth history	24.1	30.4	28.7	NA	NA	NA
SRS CBR	NA	NA	NA	24.0	32.2	29.6

Note: Rates from the NFHS are for the period 1-36 months before the interview except for the CBR from the household birth record which is based on the period 1-24 months before the interview. Rates for the age group 45-49 might be slightly biased due to truncation.
TFR: Total Fertility Rate for ages 15-44 and 15-49, expressed per woman.
GFR: General Fertility Rate (births to Women age 13-49 divided by woman-years lived between age 15 and 49, expressed per 1,000 women.
CBR: Crude Birth Rate, expressed per 1,000 population.
NA: Not applicable.
1 Three years preceding the survey. *Source of SRS data*: Office of the Registrar General (1994)

General Fertility Rate

The general fertility rate (GFR) in the NFHS is calculated by dividing the total number of births to women age 13-49 occurring during the three years preceding the survey by the number of woman-years lived between the ages of 15 and 49 during the same period, and multiplying the result by 1,000. The estimated GFR for 1990-92 is 123 births per 1,000 women for India as a whole, almost the same as the SRS GFR for 1990-92 (121). The observed GFR in the NFHS is 26 per cent lower in urban areas (98) than in rural areas (133). The 1990-92 SRS estimate for urban areas (93) is 28 per cent lower than the estimate for rural areas (129).

Age-Specific and Total Fertility Rates

Both the GFR and the CBR are crude summary measures of the rate at which the population is replacing itself. A more precise picture of fertility can be obtained by examining the age-specific fertility rates (ASFRs) and the total fertility rate (TFR), because they are not affected by the age structure of the population. Both the ASFRs and the TFR from the NFHS, as shown in Table 5.1, are based on births during the three-year period preceding the survey. The numerator of each age-specific fertility rate is live births in a five-year age group, and the denominator is the number of woman-years lived in the same five-year age interval during the three-year time period. The TFR is a summary measure that is calculated as five times the sum (over five-year age groups) of the age-specific fertility rates. The TFR is interpreted as the number of children a woman would bear during her reproductive years (alternatively, 15-44 or 15-49) if she were to experience the age-specific fertility rates prevailing during the three-year period preceding the survey.

A TFR of 3.4 children per woman is observed for the period 1990-92 for both the 15-44 age range and the 15-49 age range, because there were very few births to women age 45-49 during the three years preceding the survey. The urban TFR (2.7 children per woman) is considerably lower than the rural TFR (3.7 children per woman). Under the present age schedule of fertility, a woman in the urban areas would have, on average, one child less (or 26 per cent fewer children) during her childbearing years than a woman in the rural areas.

The age-specific fertility rates follow the expected pattern. Fertility peaks in the 20-24 age group, reflecting a pattern of early marriage and childbearing. This is true for both the urban and rural areas (see Figure 5.1). Fertility rates decline steadily after age 25, reaching very low levels for women in their forties. Fertility is highly concentrated in the 15-29 age group. Eighty per cent of urban fertility and 75 per cent of rural fertility is concentrated in this age group. Current fertility in India is characterized by a substantial amount of early childbearing; 17 per cent of total fertility is accounted for by births to women in the age group 15-19. Births to women age 35 years and above account for only 9 per cent of the TFR. Births to women age 40-49 account for even less of the TFR: 2 per cent in urban areas and 3 per cent in rural areas. The age-specific fertility rates are considerably higher in rural than in urban areas in every age group, although the relative differentials are smaller in the prime childbearing years (age 20-29) than at either younger or older ages.

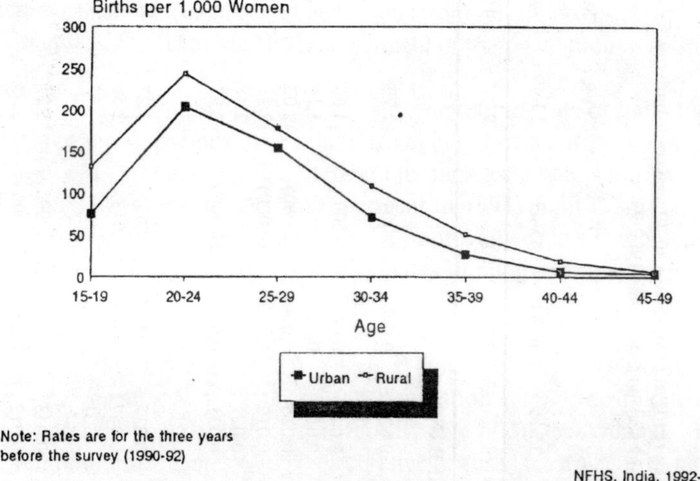

Figure 5.1 :Age-Specific Fertility Rates by Residence

The TFR from the NFHS for 1990-92 in Table 5.1 is identical to the 1990-92 SRS estimate in urban areas (2.7) and 8 per cent lower than the SRS estimate in rural areas. For the country as a whole, the NFHS TFR is also 8 per cent lower than the SRS TFR. Given the sampling variability in both surveys and the differences in methodology, the correspondence between the SRS and NFHS estimates should be considered to be reasonable.

It is instructive to extend the comparison of NFHS and SRS results from total fertility rates to the corresponding age-specific fertility rates, as shown in Table 5. 1 and Figure 5.2. The estimates are nearly identical in the highest fertility age group (age 20-24), but the NFHS estimate is considerably higher than the SRS estimate at age 15-19 and considerably lower than the SRS estimates for women age 25-49. The difference for the 15-19 age group may be due to the fact that the SRS rates are *de jure* while the NFHS rates are *de facto*. Thus, in calculating fertility estimates, the SRS excludes births occurring within the sample

Table 5.2 Fertility by state

Age-specific and total fertility rates (TFR), average number of children ever born (CEB) for women age 40-49, and crude birth rate for the three-year period prior to the survey, according to residence and state, India, 1992-93

State	Age-specific fertility rates							TFR	Mean CEB for women age 40-49	Crude birth rate
	15-19	20-24	25-29	30-34	35-39	40-44	45-49	15-49		
1	2	3	4	5	6	7	8	9	10	11
					URBAN					
India	0.075	0.203	0.154	0.071	0.027	0.006	0.004	2.70	4.16	24.1
North										
Delhi	0.061	0.223	0.186	0.085	0.041	0.005	0.000	3.00	4.15	26.2
Haryana	0.075	0.274	0.181	0.063	0.019	0.015	*	3.14	4.35	26.7
Himachal Pradesh	0.023	0.184	0.124	0.059	0.015	0.000	(0.000)	2.03	3.41	20.2
Jammu Region of J & K	0.026	0.144	0.165	0.081	0.010	0.000	(0.000)	2.13	3.89	21.2
Punjab	0.041	0.224	0.147	0.059	0.021	0.003	*	2.48	3.92	21.0
Rajasthan	0.063	0.184	0.181	0.087	0.031	0.000	(0.007)	2.77	4.14	22.3
Central										
Madhya Pradesh	0.092	0.239	0.188	0.077	0.037	0.012	(0.009)	3.27	4.58	27.1
Uttar Pradesh	0.062	0.240	0.204	0.125	0.057	0.014	0.013	3.58	5.18	28.5
East										
Bihar	0.089	0.224	0.182	0.090	0.053	0.012	0.000	3.25	4.59	27.5
Orissa	0.070	0.182	0.147	0.084	0.012	0.011	(0.000)	2.53	4.64	23.9
West Bengal	0.083	0.158	0.107	0.058	0.016	0.000	(0.007)	2.14	3.64	18.5

Northeast										
Arunachal Pradesh	*	*	*	*	**	*	*	NC	*	NC
Assam	0.070	0.167	0.159	0.054	0.046	0.011	(0.000)	2.53	4.16	23.2
Manipur	0.030	0.122	0.121	(0.133)	(0.035)	(0.000)	*	NC	(4.51)	NC
Meghalaya	0.046	(0.207)	(0.194)	*	*	*	*	NC	(4.55)	NC
Mizoram	0.053	0.125	0.154	0.089	(0.029)	(0.006)	(0.000)	NC	4.06	NC
Nagaland	0.026	(0.145)	(0.126)	*	(0.035)	*	*	NC	(3.71)	NC
Tripura	(0.057)	(0.089)	(0.121)	(0.062)	*	*	*	NC	*	NC
West										
Goa	0.019	0.092	0.124	0.083	0.032	0.008	0.002	1.80	3.56	16.4
Gujarat	0.063	0.227	0.154	0.065	0.011	0.006	(0.004)	2.65	4.01	24.6
Maharashtra	0.088	0.196	0.151	0.054	0.014	0.003	0.000	2.54	3.94	24.2
South										
Andhra Pradesh	0.085	0.210	0.104	0.049	0.019	0.003	(0.000)	2.35	3.88	22.3
Karnataka	0.094	0.169	0.127	0.057	0.020	0.002	0.009	2.38	4.04	22.7
Kerala	0.033	0.149	0.121	0.036	0.013	0.003	0.000	1.78	3.31	18.0
Tamil Nadu	0.063	0.188	0.149	0.051	0.017	0.004	0.000	2.36	4.10	23.4
					RURAL					
India	0.131	0.243	0.177	0.108	0.051	0.019	0.006	3.67	5.13	30.4
North										
Delhi	(0.131)	(0.231)	(0.160)	*	*	*	*	NC	4.91	NC

Cont...

1	2	3	4	5	6	7	8	9	10	11
Haryana	0.166	0.331	0.202	0.100	0.043	0.015	(0.004)	4.32	5.51	35.1
Himachal Pradesh	0.080	0.267	0.179	0.044	0.036	0.008	0.000	3.07	4.54	29.0
Jammu Region of J & K	0.058	0.243	0.216	0.093	0.045	0.011	0.007	3.36	5.37	29.3
Punjab	0.074	0.242	0.194	0.078	0.021	0.005	0.003	3.09	4.29	26.5
Rajasthan	0.124	0.264	0.181	0.113	0.063	0.017	0.011	3.87	5.22	28.1
Central										
Madhya Pradesh	0.173	0.260	0.192	0.115	0.051	0.020	0.011	4.11	5.42	32.9
Uttar Pradesh	0.128	0.289	0.264	0.195	0.105	0.044	0.014	5.19	6.19	37.9
East										
Bihar	0.127	0.244	0.191	0.150	0.083	0.029	0.005	4.14	5.36	32.9
Orissa	0.089	0.209	0.166	0.089	0.036	0.010	0.000	3.00	4.93	27.0
West Bengal	0.140	0.219	0.152	0.084	0.039	0.012	0.005	3.25	5.28	28.4
Northeast										
Arunachal Pradesh	0.118	0.246	0.194	0.150	0.086	(0.045)	*	4.38	4.88	34.6
Assam	0.122	0.205	0.200	0.128	0.057	0.023	(0.000)	3.68	6.01	31.4
Manipur	0.033	0.170	0.195	0.124	0.067	(0.016)	*	3.03	4.97	25.5
Meghalaya	0.086	0.176	0.176	0.125	0.116	0.053	(0.029)	3.80	5.03	31.9
Mizoram	0.039	0.157	0.129	(0.082)	(0.033)	(0.020)	(0.000)	(2.30)	4.43	(19.6)
Nagaland	0.064	0.199	0.212	0.150	0.067	0.019	0.008	3.60	4.28	34.2
Tripura	0.091	0.185	0.126	0.090	0.058	0.031	(0.000)	2.91	5.70	24.5
West										
Goa	0.011	0.099	0.172	0.084	0.030	0.001	0.000	1.99	3.94	17.8

Gujarat	0.096	0.264	0.158	0.080	0.027	0.005	0.004	3.17	4.64	28.4
Maharashtra	0.183	0.252	0.118	0.052	0.010	0.009	0.000	3.12	4.53	27.9
South										
Andhra Pradesh	0.164	0.198	0.101	0.046	0.020	0.005	0.000	2.67	4.12	24.7
Karnataka	0.147	0.226	0.138	0.069	0.026	0.009	0.002	3.08	4.99	27.5
Kerala	0.040	0.164	0.123	0.063	0.019	0.008	0.001	2.09	3.82	20.3
Tamil Nadu	0.099	0.212	0.121	0.051	0.020	0.004	0.000	2.54	4.27	23.5
					TOTAL					
India	0.116	0.231	0.170	0.097	0.044	0.015	0.005	3.39	4.84	**28.7**
North										
Delhi	0.066	0.224	0.184	0.086	0.040	0.005	0.000	3.02	4.19	26.6
Haryana	0.143	0.316	0.196	0.088	0.036	0.015	0.003	3.99	5.21	32.9
Himachal Pradesh	0.075	0.259	0.172	0.046	0.034	0.007	0.000	2.97	4.42	28.2
Jammu Region of J & K	0.054	0.223	0.206	0.090	0.038	0.009	0.005	3.13	5.05	27.9
Punjab	0.065	0.238	0.180	0.072	0.021	0.005	0.002	2.92	4.18	25.0
Rajasthan	0.112	0.247	0.181	0.107	0.055	0.014	0.010	3.63	5.00	27.0
Central										
Madhya Pradesh	0.153	0.255	0.191	0.106	0.047	0.018	0.010	3.90	5.22	31.6
Uttar Pradesh	0.113	0.279	0.251	0.177	0.094	0.037	0.014	4.82	5.97	35.9
East										
Bihar	0.121	0.241	0.190	0.141	0.078	0.026	0.004	4.00	5.23	32.1

Cont...

1	2	3	4	5	6	7	8	9	10	11
Orissa	0.086	0.204	0.163	0.089	0.031	0.010	O.000	2.92	4.88	26.5
West Bengal	0.123	0.202	0.138	0.075	0.031	0.008	0.005	2.92	4.72	25.5
Northeast										
Arunachal Pradesh	0.115	0.246	0.194	0.139	0.081	(0.039)	*	4.25	4.86	34.6
Assam	0.116	0.200	0.195	0.117	0.055	0.021	0.000	3.53	5.74	30.4
Manipur	0.037	0.152	0.170	0.128	0.057	0.010	(0.000)	2.76	4.80	24.4
Meghalaya	0.079	0.182	0.180	0.117	0.115	0.051	0.022	3.73	4.92	31.9
Mizoram	0.046	0.140	0.143	0.085	0.031	0.014	0.000	2.30	4.26	20.8
Nagaland	0.057	0.188	0.196	0.131	0.059	0.015	0.006	3.26	4.16	31.3
Tripura	0.085	0.166	0.125	0.081	0.052	0.026	(0.000)	2.67	5.44	23.1
West										
Goa	0.016	0.096	0.148	0.083	0.031	0.005	0.001	1.90	3.74	17.2
Gujarat	0.086	0.251	0.157	0.074	0.021	0.005	0.004	2.99	4.42	27.2
Maharashtra	0.141	0.227	0.132	0.053	0.012	0.006	0.000	2.86	4.25	26.3
South										
Andhra Pradesh	0.144	0.202	0.101	0.047	0.019	0.005	0.000	2.59	4.05	24.2
Karnataka	0.129	0.206	0.134	0.064	0.024	0.006	0.005	2.85	4.65	25.9
Kerala	0.038	0.160	0.123	0.054	0.017	0.006	0.001	2~00	3.65	19.6
Tamil Nadu	0.087	0.203	0.132	0.051	0.019	0.004	0.000	2.48	4.21	23.5

NC: Not calculated because there are too few women in this category.

( ) Based on 125-249 woman-years of exposure for age-specific fertility rates and 25-49 unweighted women age 40-49 for CEB.

* Rate not shown; based on fewer than 125 woman-years of exposure for age-specific fertility rates and fewer than 25 unweighted women age 40-49 for CEB.

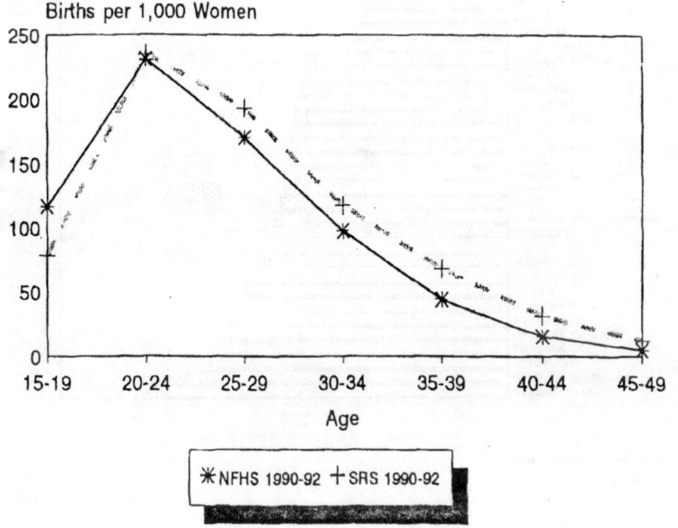

Figure 5.2 Age-Specific Fertility Rates by NFHS and SRS

unit to visitors, but includes births to usual residents outside the sample unit. Because young women typically return to their parental household to have their first baby, the SRS may not be able to obtain complete information on recent births to usual residents who are temporarily absent. Thus, it is not surprising that the NFHS fertility estimate for the 15-19 age group is somewhat higher than the SRS estimate. More difficult to explain are the differences in the older age groups. The very low fertility rates for women in the highest age groups in India are reasonable, because many women at these ages have been sterilized or are menopausal. Moreover, terminal abstinence from sexual intercourse is commonly practised by couples once their daughter. attains menarche or once any of their children gets married or has a child. A complete explanation of the differences in fertility estimates at older ages from the two data sets must await further analysis.

FERTILITY DIFFERENTIALS AND TRENDS

There are wide variations in fertility levels among the states (Table 5.2 and Figure 5.3). Fertility is considerably below thenational average in South India and West India, where two states (Kerala and Goa, have achieved below-replacement fertility[1]. Goa has a unique pattern of childbearing, with very low fertility before age 25 as a result of the high

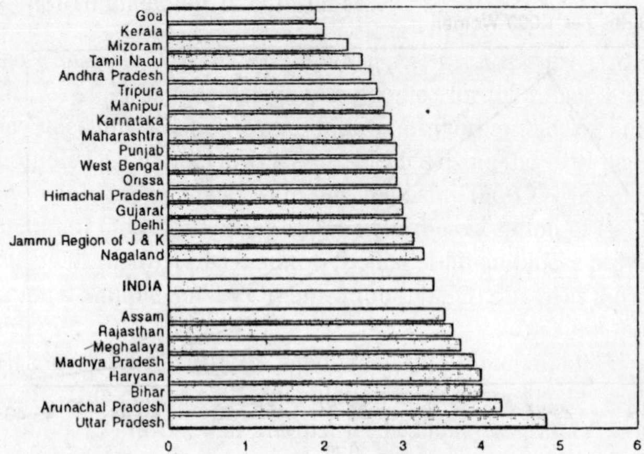

Figure 5.3 Total Fertility Rate (TFR) by State

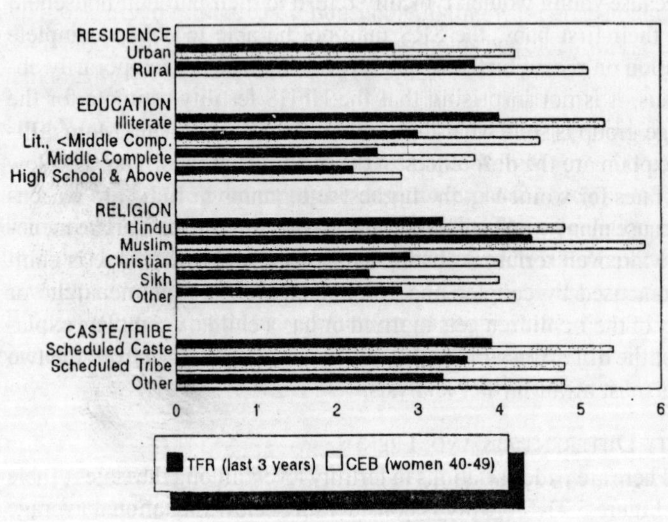

Figure 5.4 Total Fertility Rate (TFR) and Mean Number of Children Ever Born (CEB)

average age at marriage and the late initiation of childbearing. At the other end of the spectrum, fertility is four children per woman or higher in Uttar Pradesh, Bihar, Haryana and Arunachal Pradesh, and the TFR also exceeds the national average in Madhya Pradesh, Meghalaya, Rajasthan and Assam. With a TFR of 4.8, Uttar Pradesh stands out as having especially high fertility (more than 40 per cent higher than the national average). Early childbearing (fertility at age 15-19) is particularly high in Madhya Pradesh, Andhra Pradesh, Haryana and Maharashtra. The highest rates of childbearing for women in their forties are found in Uttar Pradesh, Bihar, Madhya Pradesh and some of the small northeastern states. Childbearing at age 40 and above is rare in Tamil Nadu, Andhra Pradesh, Delhi, Maharashtra, Goa, Himachal Pradesh, Punjab, and Kerala, all of which have age-specific fertility rates of 7 or fewer children per 1,000 women at these ages. In Maharashtra, fertility begins early and ends early. In fact, Maharashtra has lower fertility rates than any other state for women age 35-49. For most states, the NFHS fertility estimates are slightly lower than the estimates from the Sample Registration System for approximately corresponding years (see individual NFHS state reports for comparative statistics). In half of the major states, the two sets of estimates are quite close (within 0.2 children). The two sets of estimates differ by more than half a child in only two states Bajasthan and Madhya Pradesh). Given other available information, it is likely that the current fertility estimates in the NFHS are too low in both of these states (see individual state reports).

In urban areas, the total fertility rate is less than 2.5 children per woman in 9 of the 19 states for which estimates are shown. In every state which has urban and rural estimates, the total fertility rate from the NFHS is lower in urban areas than in rural areas. There is, however, a convergence of urban and rural fertility rates for states with low fertility. In the four states with the lowest overall fertility (Goa, Kerala, Tamil Nadu and Andhra Pradesh), rural fertility is only 12 per cent higher than urban fertility, on average. In the remaining states, rural fertility exceeds urban fertility by an average of 35 per cent, varying from 19 per cent in Orissa to 58 per cent in Jammu.

Table 5.3 and Figure 5.4 show current and cohort fertility by selected background characteristics. Current fertility is measured by the total fertility rate for the three years prior to the survey. Cohort fertility is measured by the mean number of children ever born to women age 40-49 at the time of the survey. Both measures are calculated from the birth history information in the Woman's Questionnaire.

Table 5.3: Fertility by background characteristics

Total fertility rate for the three years preceding the survey, and mean number of children ever born to women age 40-49, by selected background characteristics, India, 1992-93

Background characteristic	Total fertility rate[1]	Mean number of children ever born to women age 40-49
Residence		
Urban	2.70	4.16
Rural	3.67	5.13
Education		
Illiterate	4.03	5.26
Literate, < middle complete	3.01	4.50
Middle school complete	2.49	3.71
High school and above	2.15	2.80
Religion		
Hindu	3.30	4.78
Muslim	4.41	5.83
Christian	2.87	4.01
Sikh	2.43	3.99
Other	2.77	4.24
Caste/tribe		
Scheduled caste	3.92	5.40
Scheduled tribe	3.55	4.81
Other	3.30	4.76
Total	3.39	4.84

1 Rate for women age 15-49 years

If there had been no change in fertility for three or more decades prior to the survey, the current and cohort indicators would be nearly identical, differences being due solely to the slightly incomplete fertility of women age 40-49. If fertility has declined, current fertility will be lower than cohort fertility, with larger differences generally indicating more rapid decline. The gap between the TFR of 3.4 and the mean number of children ever born of 4.8 indicates that a substantial fertility decline has taken place in India. In absolute terms, the total fertility rate is 1.5 children lower than the average number of children ever born in both urban and rural areas. But the larger relative decline in urban areas (35 per cent) than in rural areas (28 per cent) indicates that fertility has been declining somewhat more rapidly in urban areas.

Differentials by education are substantial, with current fertility

Table 5.4: Fertility by religion and education
Total fertility rate (TFR) for the three years preceding the survey, and mean number of children ever born (CEB) to women age 40-49, by religion and education, India, 1992-93

	Illiterate		Literate, < middle complete		Middle school complete		High school and above	
Religion	TFR	CEB	TFR	CEB	TFR	CEB	TFR	CEB
Hindu	3.93	5.18	2.93	4.44	2.45	3.n	2.07	2.79
Muslim	5.03	6.06	3.61	5.49	3.05	4.59	2.97	4.04
Christian	3.30	4.68	2.86	4.23	2.50	4.00	2.79	2.81
Sikh	3.43	4.43	2.80	3.73	2.06	3.53	1.68	2.64
Other	3.57	4.63	2.59	4.44	2.59	3.25	2.14	2.88
Total	4.03	5.26	3.01	4.50	2.49	3.71	2.15	2.80

Note: TFR is for women age 15-49 years.

declining steadily from 4.0 children per woman for illiterate women to 2.2 children per woman for women with at least a high school education. Cohort fertility also is higher among illiterate women than among women with at least a high school education (5.3 children compared to 2.8 children). Fertility has declined rapidly in all education groups, but it has declined most rapidly among literate women with less than a high school education. Differences in current fertility by religion and caste/tribe are less pronounced, but still substantial. Although fertility has declined substantially in all caste/tribe groups, women from scheduled castes still have higher fertility than other groups. The fertility of scheduled tribe women is also slightly higher than the fertility of women who do not belong to either scheduled castes or scheduled tribes.

Muslims have considerably higher fertility than any other religious group. On average, Muslim women have 1.1 children more than Hindu women. However, even among Muslims there has been a considerable decline in fertility over time. The lowest fertility levels (under three children per woman) are exhibited by Christians, Sikhs, and women from other religions primarily Buddhists and Jains). Religious differentials may be due to socioeconomic differences among the different religious groups rather than religious affiliation itself. A complete examination of factors responsible for the religious differentials requires a multivariate analysis of the determinants of fertility, which is beyond the scope of this report. Some insight into the role of socioeconomic factors may be gained, however, by examining religious differentials in fertility within education groups (Table 5.4). Within each education group, Muslims have substantially higher fertility than Hindus. In the first three education groups, the Muslim TFR is 23-28 per cent higher than the Hindu TFR. The differential is even larger (43 per cent) for the relatively small number of women in the highest education group. The differential between Muslim and Hindu fertility overall (see Table 5.3) is 34 per cent. Thus, controlling for the effects of education does decrease religious differentials in fertility to some extent for women with less than a high school education, but religion is still strongly related to fertility even within education groups. It should be noted, however, that according to both measures fertility generally declines sharply with increasing education in every religious group, including Muslims.

The most direct way of observing fertility trends is to examine changes in age-specific rates over time. Table 5.5 shows age-specific fertility rates for the 20-year period preceding the survey, calculated from the birth history information. Because birth histories are obtained only for women under age 50 at the time of the survey, no rates are available for women age 45 and over for the period 5-9 years prior to the survey, or for women age 40 and over 10-14 years prior to the survey, or for women age 35 and over 15-19 years prior to the survey. In every age group, fertility fell steadily from the period 10-14 years before the survey to the period 0-4 years before the survey. There was a general tendency for the fertility decline to accelerate during the most recent period in both urban and rural areas. Over the last 15 years, the rate of fertility decline was slightly faster at age 15-19 than at age 20-24, probably because of the rising age at marriage. The rapidity of the fertility decline increases with age after age 20-24 as is typical during the fertility transition.

The TFR for the five years before the NFHS (roughly 1988-92) is 9 per cent lower than the average TFR from the SRS for 1988-92. On the other hand, at ages 15-44 the average SRS TFR for 1983-87 is 9 per cent lower than the NFHS TFR for the period 5-9 years before the survey. This suggests that there was some age displacement of NFHS births out of the most recent five-year period. The average 10-year fertility rate estimates from the NFHS and the SRS for 1983-92 are virtually identical.

Further evidence of a decline in fertility over time is shown in Table 5.6, which gives fertility rates over the last 20 years by the number of years since women started living with their husbands[2]. This measure controls to some extent for changing age at marriage and may help to elucidate the trends in Table 5.5. In almost all marital duration groups, fertility has fallen steadily over time. The rapidity of the fertility decline increases dramatically with marital duration, being most pronounced for women married 20 years or more. The absence of any marked fertility decline in the group married for 0-4 years is typical of populations in which contraception is initiated only after the first birth or later.

For women married at least five years, marital fertility is lower in urban than in rural areas in every five-year time period. The opposite relationship is observed for women who have been married for less than five years. This pattern is not uncommon in populations in which the age at marriage is higher in urban areas than in rural areas, as is the case in India. Women who marry at later ages often have their first birth sooner after marriage and concentrate their births earlier in their marriage.

5.2 Outcome of Pregnancies

Table 5.7 shows the outcome of all lifetime pregnancies reported by ever-married women according to their current age and current place of residence. Information on still births and spontaneous and induced abortions was obtained in the reproduction section of the Woman's Questionnaire. In any survey, it is more difficult to collect retrospective information on pregnancies than on live births, particularly on pregnancies spontaneously aborted within thefirst few months after conception. The total number of pregnancies and the percent of all pregnancies that end in spontaneous abortions are almost certainly underestimated, and should not be subject to very intensive interpretation. Stillbirths are probably much more accurately reported than abortions. Reports of induced abortions may be suppressed by respondents, or induced abortions may be reported as spontaneous abortions, so that the actual incidence of induced abortions may be much higher than is reported.

Table 5.5 Fertility trends

Age-specific fertility rates for five-year periods preceding the survey by residence, India, 1992

Maternal age at birth	Years preceding survey 0-4	5-9	10-14	15-19
	URBAN			
15-19	0.079	0.114	0.128	0.129
20-24	0.204	0.249	0.262	0.266
25-29	0.155	0.189	0.216	0.226
30-34	0.072	0.100	0.129	[0.165]
35-39	0.027	0.042	[0.068]	U
40-44	0.006	[0.017]	U	U
45-49	[0.004]	U	U	U
	RURAL			
15-19	0.137	0.181	0.190	0.181
20-24	0.246	0.306	0.305	0.299
25-29	0.179	0.233	0.253	0.260
30-34	0.107	0.146	0.171	[0.206]
35-39	0.051	0.080	[0.116]	U
40-44	0.019	[0.038]	U	U
45-49	[0.007]	U	U	U
	TOTAL			
15-19	0.121	0.162	0.172	0.166
20-24	0.234	0.289	0.292	0.288
25-29	0.172	0.220	0.241	0.250
30-34	0.097	0.131	0.159	[0.195]
35-39	0.043	0.069	[0.103]	U
40-44	0.015	[0.033]	U	U
45-49	[0.006]	U	U	U

Note: Age-specific fertility rates are per woman.

U.: Not available.

[ ] Truncated, censored.

Table 5.6: Fertility by marital duration

fertility rates for ever-married women by duration since first effective marriage (in years) for five-year periods preceding the survey, India, 1992-93

Duration of effective marriage	Years preceding survey			
	0-4	5-9	10-14	15-19
URBAN				
0 - 4	0.304	0.329	0.325	0.307
5 - 9	0.186	0.228	0.263	0.272
10-14	0.093	0.138	0.170	0.215
15-19	0.046	0.071	0.118	0.160
20-24	0.019	0.044	0.070	(0.141)
25-29	0.006	0.016	(0.113)	*
RURAL				
0 - 4	0.287	0.320	0.308	0.281
5 - 9	0.240	0.300	0.304	0.302
10-14	0.152	0.207	0.229	0.249
15-19	0.089	0.129	0.159	0.198
20-24	0.044	0.076	0.115	0.151
25-29	0.018	0.038	0.117	*
TOTAL				
0 - 4	0.291	0.322	0.312	0.288
5 - 9	0.226	0.280	0.293	0.294
10-14	0.136	0.188	0.213	0.240
15-19	0.077	0.113	0.149	0.190
20-24	0.037	0.068	0.106	0.149
25-29	0.015	0.034	0.117	

Note: Duration-specific fertility rates are per woman. The duration of effective marriage is defined as the difference between the woman's age at the specified time period and the age she began living with her husband.

( ) Based on 125-249 unweighted woman-years of exposure.

*** Rate not shown; based on fewer than 125 unweighted woman-years of exposure.**

Of the 301,400 pregnancies reported by sample women, 92 per cent resulted in live births, 2 per cent in stillbirths, 1 per cent in induced abortions, and 5 per cent in spontaneous abortions. There is relatively little variation in the outcome of pregnancies by the current age of the mother, although the proportion of live births increases somewhat with an increase in age, and spontaneous abortions are particularly common for young women. Women currently living in urban areas report somewhat higher pregnancy wastage than do rural women.

In view of the problems of under reporting early spontaneous abortions, it is useful to consider induced abortions and stillbirths in relation to live births rather than to total pregnancies. By this measure, there were 2.5 stillbirths and 1.4 induced abortions for every 100 live births in the country as a whole.

5.3 Children Ever Born and Living

The distribution of women age 15-49 by number of children ever born is shown in Table 5.8, both for currently married women and for all women (including never-married women). The table also shows the mean number of children ever born and surviving. Women of childbearing age in India, both ever-married and never-married, have borne an average of 2.5 children and have an average of 2.2 currently living children. Women who are currently married have borne 3.1 children, on average, of whom 2.7 children are still living. The mean number of children ever born increases steadily with age among all women as well as among currently married women, reaching a high of more than five children for women age 45-49. Currently, early childbearing is relatively rare in India. Only 19 per cent of all women in the 15-19 age group have ever had a child.

It is not uncommon in sample surveys to find mean numbers of children ever born for older age groups declining, which may indicate deteriorating completeness of reporting of children ever born as women reach the end of the reproductive age span. Although the steady increase with age in the NFHS mean number of children ever born does not provide conclusive evidence that births have been completely reported by older women, there is no indication of under reporting, either in the pattern or the level of fertility.

The distribution of women age 45-49 by number of children ever born is of particular interest since these women have nearly completed their childbearing. The distribution of children ever born to this cohort, therefore, approximates their completed parity distribution. The majority of women in this age group have had five or more live births and 17 per cent have had at least eight live births.

The parity distribution of older currently married women provides a measure of primary sterility, which is the proportion of couples who are unable to have children. In India, only 2 per cent of currently married women age 45-49 (as well as women age 40-44) have never had a live birth.

Differentials in the number of children ever born and children still living by background characteristics, shown in Table 5.9, provide additional information on fertility patterns in India. To avoid the confounding influence of different age distributions of women in different groups, the mean values in the table are age-standardized according to the age distribution of all currently married women. The differentials by background characteristics seen in Table 5.9 are similar to those observed earlier in Table 5.3. Fertility is higher among illiterate women and those with low educational attainment, Muslims and scheduled caste women.

Table 5.7: Outcome of Pregnancy

Per cent distribution of all pregnancies of ever-married women by their outcome, according to age of the woman and residence, India, 1992-93

Current age	Spontaneous abortion	Induced abortion	Still-birth	Live birth	Total per cent	Number of pregnancies
			Outcome of pregnancy			
			URBAN			
15-19	9.5	3.3	1.9	85.3	100.0	968
20-24	6.4	2.2	1.9	89.5	100.0	6842
25-29	6.1	2.5	2.0	89.4	100.0	12727
30-34	4.9	3.1	1.9	90.2	100.0	14710
35-39	5.4	2.7	1.9	89.9	100.0	14976
40-44	5.1	2.1	1.9	90.9	100.0	12960
45-49	5.2	1.3	2.0	91.5	100.0	10723
Total	5.5	2.4	1.9	90.2	100.0	73922
			RURAL			
15-19	6.8	1.4	2.5	89.3	100.0	5357
20-24	5.2	0.9	2.6	91.3	100 0	25640
25-29	4.5	1.2	2.4	92.0	100 0	40551
30-34	4.1	0.9	2.4	92.6	100.0	43904
35-39	3.8	1.0	2.4	92.9	100.0	42069
40-44	3.7	0.7	2.3	93.2	100.0	36532
45-49	3.6	0.6	2.2	93.5	100.0	33397
Total	4.2	0.9	2.4	92.5	100.0	227478
			TOTAL			
13-14	(11.9)	(—)	(—)	(88.1)	100.0	40
15-19	7.3	1.7	2.4	88.7	100.0	6325
20-24	5.5	1.2	2.5	90.9	100.0	32481
25-29	4.9	1.5	2.3	91.4	100.0	53278
30-34	4.3	1.4	2.2	92.0	100.0	58613
35-39	4.2	1.4	2.3	92.1	100.0	57045
40-44	4.1	1.1	2.2	92.6	100.0	49492
45-49	4.0	0.8	2.2	93.0	100.0	44121
Total	4.5	1.3	2.3	92.0	100.0	301400

Note: The urban and rural totals include 12 and 28 pregnancies to women age 13-14 respectively, which are not shown separately.

( ) Based on 25-49 unweighted cases — Less than 0.05 per cent

Table 5.8 Children ever born and living

Percent distribution of all women and currently married women age 15-49 by number of children ever born and mean number of children ever born (CEB) and living, according to age and residence, India, 1992-93

Age	Children ever born 0	1	2	3	4	5	6	7	8	9	10+	Total percent	Number of women	Mean CEB	Mean children living
1	2	3	4	5	6	7	8	9	10	11	12	13	14	15	16
							URBAN All Women								
15-19	89.6	8.1	1.9	0.3	—	—	—	—	—	—	—	100.0	6299	0.13	0.12
20-24	47.3	22.2	19.0	8.5	2.2	0.6	0.2	—	—	—	—	100.0	6198	0.99	0.92
25-29	16.1	17.5	27.2	19.6	11.9	5.4	1.6	0.5	0.1	—	—	100.0	5166	2.20	2.02
30-34	7.5	10.1	24.6	22.8	17.1	9.9	4.7	1.9	0.8	0.3	0.3	100.0	4429	2.99	2.72
35-39	5.8	6.4	19.1	22.9	17.9	12.1	7.2	4.5	2.0	1.3	0.7	100.0	3781	3.56	3.20
40-44	4.9	4.9	15.9	20.1	18.9	13.5	7.9	6.8	3.4	2.2	1.5	100.0	2955	3.99	3.49
45-49	4.7	6.2	12.1	17.3	15.6	14.1	10.6	7.5	5.6	3.0	3.2	100.0	2232	4.39	3.73
Total	32.9	12.1	16.9	14.2	10.0	6.2	3.4	2.1	1.1	0.6	0.5	100.0	31061	2.15	1.92
							Currently married women								
15-19	52.4	37.1	8.9	1.4	0.2	—	—	—	—	—	—	100.0	1339	0.60	0.55
20-24	22.5	32.6	28.0	12.4	3.3	0.9	0.4	—	—	—	—	100.0	4116	1.46	1.35
25-29	7.3	19.0	30.0	21.8	13.3	6.0	1.8	0.6	0.1	—	0.1	100.0	4553	2.44	2.24
30-34	3.8	9.7	25.6	24.0	18.2	10.1	5.1	2.0	0.8	0.4	0.3	100.0	4083	3.14	2.86
35-39	3.7	5.9	19.2	23.4	18.6	12.6	7.6	4.8	2.2	1.3	0.8	100.0	3493	3.68	3.32
40-44	2.4	4.6	15.6	20.8	19.7	13.9	8.4	6.9	3.6	2.4	1.7	100.0	2603	4.14	3.64
45-49	2.4	5.9	13.0	17.4	16.0	14.4	10.8	8.0	5.6	3.1	3.4	100.0	1849	4.51	3.88
Total	10.7	16.1	22.7	19.0	13.4	8.1	4.5	2.7	1.4	0.8	0.7	100.0	22036	2.85	2.56

RURAL															
All women															
15-19	78.4	15.9	4.9	0.8	0.1	—	—	—	—	—	—	100.0	16914	0.28	0.25
20-24	28.0	25.5	25.7	14.5	5.0	1.1	0.3	0.1	—	—	—	100.0	15846	1.48	1.31
25-29	8.5	10.5	22.3	27.0	17.6	9.2	3.4	1.2	0.3	0.1	—	100.0	13121	2.84	2.48
30-34	4.1	5.1	12.8	22.3	21.2	15.6	9.8	5.8	2.2	0.7	0.3	100.0	10483	3.88	3.28
35-39	3.6	3.8	10.7	17.7	18.6	16.7	11.5	7.7	5.2	2.4	2.1	100.0	8794	4.44	3.66
40-44	3.0	3.9	8.0	13.6	16.1	16.5	14.0	9.7	7.1	4.3	3.9	100.0	6870	4.96	3.99
45-49	3.4	3.3	5.7	10.3	15.5	16.1	14.6	11.8	8.4	5.4	5.6	100.0	5866	5.33	4.16
Total	25.6	12.1	14.1	14.6	11.5	8.4	5.6	3.6	2.2	1.2	1.0	100.0	77893	2.70	2.26
Currently married women															
15-19	52.3	35.0	10.8	1.7	0.2	—	—	—	—	—	—	100.0	7558	0.63	0.55
20-24	16.6	29.0	29.9	16.9	5.8	1.3	0.3	0.1	—	—	—	100.0	13388	1.72	1.52
25-29	5.0	10.1	23.2	28.3	18.5	9.7	3.6	1.3	0.3	0.1	—	100.0	12254	2.97	2.60
30-34	2.4	4.2	12.6	22.9	21.8	16.3	10.3	6.1	2.4	0.7	0.3	100.0	9818	4.00	3.39
35-39	2.5	3.0	10.0	18.0	19.1	17.2	11.9	8.1	5.4	2.5	2.2	100.0	8104	4.57	3.77
40-44	2.2	2.7	7.1	13.3	16.6	16.8	14.6	10.2	7.5	4.6	4.2	100.0	6122	5.13	4.15
45-49	2.4	2.5	5.2	9.9	15.6	16.5	14.9	12.3	8.8	5.8	6.1	100.0	5047	5.50	4.31
Total	12.0	14.0	16.7	17.5	13.7	10.0	6.6	4.3	2.6	1.4	1.3	100.0	62291	3.21	2.69
TOTAL															
All women															
15-19	81.4	13.8	4.1	0.6	0.1	—	—	—	—	—	—	100.0	23150	0.24	0.21
20-24	33.5	24.5	23.8	12.8	4.2	1.0	0.3	—	—	—	—	100.0	22057	1.34	1.20
25-29	10.7	12.5	23.7	24.9	16.0	8.1	2.9	1.0	0.2	0.1	—	100.0	18296	2.66	2.35
30-34	5.1	6.6	16.3	22.4	20.0	13.9	8.3	4.6	1.8	0.6	0.3	100.0	14915	3.62	3.11
35-39	4.2	4.6	13.2	19.3	18.4	15.3	10.2	6.8	4.2	2.1	1.7	100.0	12577	4.18	3.52
40-44	3.9	4.2	10.3	15.5	16.9	15.5	12.1	8.8	5.9	3.7	3.1	100.0	9859	4.65	3.83

Cont...

1	2	3	4	5	6	7	8	9	10	11	12	13	14	15	16
45-49	3.7	4.1	7.5	12.2	15.6	15.5	13.5	10.6	7.6	4.7	5.0	100.0	8088	5.07	4.05
Total	27.7	12.1	14.9	14.5	11.1	7.8	5.0	3.2	1.9	1.0	0.9	100.0	108940	2.54	2.16
							Currently married women								
15-19	52.3	35.3	10.5	1.7	0.2	—	—	—	—	—	—	100.0	8897	0.62	0.55
20-24	18.0	29.9	29.5	15.9	5.2	1.2	0.3	0.1	—	—	—	100.0	17504	1.66	1.48
25-29	5.6	12.5	25.1	26.5	17.1	8.7	3.1	1.1	0.2	0.1	—	100.0	16807	2.83	2.50
30-34	2.8	5.8	16.4	23.2	20.7	14.5	8.8	4.9	1.9	0.6	0.3	100.0	13901	3.75	3.24
35-39	2.9	3.9	12.8	19.7	18.9	15.8	10.6	7.1	4.4	2.2	1.8	100.0	11596	4.30	3.63
40-44	2.2	3.3	9.7	15.6	17.6	15.9	12.8	9.2	6.3	4.0	3.5	100.0	8725	4.84	4.00
45-49	2.4	3.4	7.3	11.9	15.7	16.0	13.8	11.1	7.9	5.1	5.4	100.0	6896	5.23	4.19
Total	11.7	14.5	18.3	17.9	13.6	9.5	6.0	3.9	2.3	1.2	1.1	100.0	84327	3.11	2.65

Note: All women includes never-married women.

— Less than 0.05 per cent.

Differentials in the mean number of children still living are smaller than differentials in the mean number of children ever born. This cdnvergence is caused by the simultaneous occurrence of high fertility and relatively high levels of infant and child mortality in some groups. For example, while women in rural area have borne almost 0.4 children more than women in urban areas, they have only 0.1 living children more than urban women. Rural women have had more children, but have lost relatively more as well.

State differentials in the number of children ever born (Table 5.10) generally parallel the differentials in current fertility rates discussed earlier. For currently married women of all ages, the average number of children ever born ranges from 2.5 in Kerala to 3.7 in Assam. Because high fertility states tend to have high mortality as well, the range is somewhat smaller in the case of the average number of children still living (from 2.3 in Kerala and Tamil Nadu to 3.2 in Nagaland). High fertility and high mortality have combined to make the average child loss quite high (0.7 children per woman) in Uttar Pradesh. In the case of Rajasthan, the difference between the average number of children ever born and living is only 0.3 children, which may reflect under reporting of dead children in the birth history.

5.4 Sex Ratio at Birth

The sex ratio at birth of children ever born. Information is available for 277,192 children born to interviewed women. In all, the sex ratio at birth is 107.0 which is on the high end of the normal range of 105-107 which has been observed in most other countries. The sex ratio at birth is particularly high (112.0) for births occurring before 1972, indicating that there is underenumeration of female births that occurred more than 20 years before the survey. Since 1972, however, the sex ratio at birth has been almost constant at an average level of 106.3-106.6 for five year periods. Therefore, there is no evidence in India of the type of rise in the sex ratio at birth over time that has been observed in countries such as Korea and China, where the preference for sons is strong and sex-selective abortions have been carried out based on the determination of the sex of unborn foetuses (Park and Cho, 1995)[3].

Table 5.9 Mean number of Children ever born and living by background characteristics Age-standardized mean number of children ever born and living for currently married women according to sex and selected background characteristics India 1992-93

Background characteristic	Children ever born			Children living		
	Male	Female	Total	Male	Female	Total
Age						
13-14	0.1	0.0	0.1	0.0	0.0	0.1
15-19	0.3	0.3	0.6	0.3	0.3	0.6
20-24	0.8	0.8	1.7	0.7	0.7	1.5
25-29	1.5	1.4	2.8	1.3	1.2	2.5
30-34	2.0	1.8	3.7	1.7	1.5	3.2
35-39	2.2	2.1	4.3	1.9	1.7	3.6
40-44	2.5	2.3	4.8	2.1	1.9	4.0
45-49	2.7	2.5	5.2	2.2	2.0	4.2
Residence						
Urban	1.5	1.4	2.8	1.3	1.2	2.6
Rural	1.6	1.5	3.2	1.4	1.3	2.7
Education						
Illiterate	1.8	1.7	3.5	1.5	1.4	2.9
Literate < middle complete	1.5	1.4	2.9	1.3	1.3	2.6
Middle school complete	1.2	1.1	2.3	1.1	1.0	2.1
High school and above	1.0	0.9	1.9	0.9	0.9	1.8
Religion						
Hindu	1.6	1.5	3.0	1.3	1.2	2.6
Muslim	1.8	1.8	3.6	1.6	1.5	3.2
Christian	1.4	1.4	2.8	1.3	1.3	2.5
Sikh	1.5	1.4	2.9	1.4	1.2	2.6
Jain	1.3	1.2	2.5	1.2	1.2	2.3
Buddhist	1.6	1.4	3.0	1.3	1.2	2.5
Other	1.5	1.4	2.9	1.3	1.2	2.5
Caste/tribe						
Scheduled caste	1.7	1.6	3.3	1.4	1.3	2.7
Scheduled tribe	1.6	1.5	3.1	1.4	1.3	2.7
Other	1.6	1.5	3.1	1.4	1.3	2.6
Total	1.6	1.5	3.1	1.4	1.3	2.6

Note: The means by residence, education religion and caste/tribe are standarized on the age distribution of all currently married women.

Table 5.10: Mean number of children ever born and living by state
Mean number of children ever born and living for currently married women, according to sex and state, India, 1992-93

	Children ever born			Children living		
State	Male	Female	Total	Male	Femate	Total
India	1.6	1.5	3.1	1.4	1.3	2.6
North						
Delhi	1.5	1.3	2.8	1.4	1.2	2.6
Haryana	1.6	1.5	3.1	1.4	1.3	2.7
Himachal Pradesh	1.5	1.4	3.0	1.4	1.3	2.7
Jammu Region of J & K	1.6	1.5	3.1	1.5	1.3	2.9
Punjab	1.5	1.4	2.9	1.4	1.3	2.7
Rajasthan	1.7	1.5	3.1	1.5	1.3	2.8
Central						
Madhya Pradesh	1.7	1.5	3.2	1.4	1.2	2.6
Uttar Pradesh	1.9	1.7	3.6	1.5	1.3	2.9
East						
Bihar	1.7	1.6	3.2	1.4	1.3	2.7
Orissa	1.6	1.5	3.0	1.3	1.2	2.5
West Bengal	1.5	1.5	3.0	1.3	1.2	2.6
Northeast						
Arunachal Pradesh	1.6	1.5	3.1	1.4	1.3	2.8
Assam	1.9	1.8	3.7	1.6	1.5	3.1
Manipur	1.8	1.6	3.4	1.6	1.5	3.1
Meghalaya	1.7	1.5	3.2	1.6	1.4	3.0
Mizoram	1.6	1.5	3.1	1.5	1.4	3.0
Nagaland	1.7	1.5	3.2	1.6	1.5	3.2
Tripura	1.7	1.5	3.3	1.5	1.3	2.8
West						
Goa	1.4	1.3	2.7	1.3	1.2	2.5
Gujarat	1.5	1.4	2.9	1.3	1.2	2.6
Maharashtra	1.5	1.4	2.9	1.3	1.3	2.6
South						
Andhra Pradesh	1.4	1.3	2.7	1.2	1.2	2.4
Karnataka	1.6	1.5	3.1	1.4	1.3	2.6
Kerala	1.3	1.2	2.5	1.2	1.2	2.3
Tamil Nadu	1.4	1.3	2.7	1.2	1.2	2.3

Table 5.11 Birth order by age of woman

Per cent distribution of births during the three years preceding the survey by order of birth and age of the woman at birth, according to residence, India, 1992-93

Maternal age at birth	Order of birth 1	2	3	4	5	6+	Total per cent	Number of births
URBAN								
13-14	(96.7)	(3.3)	(—)	(—)	(—)	(—)	100.0	41
15-19	67.9	24.6	6.1	1.1	0.3	—	100.0	1474
20-24	35.2	34.4	20.0	7.1	2.4	0.9	100.0	3533
25-29	15.8	26.3	21.3	18.4	11.9	6.4	100.0	2272
30-34	7.4	15.4	16.3	18.3	14.7	28.0	100.0	910
35-39	4.0	6.3	8.3	14.3	6.9	60.2	100.0	285
40-44	6.3	4.3	3.0	9.1	7.3	70.0	100.0	48
Total	31.8	27.2	16.9	10.5	6.0	7.6	100.0	8580
RURAL								
13-14	93.2	6.8	—	—	—	—	100.0	231
15-19	63.5	28.2	7.2	0.9	0.2	—	100.0	6824
20-24	24.6	33.6	25.1	11.6	3.9	1.2	100.0	10869
25-29	6.7	14.4	24.4	23.9	17.2	13.6	100.0	6523
30-34	1.6	5.0	11.1	15.9	18.5	47.9	100.0	3214
35-39	0.5	2.3	5.1	8.3	12.5	71.3	100.0	1244
40-44	0.3	0.4	1.7	5.6	11.4	80.6	100.0	366
45-49	0.2	—	1.1	6.9	6.2	85.6	100.0	65
Total	26.3	22.9	17.9	12.0	8.0	12.9	100.0	29336
TOTAL								
13-14	93.7	6.3	—	—	—	—	100.0	273
15-19	64.3	27.6	7.0	1.0	0.2	—	100.0	8298
20-24	27.2	33.8	23.9	10.5	3.5	1.1	100.0	14403
25-29	9.0	17.5	23.6	22.4	15.8	11.7	100.0	8794
30-34	2.9	7.3	12.2	16.4	17.6	43.5	100.0	4124
35-39	1.2	3.0	5.7	9.4	11.5	69.2	100.0	1529
40-44	1.0	0.8	1.8	6.0	10.9	79.4	100.0	414
45-49	0.2	1.3	2.2	8.0	6.7	81.5	100.0	82
Total	27.5	23.9	17.6	11.6	7.6	11.7	100.0	37916

Note: Table is based on children born in the period 1-36 months prior to the survey. Urban total includes 17 births to women age 45-49, which are not shown separately.

( ) Based on 25-49 unweighted cases.

— Less than 0.05 per cent.

Table 5.12 Birth order by education of woman

Per cent distribution of births during the three years preceding the survey by order of birth and age of the woman at birth, according to education, India, 1992-93

Maternal age at birth	Order of birth 1	2	3	4	5	6+	Total per cent	Number of births
				ILLITERATE				
13-14	94.9	5.1	—	—	—	—	100.0	213
15-19	60.1	29.9	8.5	1.2	0.3	—	100.0	5598
20-24	19.9	31.6	27.8	13.9	5.0	1.7	100.0	8697
25-29	4.0	11.2	23.4	26.0	19.5	15.8	100.0	5678
30-34	1.2	3.4	9.6	16.8	18.9	50.1	100.0	3052
35-39	0.3	2.0	3.8	7.8	11.4	74.6	100.0	1271
40-44	0.3	0.1	1.5	5.2	10.8	82.2	100.0	366
45-49	0.2	1.5	2.5	7.2	5.4	83.3	100.0	75
Total	22.3	20.9	18.3	13.6	9.3	15.6	100.0	24949
				LITERATE, < MIDDLE SCHOOL COMPLETE				
13-14	(86.8)	(13.2)	(—)	(—)	(—)	(—)	100.0	47
15-19	68.6	25.7	5.1	0.5	—	—	100.0	1570
20-24	28.0	37.5	23.5	8.6	2.1	0.4	100.0	2644
25-29	7.5	17.3	28.3	24.8	14.9	7.3	100.0	1333
30-34	3.5	7.0	15.4	17.4	19.1	37.6	100.0	539
35-39	0.7	3.1	10.5	19.5	12.2	54.0	100.0	157
40-44	(—)	(6.3)	(1.4)	(7.6)	(8.7)	(75.9)	100.0	33
Total	31.3	26.5	18.6	10.9	6.0	6.7	100.0	6328
				MIDDLE SCHOOL COMPLETE				
15-19	76.5	20.1	2.5	0.4	0.5	—	100.0	683
20-24	35.5	42.8	18.0	3.4	0.3	—	100.0	1343
25-29	15.8	26.5	28.2	15.7	10.2	3.7	100.0	523
30-34	3.8	11.7	18.7	20.5	19.8	25.5	100.0	157
35-39	(11.5)	(2.2)	(15.5)	(2.2)	(15.8)	(52.8)	100.0	34
Total	40.1	31.5	16.0	6.0	3.5	2.9	100.0	2757
				HIGH SCHOOL AND ABOVE				
15-19	82.5	16.1	1.4	—	—	—	100.0	446
20-24	56.5	32.0	9.2	1.5	0.5	0.3	100.0	1719
25-29	30.2	41.9	17.5	6.6	2.6	1.1	100.0	1260
30-34	15.3	37.1	26.1	10.7	4.2	6.6	100.0	376
35-39	13.4	23.1	24.7	20.6	8.2	10.0	100.0	67
Total	46.1	33.6	12.9	4.3	1.7	1.3	100.0	3882

Note: Table is based on children born in the period 1-36 months prior to the survey. Total for literate, < middle school complete includes 5 births to women age 45-49, total for middle school complete includes 11 and 5 births to women age 13-14 and 40-44, respectively, and total for high school and above includes 1, 12 and 2 births to women age 13-14, 40-44 and 45-49, respectively, which are not shown separately.

( ) Based on 25-49 unweighted cases.

— Less than 0.05 per cent.

Table 5.13: Birth order by state

Per cent distribution of births during the three years preceding the survey by order of birth and state, India, 1992-93

State	Order of birth 1	2	3	4	5	6+	Total per cent
India	27.5	23.9	17.6	11.6	7.6	11.7	100.0
North							
Delhi	28.0	27.7	17.5	12.7	6.7	7.5	100.0
Haryana	28.4	24.1	19.4	11.6	6.5	10.2	100.0
Himachal Pradesh	30.8	26.5	21.3	10.9	4.6	5.9	100.0
Jammu Region of J & K	31.6	24.3	18.6	10.9	6.0	8.6	100.0
Punjab	29.2	28.1	20.1	11.3	6.1	5.2	100.0
Rajasthan	27.0	22.3	17.1	12.4	9.0	12.1	100.0
Central							
Madhya Pradesh	26.5	23.7	16.9	12.0	8.3	12.6	100.0
Uttar Pradesh	22.9	19.6	16.4	12.5	9.6	19.0	100.0
East							
Bihar	23.5	20.1	16.3	14.3	9.8	16.0	100.0
Orissa	27.4	24.6	19.8	12.8	6.8	8.6	100.0
West Bengal	29.2	24.6	17.2	11.0	7.5	10.4	100.0
Northeast							
Arunachal Pradesh	26.1	19.3	17.9	15.4	8.4	12.8	100.0
Assam	22.4	19.4	17.3	13.8	8.5	18.5	100.0
Manipur	27.5	20.5	18.9	13.5	7.5	12.1	100.0
Meghalaya	24.9	21.6	15.6	11.0	9.3	17.6	100.0
Mizoram	30.4	24.6	20.3	14.2	4.1	6.4	100.0
Nagaland	27.8	24.1	16.4	10.4	10.4	10.8	100.0
Tripura	29.0	25.2	16.1	11.1	8.1	10.6	100.0
West							
Goa	38.1	29.7	17.7	7.9	3.5	3.1	100.0
Gujarat	33.2	24.8	17.8	11.0	6.3	6.9	100.0
Maharashtra	29.9	27.3	19.9	11.8	5.1	6.1	100.0
South							
Andhra Pradesh	30.6	27.3	20.6	10.7	5.5	5.3	100.0
Karnataka	30.9	26.7	17.8	9.0	6.4	9.2	100.0
Kerala	39.5	34.5	15.5	4.2	2.5	3.8	100.0
Tamil Nadu	35.7	32.0	18.2	6.9	4.1	3.1	100.0

Note: Table is based on Children born in the period 1-36 months prior to the survey.

5.5 Birth Order

Birth order analysis is important in understanding trends and differentials in fertility. Information on birth order can also be used to gauge the extent to which couples are following the 2-child family norm promoted by the family welfare programme. The birth order of children born during the three years before the survey is shown in Table 5.11. Overall, 28 per cent of all births were first births and 24 per cent were second births. As one would expect, the number of births at each order is greater than the number at the next higher order. Also as expected, younger women have more lower order births and older women have more higher order births. First births, as a per cent of all births, decline rapidly with increasing age of the mother and third and higher order births increase with increasing age of the mother. Predictably, the birth order distribution is more skewed toward lower order births in urban than in rural areas. Even in urban areas, however, 14 per cent of all births were of order five and above. The birth order distribution in the NFHS is similar to the estimates produced by the Sample Registration System for live births in 1991, although the NFHS reports a slightly higher percentage of high order births (Office of the Registrar General, 1993a).

The birth order distribution for illiterate women differs dramatically with a substial amount of education (Table 5.12). Eighty per cent of recent births to women with a high school education are first or second births and only 7 per cent are fourth or higher order births. For illiterate women, only 43 per cent of births are first and second order, whereas 39 per cent are fourth or higher order.

5.6 Birth intervals

Birth Intervals are an important measure of the pace of child-bearing. Past research has shown that children born too close to a previous birth have an increased risk of dying, especially if the interval between births is less than 24 months (Govindasamy *et al.*, 1993; Hobcraft *et al.*, 1983). Table 5.14 presents the percentage distribution of second and higher order births in the five years prior to the survey by the interval since the previous birth. Intervals between marriage and first birth, which do not include an interval of postpartum amenorrhoea, are excluded to make comparisons of the intervals over different characteristics of women more meaningful. Overall, 12 per cent of the births occurred within 18 months of the previous birth and 27 per cent occurred within 24 months. The median birth interval is 32 months or about 2.6 years.

Tabte 5.14 Birth Intervals

Per cent distribution of births during the five years preceding the survey by interval since previous birth, according to demographic and bakground characteristics, India, 1992-93

Characteristic	Months since previous birth <12	12-17	18-23	24-35	36-47	48+	Total percent	Median month since previous birth	Number of births
Age of the Mother									
15-19	3.6	18.4	23.2	40.3	11.7	2.9	100.0	24.8	1263
20-24	2.7	12.6	18.5	38.8	19.2	8.2	100.0	27.8	12445
25-29	1.9	9.3	15.7	33.7	21.8	17.5	100.0	31.8	16093
30-34	1.4	7.5	11.9	30.7	21.9	26.6	100.0	35.4	9331
35-39	1.6	7.4	10.7	26.8	21.7	31.8	100.0	37.3	4060
40-44	1.3	5.7	6.2	26.6	21.4	38.8	100.0	40.0	1338
45-49	0.9	3.6	4.9	23.8	21.9	45.0	100.0	43.6	369
Order of proior birth									
1	1.9	10.9	16.8	33.3	19.5	17.6	100.0	30.7	14701
2	2.1	9.0	14.3	35.1	21.2	18.3	100.0	31.7	10883
3	1.8	9.0	14.6	33.8	21.2	19.5	100.0	31.9	7259
4	2.1	9.4	14.1	32.3	22.0	20.2	100.0	32.8	4758
5	1.7	8.8	14.7	33.2	22.0	19.6	100.0	32.9	2984
6+	2.4	10.2	13.5	33.9	21.5	18.5	100.0	31.9	4315
Sex of proior birth									
Male	1.9	9.5	15.0	33.2	21.2	19.2	100.0	32.1	22381
Female	2.1	10.0	15.1	34.3	20.5	18.0	100.0	31.3	22518
Survival of prior birth									
Still living	1.4	8.1	14.8	34.4	21.8	19.4	100.0	32.5	39043

Deceased	5.8	20.8	16.7	29.3	14.2	13.2	100.0	25.7	5856
Residence									
Urban	2.3	10.5	16.0	32.1	19.1	20.0	100.0	31.0	9563
Rural	1.9	9.6	14.8	34.2	21.3	18.2	100.0	31.8	35337
Education of the Mother									
Illiterate	2.1	9.5	14.2	34.0	21.6	18.6	100.0	32.0	32113
Lit., < middle complete	1.5	10.3	16.9	35.5	19.3	16.5	100.0	30.6	7041
Middle school complete	1.6	10.7	18.3	32.6	19.1	17.7	100.0	29.6	2559
High school and above	2.1	11.1	17.1	28.3	17.7	23.6	100.0	31.7	3186
Religion									
Hindu	1.9	9.6	14.7	33.6	21.1	19.1	100.0	32.0	35344
Muslim	2.7	10.2	16.2	34.6	20.2	16.1	100.0	30.3	7411
Christian	1.7	8.8	17.9	33.6	18.2	19.8	100.0	31.1	829
Sikh	2.0	14.8	17.9	31.5	18.9	14.9	100.0	28.8	710
Jain	0.1	12.6	10.9	31.0	19.9	25.4	100.0	35.0	101
Buddhist	1.4	9.6	17.7	38.7	17.7	14.8	100.0	30.0	300
Other	2.1	8.1	17.0	36.7	13.9	22.1	100.0	30.3	205
Caste/tribe									
Scheduled caste	2.1	10.1	15.0	33.5	21.0	18.3	100.0	31.4	6280
Scheduled tribe	2.0	9.9	14.6	35.9	19.9	17.6	100.0	31.2	4361
Other	2.0	9.7	15.2	33.5	20.9	18.7	100.0	31.7	34258
Totat	2.0	9.8	15.1	33.8	20.8	18.6	100.0	31.6	44900

Note: First order births are excluded. The interval for multiple births is the number of months since the preceding pregnancy that ended in a live birth. There were no reported second or higher order births to women age 13-14.

Table 5.15: Birth Intervals by State

Per cent distribution of births during the five years preceding the survey by interval since previous birth, according to state, India, 1992-93

Characteristic	Months since previous birth						Total per cent	Median month since previous birth
	<12	12-17	18-23	24-35	36-47	48+		
1	2	3	4	5	6	7	8	9
India	2.0	9.8	15.1	33.8	20.8	18.6	100.0	31.6
North								
Delhi	2.3	11.8	16.3	31.0	18.3	20.2	100.0	30.6'
Haryana	2.1	13.7	17.6	34.7	18.7	13.2	100.0	28.1
Himachal Pradesh	1.9	12.7	18.7	37.4	16.9	12.4	100.0	28.3
Jammu Region of J & K	1.8	12.5	14.3	34.0	21.3	16.0	100.0	30.9
Punjab	2.4	13.7	17.1	32.8	18.1	15.9	100.0	29.3
Rajasthan	2.2	8.8	13.1	33.4	21.9	20.6	100.0	32.5
Central								
Madhya Pradesh	1.9	9.4	13.8	35.4	21.3	18.3	100.0	32.1
Uttar Pradesh	2.6	10.4	14.5	32.2	21.6	18.6	100.0	32.1
East								
Bihar	1.7	8.8	13.6	31.7	23.4	20.8	100.0	33.9
Orissa	1.9	9.7	13.8	32.6	21.6	20.5	100.0	32.7
West Bengal	1.3	8.8	14.4	35.4	20.7	19.4	100.0	31.7

Northeast								
Arunachal Pradesh	0.8	8.5	19.6	36.3	16.4	18.4	100.0	29.8
Assam	0.8	12.4	16.6	34.9	19.8	15.4	100.0	29.8
Manipur	1.3	10.1	14.5	35.6	20.4	18.1	100.0	31.6
Meghalaya	0.9	11.4	22.1	36.1	16.9	12.5	100.0	27.5
Mizoram	1.5	13.4	20.7	34.9	13.2	16.3	100.0	27.6
Nagaland	2.8	10.5	20.2	37.8	16.7	11.9	100.0	28.1
Tripura	0.6	8.7	12.7	34.1	20.4	23.6	100.0	33.9
West								
Goa	1.2	8.8	13.8	27.9	20.0	28.2	100.0	35.2
Gujarat	1.9	10.2	17.2	36.9	19.3	14.5	100.0	30.0
Maharashtra	2.8	9.0	18.8	36.1	19.6	13.6	100.0	28.7
South								
Andhra Pradesh	1.8	8.0	12.9	33.7	21.2	22.5	100.0	33.4
Karnataka	2.0	9.7	16.9	36.9	18.4	16.2	100.0	29.9
Kerala	1.4	8.3	13.5	28.5	19.7	28.6	100.0	34.9
Tamil Nadu	0.9	9.7	16.5	33.1	18.5	21.3	100.0	31.6

Note: First order births are excluded. The interval for multiple births is the number of months since the preceding pregnancy that ended in a live birth.

Table 5.16 Age at first birth
Per cent distribution of women by age at first birth, according to current age and residence, India, 1992-93

Current ages[1]	No birth[2]	Age at first birth <15	15-17	18-19	20-21	22-24	25+	Total per cent
				URBAN				
15-19	89.6	1.6	5.9	2.9	NA	NA	NA	100.0
20-24	47.3	2.6	13.5	17.5	14.1	5.0	NA	100.0
25-29	16.1	4.0	18.3	19.2	17.7	17.1	7.7	100.0
30-34	7.5	3.6	19.9	20.7	18.2	17.2	12.9	100.0
35-39	5.8	4.2	20.7	21.3	17.4	17.7	13.0	100.0
40-44	4.9	4.5	23.4	21.3	18.3	15.6	12.2	100.0
45-49	4.7	5.8	22.5	21.3	18.5	15.8	11.3	100.0
20-49	18.4	3.8	18.7	19.8	17.0	13.9	8.4	100.0
25-49	8.8	4.2	20.5	20.6	17.9	16.8	11.2	100.0
				RURAL				
15-19	78.4	3.4	13.5	4.8	NA	NA	NA	100.0
20-24	28.0	6.1	27.0	21.4	13.2	4.3	NA	100.0
25-29	8.5	6.5	30.9	23.3	16.4	11.1	3.3	100.0
30-34	4.1	6.5	30.6	24.7	17.2	11.6	5.3	100.0
35-39	3.6	7.2	31.4	23.5	16.1	11.8	6.6	100.0
40-44	3.0	6.9	30.0	24.7	17.8	11.6	6.0	100.0
45-49	3.4	7.4	29.5	22.5	16.1	13.2	7.9	100.0
20-49	11.0	6.6	29.7	23.2	15.8	9.8	4.0	100.0
25-49	5.0	6.8	30.6	23.8	16. 7	11.7	5.4	100 0
				TOTAL				
15-19	81.4	2.9	11.4	4.3	NA	NA	NA	100.0
20-24	33.5	5.1	23.2	20.3	13.4	4.5	NA	100.0
25-29	10.7	5.8	27.3	22.2	16.8	12.8	4.6	100.0
30-34	5.1	5.7	27.4	23.5	17.5	13.2	7.6	100.0
35-39	4.2	6.3	28.2	22.8	16.5	13.5	8.5	100.0
40-44	3.9	6.1	27.9	23.6	17.9	12.8	7.8	100.0
45-49	3.7	7.0	27.6	22.2	16.8	13.9	8.9	100.0
20-49	13.2	5.8	26.5	22.2	16.1	10.9	5.3	100.0
25-49	6.2	6.1	27.6	22.8	17.1	13.2	7.1	100.0

NA: Not applicable.
1 The current age groups include both never-married and ever-married women.
2 Never-married women are included in this category.

The relatively short median birth interval for women age 15-19 at the time of the survey probably results from a selection effect. Only women who have had two or more births are included in this table, and women age 15-19 with two or more births are likely to have considerably higher fecundability than women at large. Differences in fecundability by age of the mother may likewise account for the generally positive gradient in the length of birth intervals by mother's age. Curiously, in view of the correlation between age of women and birth order, there is little variation in median intervals according to the birth order of the previous birth. This is because women With large numbers of births are probably more fecund, and therefore have shorter median intervals than other women.

The median birth interval is seven months shorter when when the last birth is deceased than when the last birth is still alive and very short birth intervals are unusually high for the former group. This probably reflects the cessation of breastfeeding when the child dies and the consequent shortening of the period of postpartum amenorrhoea.

Birth intervals vary little by the sex of the prior birth, residence, education, or caste/tribe. Jains have particularly long birth intervals (a median of 35 months) and birth intervals are shortest for Sikhs, who have low fertility but a more rapid pace of childbearing than other groups. Interestingly, median birth intervals are relatively high in both the highest and lowest fertility states (see Table 5.15). This phenomenon is probably due to the older average age of women having children in high fertility states and a number of factors in low- fertility states, such as high levels of child survivorship and more frequent use of temporary methods of contraception.

5.7 AGE AT FIRST AND LAST BIRTH

The onset of childbearing is an important demographic indicator. Postponement of first births, reflecting a rise in the age at marriage, can make an important contribution to overall fertility decline. Table 5. 16 shows the distribution of women by age at first birth. Nearly half of all women age 20-49 had their first birth at age 15-19 and more than one-quarter had their first birth at age 20-24. Very early childbearing (below age 15) is relatively rare in all of the age groups and the incidence has dropped fairly steadily across cohorts of women. Childbearing before age 15 is negligible in the 15-19 age group. Childbearing before age 20 has also declined slightly, with the proportion of women having their first child before age 20 dropping below 50 per cent for the first time in the 20-24 age group. Urban women are much less likely than rural women to have their first birth before age 18 and much more likely to have their first birth after age 22.

Table 5.17 :Median age at first birth by background characteristics
Median age at first birth among women age 20-49 years, by current age and selected background characteristics, India, 1992-93

Background characteristic	Current age 20-24	25-29	30-34	35-39	40-44	45-49	20-49	25-49
Residence								
Urban	NC	20.9	20.6	20.4	20.1	20.0	NC	20.5
Rural	19.6	19.0	19.0	18.9	19.0	19.1	19.1	19.0
Education								
Illiterate	18.8	18.5	18.7	18.6	18.8	19.0	18.7	18.7
Lit., < middle complete	NC	19.5	19.3	19.3	19.2	19.5	19.5	19.4
Middle school complete	NC	20.6	20.2	20.5	20.1	21.0	NC	20.4
High school and above	NC	23.6	23.1	23.3	23.1	23.1	NC	23.3
Religion								
Hindu	NC	19.5	19.4	19.3	19.3	19.3	19.5	19.4
Muslim	19.5	18.8	18.8	18.6	18.7	18.8	18.9	18.7
Christian	NC	21.9	22.2	21.7	21.6	20.9	NC	21.7
Sikh	NC	21.8	21.3	20.9	21.3	21.5	NC	21.4
Other	NC	19.8	20.4	19.2	19.7	19.6	NC	19.8
Caste/tribe								
Scheduled caste	19.2	18.6	18.7	18.7	18.8	19.0	18.8	18.7
Scheduled tribe	19.2	19.0	18.9	18.8	19.2	19.3	19.1	19.0
Other	NC	19.7	19.6	19.5	19.4	19.4	19.7	19.6
Total	NC	19.5	19.4	19.3	19.3	19.4	19.6	19.4

NC: Median is not calculated when less than 50 per cent of the women age x to x+n have had a birth by age x.

Table 5.17 shows the median age at first birth by selected background characteristics. The median age at first birth for any group of women is the age by which half of them have had their first birth. For women in the younger age groups, the number who will eventually become mothers is not known since some first births to the cohort will occur only in the future. The medians are, therefore, calculated as the ages by which half of all women in the cohort have had a first birth, rather than the age by which half of all mothers in the cohort have had a first birth. This statistic may be computed without knowing how many women in the cohort will eventually have a first birth. The medians are, of course, undefined for cohorts in which fewer than half of the women have had a first birth. This is the reason why no medians are shown for women age 20-24 and 20-49 for some background characteristics in Table 5.17.

For women age 25-49, the median age at first birth has been almost constant at 19.3-19.5 years. Although the median age at first marriage is 1.2 years higher for women age 25-29 than for women age 45-49 (see Table 4.5), and the median age at first cohabitation is 0.8 years higher (see Table 4.9), the median age at first birth is almost the same for these two age groups. This means that the interval between marriage and first cohabitation and the interval between first cohabitation and first birth have both been decreasing over time, as the age at first marriage and first cohabitation have been increasing.

On average, median ages at first birth are 1-2 months higher in urban than in rural areas. In all age groups, better educated women have a considerably higher median age at first birth than do less educated women: the median at age 25-49 is 23 years of age among women with at least a high school education but only 19 years of age among illiterate women. Among the religious groups, Muslims have the youngest median age at first birth and Christians and Sikhs the oldest, with Hindus falling in between. Although the median age at first marriage is the same for Hindus and Muslims (see Table 4.5), Muslims begin childbearing at a slightly younger age than Hindus, reflecting the shorter gap between marriage and childbearing among Muslim women. Scheduled castes and tribes begin childbearing slightly earlier than non-SC/ST group, but the differences are small.

For all women age 25-49, the median age at first birth is four years higher than average in Goa and three years higher than average in Manipur and Mizoram (Table 5.18). Particularly young ages at first birth are common in Andhra Pradesh, West Bengal, Assam, Madhya Pradesh, and Karnataka. The difference between the median age at first birth and the median age at first marriage for women age 25-49 (Table 4.6) is less than three years in every state except the early marriage states of Rajasthan, Uttar Pradesh, Bihar, Haryana and Madhya Pradesh (where the difference ranges from 3.7 to 4.7 years). This result is consistent with the findings of Basu (1993) of particularly long first birth intervals related to cultural practices in North India. This finding may also be related to adolescent subfecundity among women who marry at very young ages. The difference hetweeo the median age at first birth and the median age at first marriage is unusually low in all of the northeastern states, where the culture is more accepting of premarital conception and even premarital births.

Table 5.18: Median age at first birth by state

Median age at first birth among women age 20-49 years, by current age and state, India, 1992-93

State	Current age 20-24	25-29	30-34	35-39	40-44	45-49	20-49	25-49
India	NC	19.5	19.4	19.3	19.3	19.4	19.6	19.4
North								
Delhi	NC	21.2	21.1	20.9	20.8	19.8	NC	20.9
Haryana	19.7	19.7	19.7	19.8	20.1	20.4	19.8	19.8
Himachal Pradesh	NC	20.6	20.0	19.6	19.7	19.6	NC	20.0
Jammu Region of J & K	NC	21.1	20.4	19.6	19.1	20.1	NC	20.2
Punjab	NC	21.0	21.0	20.8	21.2	21.5	NC	21.0
Rajasthan	20.0	19.1	19.4	20.0	20.0	20.6	19.8	19.7
Central								
Madhya Pradesh	19.2	19.0	18.5	18.8	18.8	19.0	18.9	18.8
Uttar Pradesh	NC	19.5	19.4	19.6	19.6	19.5	19.7	19.5
East								
Bihar	19.5	19.1	19.1	19.2	18.9	18.8	19.1	19.0
Orissa	NC	19.8	19.2	18.5	18.7	19.2	19.5	19.1
West Bengal	19.3	19.0	18.7	18.4	18.1	18.6	18.8	18.6
Northeast								
Arunachal Pradesh	NC	20.0	19.7	20.0	20.7	21.2	NC	20.1
Assam	NC	19.1	18.9	19.0	18.3	18.7	19.2	18.8
Manipur	NC	24.0	23.0	21.9	21.6	21.8	NC	22.4
Meghalaya	NC	20.2	19.6	20.0	19.9	21.9	NC	20.3
Mizoram	NC	22.6	21.1	22.1	21.9	22.3	NC	22.0
Nagaland	NC	21.9	20.1	21.3	21.0	21.4	NC	21.2
Tripura	NC	19.7	20.3	19.1	18.8	18.9	19.7	19.4
West								
Goa	NC	NC	24.3	22.9	21.8	22.5	NC	23.7
Gujarat	NC	20.4	20.5	20.1	20.1	20.0	NC	20.2
Maharashtra	19.6	19.0	19.1	18.9	19.0	19.0	19.2	19.0
South								
Andhra Pradesh	18.5	17.9	18.0	17.6	18.2	18.1	18.0	17.9
Karnataka	19.9	18.9	18.9	18.9	18.9	18.7	19.1	18.9
Kerala	NC	22.3	22.1,	21.4	21.0	20.9	NC	21.6
Tamil Nadu	NC	20.7	20.5	20.1	19.5	19.2	NC	20.1

NC: Median is not calculated when less than 50 per cent of the women age x to x+n have had a birth by age x

The age at last birth is another important determinant of overall fertility levels. Table 5.19 shows the distribution of women by age at last birth for women age 40-44 and 45-49. Although a few of these women may have another birth later on, the very low fertility rates for women in their forties seen earlier suggest that childbearing is virtually complete for this cohort. Nearly half of women age 40-49 completed their childbearing by age 30 and three-quarters had their last birth before age 35. The median ages at last birth for women age 40-44 and 45-49 at the time of the survey are 30.0 and 31.4 years, respectively.

Differentials in the age at last birth by background characteristics are shown in Table 5.20. Rural residents, illiterate women, Muslims and women from scheduled castes and scheduled tribes are most likely to continue childbearing into their late thirties and their forties. Among all of the groups examined, the highest median age at last birth is for Muslims (32.8 years) and the lowest is for women who have completed middle school (27.9 years).

Differences between the median age at last birth and the median age at first birth for women in their forties are shown in Table 5.21. The difference between the median age at first birth and the median age at last birth gives an estimated reproductive life of 11 years for women who are approaching the end of their childbearing years. This span is likely to be considerably shorter for younger cohorts, who have begun their childbearing at a later average age and who can be expected to have their last birth at a younger age as fertility levels continue to decline. The reproductive life span is relatively short in South and West India. In fact, women in Goa and Kerala concentrated their births within a period of only 8 years. The reproductive life span is 6 years longer in Uttar Pradesh, Bihar and Tripura, where women have had their births over a period of 14 years.

5.8 Childbearing at Young Ages

Fertility among teenagers (those under age 20) is drawing increasing attention from policymakers. Table 5.22 shows the percentages of ever-married women age 13-19 who are either mothers or are pregnant with their first child. The sum of these two percentages represents the proportion of young ever-married women who have begun childbearing. Overall, 58 per cent of ever-married teenage women have started their childbearing (46 per cent have already become mothers and 12 per cent are pregnant with their first child). However, because the proportion in this age group who have never married has been rising over time, childbearing among teenage women is likely to be less common now

Table 5.19: Age at last birth

Per cent distribution of ever-married women age 40-49 by age at last birth, according to current age and residence, India, 1992-93

Current age	Age at last birth								Total per cent	Median age at last birth	Number of women
	No birth	<20	20-24	25-29	30-34	35-39	40-44	45-49			
URBAN											
40-44	3.0	2.6	19.0	32.7	29.1	11.8	1.9	NA	100.0	28.9	2899
45-49	3.2	2.8	13.3	31.8	30.0	14.5	3.5	0.9	100.0	29.8	2197
40-49	3.1	2.7	16.6	32.3	29.5	13.0	2.5	0.4	100.0	29.3	5096
RURAL											
40-44	2.7	3.2	13.1	27.9	29.5	18.8	4.9	NA	100.0	30.5	6850
45-49	3.0	2.3	9.6	24.1	27.7	22.9	9.0	1.5	100.0	32.1	5838
40-49	2.8	2.7	11.5	26.2	28.7	20.7	6.8	0.7	100.0	31.2	12688
TOTAL											
40-44	2.8	3.0	14.9	29.3	29.3	16.7	4.0	NA	100.0	30.0	9748
45-49	3.0	2.4	10.6	26 2	28.4	20.6	7.5	1.3	100.0	31.4	8036
40-49	2.9	2.7	13.0	27.9	28.9	18.5	5.5	0.6	100.0	30.6	17784

NA: Not applicable.

than in the past. Only 25 per cent of married women age 13-16 are mothers compared with 52 per cent of those age 17-19. The percentage of ever-married women who have begun childbearing is slightly higher in urban areas than in rural areas, but since a smaller proportion of urban women are married, overall childbearing is higher among teenage women in rural areas. There is no difference in the percentage of ever-married women who have begun childbearing between illiterate women and literate women with less than a middle school education, but married women who have completed high school are less likely to have begun childbearing. Differentials by religion and caste/tribe are not large. The percentage who have begun childbearing is slightly higher among scheduled tribe women and Christians and Muslims.

Table 5.23 contains similar information for ever-married teenage women in each state. The percentage who have begun childbearing is much higher than average in all of the northeastern states, as well as Goa, Maharashtra and Karnataka. Once again, however, these percentages should be considered in relation to the proportion of teenage women who have ever been married if one wants to examine the percentage of all teenage women who have begun childbearing (see the last column of Table 5.23). Overall, only 17 per cent of teenage women in India have begun childbearing. For individual states, the picture is quite different for all women than for ever-married women. Teenage childbearing is particularly high in Madhya Pradesh and Andhra Pradesh. On the other hand, less than 5 per cent of teenage women have begun childbearing in Goa and Manipur.

5.9 Postpartum Amenorrhoea, Abstinence and Nonsusceptibility

The importance of lactational amenorrhoea and postpartum abstinence as determinants of fertility is well recognized. The duration of postpartum amenorrhoea (delayed resumption of ovulation) following a birth is closely associated with the duration of breastfeeding, which tends to suppress the resumption of ovulation. Conception can also be delayed by prolonged postpartum abstinence. The total period of protection from amenorrhoea or abstinence or both is defined as the nonsusceptible duration. The percentage of births during the last three years whose mothers are presently postpartum amenorrhoeic, abstaining or nonsusceptible is presented in Table 5.24. The mean and median durations and the prevalence/incidence mean duration are also shown in the table. Estimates of means and medians are based on a smoothed distribution of the current status proportion in each months-since-birth group. The preva-

Table 5.20 :Age at last birth by background characteristics
Per cent distribution of ever-marrid women age 40-49 by age at last birth, according to current age and selected background characteristics, India, 1992-93

Background characteristic	No birth	Age at last birth							Total per cent	Median age at last birth	Number of women
		<20	20-24	25-29	30-34	35-39	40-44	45-49			
Residence											
Urban	3.1	2.7	16.6	32.3	29.5	13.0	2.5	0.4	100.0	29.3	5096
Rural	2.8	2.7	11.5	26.2	28.7	20.7	6.8	0.7	100.0	31.2	12688
Education											
Illiterate	2.9	3.1	10.7	24.6	29.1	21.7	7.1	0.8	100.0	31.6	12370
Lit.< middle complete	2.5	2.3	17.7	32.6	28.9	13.2	2.7	0.2	100.0	29.3	3146
Middle school Complete	3.7	2.0	20.7	40.8	23.9	7.9	1.0	—	100.0	27.9	832
High school and above	3.1	0.6	17.3	39.0	30.4	8.1	1.3	0.2	100.0	28.7	1436
Religion											
Hindu	2.9	2.8	13.5	28.6	28.5	17.8	5.3	0.6	100.0	30.4	14579
Muslim	3.2	2.9	8.5	20.1	28.5	26.8	9.3	0.8	100.0	32.8	1936
Christian	2.2	2.4	11.8	32.6	33.4	13.2	3.9	0.5	100.0	30.1	565
Sikh	1.6	0.4	15.3	33.6	34.2	13.6	1.4	—	100.0	29.9	366
Jain	5.1	—	19.1	33.1	31.4	9.4	1.9	—	100.0	29.4	111

Buddhist	3.1	2.8	10.1	30.2	38.9	14.1	0.6	0.2	100.0	30.4	150
Other	6.7	1.4	9.2	31.7	30.7	14.4	5.3	0.6	100.0	30.2	76
Caste/tribe											
Scheduled caste	2.2	2.8	9.8	24.4	30.4	22.3	7.2	1.0	100.0	31.9	2041
Scheduled tribe	3.7	3.9	13.9	27.3	24.0	19.3	7.1	0.8	100.0	30.2	1438
Other	2.9	2.6	13.3	28.5	29.2	17.8	5.2	0.5	100.0	30.4	14305
Total	2.9	2.7	13.0	27.9	28.9	18.5	5.5	0.6	100.0	30.6	17784

— Less than 0.05 per cent.

lence/incidence mean is obtained by dividing the number of mothers who are nonsusceptible by the average number of births per month over a 36-month period. Ninety-two per cent of all women who had a birth in the month prior to the survey were still amenorrhoeic when interviewed. The proportion amenorrhoeic gradually decreases as the number of months since birth increases, to half of women 8 months after the birth, and one-quarter of women 13-14 months after the birth. The proportions of mothers abstaining from sexual intercourse are much lower than the proportions amenorrhoeic. Half of women were still abstaining 3 months after the birth and nearly one-quarter of women were still abstaining 6 months after the birth.

Table 5.21: Median age at first birth and median age at last birth
Median age at first birth and median age at last birth for women age 40-49, by state, India, 1992-93

State	Median age at first birth	Median age at last birth	Difference
India	19.3	30.6	11.3
North			
Delhi	20.1	29.7	9.6
Haryana	20.2	31.2	11.0
Himachal Pradesh	19.6	29.3	9.7
Jammu Region of J & K	19.6	31.1	11.5
Punjab	21.4	30.0	8.6
Rajasthan	20.3	32.1	11.8
Central			
Madhya Pradesh	18.9	31.1	12.2
Uttar Pradesh	19.6	33.8	14.2
East			
Bihar	18.8	32.7	13.9
Orissa	18.8	30.9	12.1
West Bengal	18.2	29.8	11.6
Northeast			
Arunachal Pradesh	20.8	33.1	12.3
Assam	18.4	31.8	13.4
Manipur	21.6	32.7	11.1
Meghalaya	20.8	31.5	10.7
Mizoram	22.0	31.8	9.8
Nagaland	21.1	30.1	9.0
Tripura	18.8	32.8	14.0

{Cont}....

West			
Goa	22.0	29.9	7.9
Gujarat	20.0	29.3	9.3
Maharashtra	18.9	28.0	9.1
South			
Andhra Pradesh	18.1	27.9	9.8
Karnataka	18.8	29.2	10.4
Kerala	20.9	29.0	8.1
Tamil Nadu	19.3	29.1	9.8

Tabte 5.22: Childbearing among ever-married women age 13-19
Percentage of ever-married women age 13-19 who are mothers or pregnant with their first chitd by selected background characteristics India 1992-93

Background characteristic	Percentage who are: Mothers	Pregnant with first child	Per cent who have begun child-bearing	Number of women
Age				
13-16	24.5	11.7	36.1	2170
17-19	52.4	11.7	64.1	7277
Residence				
Urban	47.1	13.8	60.9	1418
Rurat	45.8	11.3	57.1	8029
Education				
llLiterate	48.1	10.2	58.3	6359
Literate <middle complete	45.1	13.7	58.8	1778
Middle school complete	39.3	15.6	54.9	787
High School and above	33.0	17.3	50.3	522
Religion				
Hindu	45.2	11.6	56.8	7858
Muslim	51.4	10.9	62.3	1261
Christian	47.3	16.0	63.4	104
Sikh	34.6	22.9	57.5	75
Buddhist	50.1	11.7	61.8	87
Other	48.2	15.5	63.7	45
Caste/tribe				
Scheduled caste	46.2	11.1	57.3	1419
Scheduled tribe	52.4	11.6	64.0	939
Other	45.1	11.8	56.9	7089
Total	46.0	11.7	57.7	9447

Note: Total incfudes 16 ever-married Jain womeu who are not shown separately.

Table 5.23: Childbearing among women age 13-19 by state
Percentage of ever-married women age 13-19 who are mothers or pregnant with their first child and percentage of ever-married women and all women age 13-19 who have begun childbearing, by state, India, 1992-93

State	Ever-married women Per centage who are: Mother	pregnant with first child	Per cent who have begun child bearing Pregnant with	All women Per cent who have begun child
India	46.0	11.7	57.7	17 0
North				
Delhi	45.5	14.3	59.7	8.0
Haryana	50.1	12.7	62.9	20.7
Himachal Pradesh	39.3	15.8	55.2	7.1
Jammu Region of J & K	37.3	12.8	50.1	6.5
Punjab	42.4	22.0	64.4	6.7
Rajasthan	35.6	9.8	45.4	13.0
Central				
Madhya Pradesh	41.9	13.0	54.9	26.5
Uttar Pradesh	41.4	8.1	49.4	14.1
East				
Bihar	39.1	9.1	48.2	18.6
Orissa	48.2	11.6	59.8	13.2
West Bengal	47.8	15.6	63.4	20.4
Northeast				
Arunachal Pradesh	50.6	18.5	69.1	14.8
Assam	59.9	10.7	70.6	17.9
Manipur	*	*	*	2.9
Meghalaya	49.3	22.4	71.6	11.5
Mizoram	(42.5)	(30.0)	(72.5)	5.7
Nagaland	(65.9)	(22.0)	(87.8)	7.3
Tripura	54.5	11.9	66.3	14.9
West				
Goa	(52.9)	(14.7)	(67.6)	1.6
Gujarat	46.9	8.8	55.7	8.9
Maharashtra	57.8	10.3	68.1	19.9
South				
Andhra Pradesh	47.4	12.7	60.1	25.4
Karnataka	57.8	13.9	71.7	20.8
Kerala	37.9	21.3	59.2	5.9
Tamil Nadu	47.9	17.1	65.0	12.0

( ) Based on 25-49 unweighted Cases.
* Per cent not shown; based on fewer than 25 unweighted cases.

Overall, nearly half (47 per cent) of women become susceptible to pregnancy within 10 months of giving birth and 70 per cent become susceptible after 15 months. The median and mean durations of nonsusceptibility are 10.2 and 11.1 months, respectively. The median duration of amenorrhoea (9.0 months) is longer than the median duration of abstinence (3.4 months). The prevalence-incidence mean suggests that on average, women remain nonsusceptible to conception for just under one year after a birth, primarily due to the effects of postpartum amenorrhoea.

Table 5.25 shows median durations of postpartum amenorrhoea, postpartum abstinence, and postpartum nonsusceptibility by selected background characteristics. Variations in postpartum abstinence are relatively small so that the duration of nonsusceptibility is determined largely by variations in the duration of postpartum amenorrhoea. The median duration of amenorrhoea is slightly longer for women age 30 and over than for women under age 30, but the median duration of abstinence does not show any consistent pattern with age. The median duration of postpartum nonsusceptibility rises consistently with the age of the mother until age 35-39. Median durations of postpartum amenorrhoea and nonsusceptibility are longer for women in rural areas than for women in urban areas, probably due to the longer period of breastfeeding in rural areas (see Table 10.5). Periods of amenorrhoea and nonsusceptibility are relatively long for illiterate women and women belonging to scheduled castes and tribes, again as a probable consequence of relatively prolonged breastfeeding in these groups. Christians, Sikhs and Jains, who have the shortest durations of breastfeeding, are also most likely to resume ovulation quickly after having a birth.

The duration of postpartum abstinence varies considerably more by state than by other characteristics (see Table 5.26). The duration of postpartum abstinence is particularly long (about 4-7 months) in most of South India and West India, as well as in Nagaland and Orissa. For three states (Nagaland, Goa and Tamil Nadu), the duration of postpartum abstinence is at least as long as the duration of postpartum amenorrhoea. The pattern in these states is quite different from the situation elsewhere in India, where the median duration of postpartum amenorrhoea is nearly three times as long as the median duration of postpartum abstinence. The duration of postpartum abstinence is about one month shorter than average in all of the states in North India, as well as Madhya Pradesh, West Bengal and some small northeastern states.

The median duration of postpartum amenorrhoea varies widely from only 4 months in Delhi, Punjab and Goa, to 10 months in Assam,

Table 5.24: Postpartum amenorrhoea. abstinence and nonsusceptibility
Per centage of births occurring during the three years preceding the survey whose mothers are postpartum amenorrhoeic, postpartum abstaining or postpartum nonsusceptible, by number of months since birth, and median and mean durations, India, 1992-93

	Per cent of births whose mothers are:			
Months since birth	Postpartum amenorrhoeic	Postpartum abstaining	Postpartum nonsusceptible	Number of births
<1	91.7	97.0	99.0	629
1	91.2	85.9	97.1	1105
2	81.3	63.1	87.8	1217
3	75.8	49.5	85.3	1234
4	70.5	35.3	76.7	1256
5	65.3	28.9	72.2	1163
6	59.0	24.4	64.9	1240
7	57.0	21.3	63.6	1206
8	49.9	19.1	57.1	1076
9	48.8	14.7	53.4	1022
10	43.6	15.0	48.4	891
11	39.4	11.5	43.3	825
12	30.5	10.9	35.6	1045
13	24.4	8.4	28.8	1238
14	25.3	9.3	30.9	1192
15	23.8	9.1	29.6	1214
16	17.2	7.5	22.1	1247
17	16.0	5.7	19.1	1158
18	13.7	7.7	19.0	1139
19	9.9	4.4	13.2	1024
20	11.0	4.7	14.5	989
21	8.6	5.3	13.1	921
2Z	8.6	5.4	12.4	795
23	6.9	3.6	9.9	814
24	5.1	5.3	9.2	1016
25	3.5	2.6	5.8	1149
26	2.4	3.6	5.6	1099
27	2.5	3.2	5.0	983
28	2.6	2.8	4.9	1077
29	2.6	4.0	6.1	934
30	2.2	3.5	5.5	997
31	1.2	1.5	2.6	889
32	1.4	2.5	3.8	903
33	1.1	2.0	2.9	887
34	1.8	3.2	4.6	882
35	2.0	2.2	4.1	803
Median	9.0	3.4	10.2	NA
Mean	9.5	5.4	11.1	NA
Prevalence/ Incidence mean	10.3	5.8	11.9	NA

{Cont.}

Note: Medians and means are based on current status. Nonsusceptible is defined as amenorrhoeic or abstaining or both.

NA: Not applicable.

Table 5.25: Median duration of postpartum nonsusceptibility by background characteristics
Median number of months of postpartum amenorrhoea, postpartum abstinence and postpartum nonsusceptibility, by selected background characteristics of mothers, for births during the three years preceding the survey, India, 1992-93

Background characteristic	Postpartum amenorrhoea	Postpartum abstinence	Postpartum nonsusceptibility	Number of births
Age				
13-14	(7.5)	(6.2)	(7.5)	35
15-19	7.2	3.5	9.5	4581
20-24	8.5	3.5	10.0	14131
25-29	9.2	3.3	10.4	10518
30-34	10.0	3.4	11.3	5167
35-39	10.7	3.4	11.7	2052
40-44	11.1	4.8	11.4	625
45-49	5.9	3.9	6.0	153
Residence				
Urban	6.7	3.3	8.0	8418
Rural	10.0	3.5	10.8	28845
Education				
Illiterate	10.8	3.5	11.4	24518
Lit., < middle complete	8.0	3.4	9.2	6222
Middle school complete	5.0	3.3	7.9	2704
High school and above	4.4	3.5	6.2	3820
Religion				
Hindu	9.3	3.6	10.3	29582
Muslim	8.3	2.9	9.2	5720
Christian	6.6	3.9	8.8	748
Sikh	4.0	3.1	4.4	653
Jain	3.7	2.8	3.7	114
Buddhist	11.8	4.0	12.1	266
Other	12.4	3.6	13.4	178
Caste/tribe				
Scheduled caste	10.7	3.7	11.0	5027
Scheduled tribe	12.0	3.5	12.3	3485
Other	8.5	3.4	9.5	28750
Total	9.0	3.4	10.2	37263

Note: Medians are based on current status. Nonsusceptible is defined aas amenorrhoeic or abstaining or both.

( ) Based on 25-49 unweighted cases.

Table 5.26 Median duration of postpartum non susceptibility be state
Median number of months of postpartum amenorrhoea, postpartum abstinence and postpartum nonsusceptibility for mothers of children born during the three years preceding the survey, by state, India, 1992-93

State	Postpartum amenorrhoea	Postpartum abstinence	Postpartum nonsusceptibility
India	9.0	3.4	10.2
North			
Delhi	4.3	1.8	4.8
Haryana	8.9	2.0	8.9
Himachal Pradesh	7.6	2.6	8.5
Jammu Region of J & K	5.7	2.5	6.3
Punjab	4.1	2.4	4.4
Rajasthan	8.0	2.0	8.6
Central			
Madhya Pradesh	8.3	2.5	9.4
Uttar Pradesh	8.9	2.9	9.5
East			
Bihar	9.9	2.9	10.6
Orissa	8.5	4.7	10.2
West Bengal	9.5	2.3	10.0
Northeast			
Arunachal Pradesh	9.3	1.8	10.6
Assam	10.2	2.9	10.9
Manipur	8.7	2.5	9.3
Meghalaya	8.7	4.0	11.0
Mizoram	5.1	1.3	6.0
Nagaland	6.3	7.2	10.7
Tripura	6.9	3.3	7.9
West			
Goa	4.1	5.6	6.7
Gujarat	8.9	2.9	4.4
Maharashtra	8.5	4.5	9.8
South			
Andhra Pradesh	9.1	4.3	10.1
Karnataka	8.6	5.3	10.0
Kerala	5.4	4.8	7.3
Tamil Nadu	5.6	5.6	9.3

Note: Medians are based on current status. Nonsusceptible is defined as amenorrhoeic or abstaining or both.

Bihar and West Bengal. Similarly, the median duration of nonsusceptibility varies from 4 months in Punjab to 11 months in Bihar and several northeastern states. These variations in the duration of postpartum nonsusceptibility are one important determinant of fertility differentials in the states of India. It is interesting to note that the median duration of nonsusceptibility is relatively low in many low fertility states. This suggests that the state differentials in fertility would be even larger in the absence of state differentials in nonsusceptibility.

5.10 Menopause

Another factor impinging on fertility is the onset of menopause. Later in life (typically beginning around age 30), the risk of pregnancy begins to decline with age. In the NFHS, menopause is defined as the lack of a menstrual period for at least six months preceding the survey for women who are neither pregnant nor postpartum amenorrhoeic. Women who report that they are menopausal are also included in this group. In India, menopause is relatively rare for women in their thirties, but its incidence increases rapidly after age 40 (Table 5.27). By age 44-45, 38 per cent of women are in menopause. This figure increases to 56 per cent for women age 46-47 and 71 per cent for women age 48-49. The onset of menopause is slightly later in urban areas than in rural areas. Among the major states, menopause takes place at relatively young ages in Maharashtra and Andhra Pradesh, and relatively old ages in Haryana and Kerala.

Notes

1 A replacement level fertility is the level at which each women, on average, is replaced by one daughter, which occurs at approximately a TFR of 2.1 children per woman.

2 Information was collected on a woman's age at effective marriage, not the year and month of her effective marriage (which would be difficult to determine accurately in most cases of, therefore, the duration since first effective' marriage is calculated as the woman's age during the specified time period minus the age at which she started living with her (first) husband. For those whose current age is the same as their age at effective marriage (marriage duration 0), the average period covered is only about six months rather than one full year. Hence, the 0-4 duration category effectively covers a period of only about 4.5 years, whereas all other duration categories cover 5 years.

3 Between 1982 and 1992, the sex ratio at birth increased from 107 to 114 in South Korea and from 108 to 119 in China.

Table 5.27 Meno Cause

Percentage of currently married women age 30-49 years who are in menopause, by age and state, India, 1992-93

State	Age						
	30-34	35-39	40-41	42-43	44-45	46-47	48-49 •
India - Urban	2.4	7.0	14.4	23.2	35.5	51.8	70.3
India - Rural	3.3	7.0	18.0	26>2	38.7	57.2	70.8
India - Total	3.0	7.0	16.9	25.3	37.8	55.8	70.6
North							
Delhi	2.5	4.1	12.1	12.1	30.1	52.1	73.7
Haryana	1.8	5.6	6.3	7.6	23.7	44.4	55.2
Himachal Pradesh	0.4	8.6	16.2	19.1	48.6	54.8	59.8
Jammu Region of J & K	0.6	4.8	8.8	20.3	36.7	56.8	66.7
Punjab	0.6	3.0	14.6	18.0	26.9	53.3	74.3
Rajasthan	2.8	5.4	12.1	20.6	36.6	45.3	59.7
Central							
Madhya Pradesh	3.5	4.3	17.7	Z2.5	32.5	58.7	55.0
Uttar Pradesh	2.3	5.6	13.6	24.6	37.2	57.9	73.1
East							
Bihar	1.5	7.8	18.8	26.3	48.2	52.9	72.5
Orissa	0.8	4.0	18.1	22.3	37.6	53.0	73.8
West Bengal	3.0	5.2	12.6	24.8	32.6	50.8	66.9

Northeast							
Arunachal Pradesh	2.6	9.2	(12.8)	*	*	*	*
Assam	5.7	11.6	16.1	44.0	40.8	68.1	(59.2)
Manipur	0.7	7.0	7.5	9.3	(25.5)	(47.2)	(53.8)
Meghalaya	0.9	2.1	(10.2)	(29.4)	(56.8)	(59.3)	(69.2)
Mizoram	0.8	0.7	5.8	(14.6)	(14.9)	(31.9)	50.8
Nagaland	10.3	7.6	6.7	*	21.1	(44.4)	40.3
Tripura	5.0	7.4	(5.4)	(21.3)	(39.4)	(51.4)	(69.4)
West							
Goa	2.1	6.6	16.0	21.1	37.4	48.1	67.1
Gujarat	3.7	7.0	16.3	23.5	38.8	62.6	70.4
Maharashtra	3.2	11.0	24.5	36.6	45.9	64.4	80.8
South							
Andhra Pradesh	8.0	15.2	26.5	41.9	52.3	66.3	82.8
Karnataka	3.7	8.1	21.6	27.3	39.2	58.5	71.3
Kerala	2.1	2.4	8.9	15.0	23.3	38.7	62.3
Tamil Nadu	1.9	4.8	17.9	18.1	30.9	49.3	70.9

Note: Percentage menopausal is defined as the percent of nonpregnant, nonamenorrhoeic currently married women whose last menstrual period occurred six or more months prior to the survey or who reported that they are menopausal.

( ) Basĕd on 25-49 unsighted cases

* Percentage not shown; based on fewer than 25 unweighted cases.

6

Family Planning

Information about knowledge of family planning and the use of contraceptive methods is of practical use to policymakers and programme administrators for formulating policies and strategies. This chapter begins with an appraisal of women's knowledge of contraceptive methods and knowledge of sources of supply of modern contraceptive methods before moving on to a consideration of current and past family planning practice. Special attention is focused on nonuse, reasons for discontinuation, and intentions to use family planning in the future. The chapter also contains information on exposure to media coverage on family planning and interspousal discussions on family planning, and concludes with an analysis of attitudes toward family planning.

6.1 Knowledge of Family Planning Methods and Sources

Each respondent was asked the following question about her knowledge of family planning, "Now I would like to talk about family planning—the various ways or methods that a couple can use to delay or avoid a pregnancy. Which ways or methods have you heard about?" The respondent was first asked to name all the methods she knew or had heard of, without any prompting. Then the interviewer read out the name and a short description of each method not mentioned, and asked if she knew the method. Thus, the woman's knowledge of contraception is measured at three levels: (a) methods the woman thinks of on her own (she can name them spontaneously without probing), (b) methods she knows when asked specifically about them (she recognizes the method after probing), and (c) methods that she has not heard of. Six modern methods (pills, IUDs, injections, condoms, female sterilization, and male sterilization) were included, as well as two traditional methods (periodic abstinence, or the rhythm method, and withdrawal). Any other methods mentioned by the respondent as a method to avoid a pregnancy, such as herbs and breastfeeding, were also recorded. For each modern method known to the respondent, either spontaneously or after probing, she was asked if she knew where a person could go to get the method. If she reported knowing about the rhythm method, she was asked if she knew where a person could obtain advice on how to use the method.

Table 6.1 presents the extent of knowledge of ever-married women and currently married women as obtained by spontaneous responses (without any probe) and probed responses. Knowledge of family planning is nearly universal in India, with 99 and 94 per cent of evermarried respondents in urban and rural areas, respectively, recognizing at least one modern method of family planning (Figure 6.1). Knowledge of at least one modern method among evermarried women is reported spontaneously by 82 per cent of urban women and 64 per cent of rural women. Effective knowledge of family planning methods is thus lower in rural than in urban areas. Ever-married and currently married women differ little in their knowledge of family planning methods, and the discussion focuses on currently married women for the sake of simplicity.

Knowledge about sterilization is widespread in India. A higher proportion of women are aware of female than male sterilization, with the gap in knowledge of the two methods being especially large in rural areas. Spontaneous knowledge is also higher for female sterilization than male sterilization in both urban and rural areas.

In contrast to widespread knowledge of sterilization, knowledge of the three officially sponsored temporary methods, namely, the IUD, the pill, and the condom, is much less widespread. Nearly one-fourth of currently married women do not know any of the modern temporary methods, this proportion being higher in rural (29 per cent) than in urban areas (9 per cent). The most well known among the modern temporary methods is the pill (reported by 66 per cent of currently married women), followed by the IUD (61 per cent) and condoms (58 per cent). Injections are the least known modern method, with only 19 per cent reporting knowledge of theme [1].

In India, traditional methods of contraception are generally less well known than modern methods. Thirty-nine per cent of currently married women report knowledge of these methods, with periodic abstinence being better known (35 per cent) than withdrawal (20 per cent). The table reveals that probing was often needed to elicit complete knowledge about contraceptive methods, especially traditional methods.

The Third All India Survey on Family Planning Practices in

Table 6.1: Knowledge of contraceptive methods and source of methods

Percentage of ever-married and current married women knowing any contraceptive method and knowing a source, by specific method and residence, India, 1992-93

Method	Ever-married women				Currently married women			
	Knowing method				Knowing method			
	Without probe	With probe	Total	Knowing source	Without probe	With probe	Total	Knowing sources
1	2	3	4	5	6	7	8	9
				URBAN				
Any method	82.5	16.1	98.5	95.4	83.3	15.4	98.7	95.6
Any modern method	82.0	16.5	98.5	95.2	82.7	15.9	98.6	95.5
Any Modern temporary method	65.5	24.9	90.4	82.3	66.7	24.5	91.2	83.3
Pill	55.0	29.6	84.6	74.1	56.1	29.4	85.5	75.1
Copper T/IUD	49.2	32.9	82.1	72.7	50.2	32.8	83.1	73.8
Injection	8.1	16.6	24.7	19.8	8.2	16.9	25.2	20.3
Condom	47.6	31.5	79.1	69.0	48.7	31.5	80.2	70.2
Female sterilization	66.5	31.1	97.6	92.9	67.1	30.6	97.7	93.1
Male sterilization	43.7	46.9	90.6	84.6	44.2	47.0	91.1	85.1
Any traditional method	15.6	32.3	48.0	NA	16.0	32.8	48.8	NA
Rhythm/periodic abstinence	11.5	31.8	43.3	31.4	11.8	32.2	44.0	31.9
Withdrawal	5.6	20.2	25.8	NA	5.8	20.6	26.4	NA
Other methods	3.7	NA	3.7	NA	3.8	NA	3.8	NA

Number of women	23455	23455	23455	23455	22077	22077	22077	22077
				RURAL				
Any method	64.9	29.6	94.5	86.7	65.5	29.3	94.7	87.0
Any modern method	63.8	30.5	94.2	86.2	64.3	30.1	94.5	86.5
Any modern temporary method	33.9	36.1	70.1	56.1	34.5	36.2	70.7	56.8
Pill	25.2	33.5	58.7	45.6	25.7	33.7	59.4	46.2
Copper T/IUD	20.6	31.7	52.4	42.2	21.0	31.9	52.9	42.7
Injection	3.8	13.2	17.0	12.6	3.8	13.4	17.2	12.8
Condom	18.3	31.2	49.4	37.4	18.7	31.5	50.2	38.0
Female sterilization	55.8	37.4	93.2	83.9	56.3	37.2	93.5	84.2
Male sterilization	32.9	48.9	81.8	71.8	33.1	49.0	82.1	72.1
Any traditional method	9.3	26.2	35.5	NA	9.5	26.5	36.0	NA
Rhythm/periodic abstinence	5.7	25.6	31.3	21.9	5.8	25.9	31.7	22.1
Withdrawal	2.2	15.4	17.6	NA	2.2	15.6	17.8	NA
Other methods	3.4	NA	3.4	NA	3.5	NA	3.5	NA
Number of women	66322	66322	66322	66322	62601	62601	62601	62601
				TOTAL				
Any method	69.5	26.1	95.5	89.0	70.1	25.7	95.8	89.2
Any modern method	68.5	26.8	95.3	88.6	69.1	26.4	95.5	88.8
Any modern temporary method	42.2	33.2	75.4	63.0	42.9	33.2	76.1	63.7
Pill	33.0	32.5	65.4	53.0	33.6	32.6	66.2	53.7
Copper T/IUD	28.1	32.0	60.1	50.2	28.6	32.1	60.8	50.8

1	2	3	4	5	6	7	8	9
Injection	4.9	14.1	19.0	14.5	5.0	14.3	19.3	14.7
Condom	25.9	31.2	57.2	45.7	26.5	31.5	58.1	46.4
Female sterilization	58.6	35.7	94.3	86.3	59.1	35.5	94.6	86.5
Male sterilization	35.7	48.4	84.1	75.1	36.0	48.5	84.5	75.5
Any traditional method	11.0	27.8	38.8	NA	11.2	28.1	39.3	NA
Rhythm/periodic abstinence	7.2	27.2	34.4	24.3	7.3	27.5	34.9	24.7
Withdrawal	3.1	16.7	19.7	NA	3.2	16.9	20.1	NA
Other methods	3.5	NA	3.5	NA	3.6	NA	3.6	NA
Number of women	89777	89777	89777	89777	84678	84678	84678	84678

NA: Not applicable.

1 For modern methods, the source refers to a place that a person could go to get the method.
For rhythmsperiodic abstinence, title source refers to a source of advice on how to use periodic abstinence.

India, conducted in 1988-89 (Operations Research Group, 1990), which studied currently married women age 15-44, reached broadly similar conclusions about women's awareness of specific methods. Comparing the two surveys and recognizing that the NFHS was done almost three years later than the Third All India Survey, the proportion of women having knowledge of condoms and male sterilization were found to be lower in the NFHS (58 and 85 per cent, respectively) than in the Third All India Survey (66 and 89 per cent). The proportion of women having knowledge of female sterilization is exactly the same in both surveys, and, the NFHS estimates of the proportion of women having knowledge of the other major methods (the IUD, the pill, periodic abstinence and withdrawal) are slightly higher (61, 66, 35 and 20, respectively) than those in the Third All India Survey (55, 60, 27 and 17, respectively).

In the NFHS, urban-rural differentials in the level of knowledge are most pronounced for the pill, the IUD, and condoms, with knowledge of these methods greater among urban than among rural women. Urban and rural women also differ in their knowledge of traditional methods. Only 36 per cent of women in rural areas know of a traditional method, compared with nearly one-half of women in urban areas.

Table 6.1 also provides information about knowledge of sources of contraceptive methods. The question about the source of a method was asked only of those women who knew about the method. Knowledge about the sources of contraceptives is generally high, with more than 89 per cent of currently married women knowing where to obtain at least one modern method of family planning. Women are most knowledgeable about a source for sterilizations, especially female sterilization. In comparison, 64 per cent of the women know where to obtain a modern temporary method. Regardless of the method, urban women are more likely to know of a contraceptive source than rural women.

Table 6.2 shows differentials in knowledge of modern contraceptive methods and sources of methods among currently married women according to background characteristics. In terms of the respondent's age, the level of knowledge increases with age through age 30-34 and stays very high through age 45-49 years. Particularly noticeable, in this context, is the relatively low level of knowledge among women age 13-14. More than one-third of women age 13-14 either do not know about any modern method of family planning or are not aware of the source of any method. The proportion of such women is also relatively high (20 per cent) among women age 15-19. The level of knowledge of at least one modern method of contraception increases with the level of education. Although the knowledge of contraception is widespread, it is low about a modern method and 16 per cent are ignorant about the source. Knowledge about a modern method is slightly higher among Sikh, Jain and Buddhist women and is lower among scheduled tribe women.

Interstate variations in the knowledge of contraception are shown in Table 6.3. Knowledge of any modern method is widespread in all states except Nagaland, where only 44 per cent of women reported having knowledge of any modern method. Knowledge of any modern method is also relatively low in two other northeastern states (Arunachal Pradesh and Meghalaya). Among the major states (with a population more than 5 million), the proportion of women knowing at least one modern method ranges from a low of 87 per cent in Rajasthan to nearly 100 per cent in Kerala and Punjab. The situation is similar in terms of knowledge of female sterilization. In fact, except in Rajasthan and Madhya Pradesh, where 85 per cent of women reported knowledge of female sterilization, in all the other major states more than 90 per cent of women know about female sterilization. Interstate variations in the knowledge of contraception are more pronounced in the case of modern temporary methods. Less than twothirds of women reported knowledge of any modern temporary method in Nagaland, Madhya Pradesh, Rajasthan, Orissa, Andhra Pradesh, Arunachal Pradesh, and Meghalaya, compared to more than 90 per cent of women in Haryana, West Bengal, Punjab, Tripura, Kerala and Delhi. Among the modern temporary methods, the pill is relatively well known. This is particularly true in Tripura and West Bengal where knowledge of the pill is much higher than knowledge of either IUDs or condoms. This is not surprising because the use of pills is also higher in these two states than in any other Indian state (see Table 6.7). In states such as Madhya Pradesh, Bihar, Rajasthan and Orissa, more than half of women report that they have not heard of the IUD. Knowledge of condoms is particularly low in Orissa, Rajasthan, Arunachal Pradesh and Nagaland. Injections, which are not included in the official family welfare programme, are the least known modern method in every state.

6.2 Contraceptive Use

Ever Use of Family Planning Methods

All respondents who knew at least one method of family planning were asked whether they had ever used each of the methods they knew. The use of contraception was further probed by asking whether they "ever used anything or tried in any way to delay or avoid getting pregnant". Table 6.4 presents the pattern of ever use by age and residence separately for evermarried and currently married women.

Table 6.2: Knowledge of methods and source by background characteristics
Percentage of currently married women knowing any contraceptive method and at least one modern method and knowing a source for a modern method by selected background characteristics, India, 1992-93

Background characteristic	Knows any method	Knows any modern modern[1]	Knows source for any modern method	Number of women
Age				
13-14	77.8	76.9	65.8	351
15-19	90.4	90.2	79.9	8897
20-24	95.1	94.8	86.4	17504
25-29	96.5	96.3	90.3	16807
30-34	97.6	97.4	92.0	13900
35-39	97.2	97.0	92.0	11596
40-44	97.0	96.9	91.1	8725
45-49	95.7	95.6	89.4	6896
Residence				
Urban	98.7	98.6	95.5	22077
Rural	94.7	94.5	86.5	62601
Education				
Illiterate	93.9	93.5	84.1	53045
Lit.,< middle complete	98.3	98.3	95.2	15476
Middle school complete	99.3	99.3	97.0	6280
High school and above	99.7	99.7	98.9	9879
Religion				
Hindu	95.6	95.4	88.7	69635
Muslim	96.8	96.6	87.5	10082
Christian	93.5	93.2	90.5	1960
Sikh	99.6	99.6	98.1	1606
Jain	99.7	99.7	99.2	418
Buddhist	97.1	97.1	95.4	665
Other	84.5	84.5	75.8	312
Caste/tribe				
Scheduled caste	95.7	95.4	86.7	10350
Scheduled tribe	85.5	85.0	75.9	7422
Other	96.9	96.7	90.6	66906
Total	95.8	95.5	88.8	84678

[1] Includes pill, copper T/IUD, injections, condoms, female sterilization and male sterilization.

Although 96 per cent of currently married women know of at least one method of family planning, only 47 per cent have ever used a method. Modern methods have been used by 42 per cent of currently

Table 6.3: Knowledge of contraceptive methods by state

Percentage of currently married women age 13-49 knowing any contraceptive method by specific method and state, India, 1992-93

State	Any meth-od	Any modern method	Any modern Temporary method	Pill	IUD	Injection	Condom	Female sterili-zation	Male sterili-zation	Any trad. method	Peri-odic absti-nence	With drawal	Other meth-ods
India	95.8	95.5	76.1	66.2	60.8	19.3	58.1	94.6	84.5	39.3	34.9	20.1	3.6
North													
Delhi	99.0	98.9	96.8	94.3	93.4	34.9	93.7	97.5	95.3	59.3	54.6	31.1	5.6
Haryana	99.4	99.4	90.6	76.2	80.0	45.8	75.9	99.2	98.2	58.7	46.5	41.9	4.2
Himachal Pradesh	99.1	98.9	88.4	70.1	73.7	45.6	74.1	98.1	95.7	61.0	49.1	37.3	9.9
Jammu Region of J & K	99.7	99.6	88.5	76.6	74.3	51.1	74.9	99.4	98.0	72.0	59.5	53.5	2.4
Punjab	99.8	99.8	94.0	83.9	87.5	47.2	82.1	99.7	99.1	64.1	56.0	41.5	1.5
Rajasthan	87.5	87.2	58.8	53.1	46.4	23.4	37.7	85.3	70.9	27.5	23.8	14.5	1.4
Central													
Madhya Pradesh	88.1	87.8	57.4	51.3	42.3	12.7	42.3	85.4	76.5	19.7	17.7	5.3	2.6
Uttar Pradesh	95.7	95.2	80.1	64.7	56.2	25.0	67.2	93.7	88.2	36.7	34.3	12.9	2.6
East													
Bihar	94.9	94.9	68.4	57.3	44.1	4.2	54.6	94.5	88.0	29.4	26.0	9.4	1.8
Orissa	92.9	92.5	60.7	52.1	48.0	7.4	34.6	91.7	72.2	33.9	27.4	9.5	7.4
West Bengal	99.1	98.8	90.9	85.6	68.2	42.5	67.6	98.0	84.8	72.5	62.0	55.4	5.0
Northeast													
Arunachal Pradesh	77.7	77.7	62.9	55.2	52.6	28.7	39.6	75.1	47.8	27.2	25.4	17.6	0.6

Assam	97.5	96.9	82.2	72.9	60.8	39.0	59.2	96.2	83.9	79.2	71.0	61.0	9.6
Manipur	93.6	93.0	87.9	77.9	81.0	5.6	60.3	87.7	87.4	72.4	71.2	44.4	3.9
Meghalaya	78.0	76.9	64.7	58.5	49.3	9.7	47.7	71.9	46.5	43.5	35.5	17.7	15.7
Mizoram	98.1	98.1	86.2	70.1	76.2	1.8	61.0	98.0	71.3	43.7	36.2	30.7	0.3
Nagaland	44.4	44.3	36.7	24.9	24.2	15.9	29.0	30.4	20.9	10.7	9.7	9.3	0.8
Tripura	99.7	99.7	95.4	93.9	65.0	42.1	68.1	99.4	89.2	85.7	75.8	68.8	7.8
West													
Goa	98.9	98.8	89.9	80.6	76.3	20.7	73.1	97.7	72.8	45.6	41.6	24.1	2.9
Gujarat	96.6	96.4	77.0	65.9	71.4	22.8	62.7	95.6	78.6	45.9	43.3	24.4	1.7
Maharashtra	97.8	97.8	76.8	67.1	70.7	8.1	57.3	97.3	83.6	23.3	21.3	8.4	2.0
South													
Andhra Pradesh	96.7	96.6	61.2	53.7	43.7	12.8	41.9	95.7	89.7	14.6	11.3	2.9	3.5
Karnataka	98.9	98.8	83.8	75.1	78.0	5.4	50.0	98.6	81.1	41.1	38.8	15.0	6.4
Kerala	99.7	99.7	96.6	87.1	90.3	13.0	91.0	99.3	90.0	72.6	66.1	50.7	2.7
Tamil Nadu	99.1	99.1	85.6	74.5	77.8	12.6	61.0	98.8	86.0	46.2	39.0	23.7	6.6

married women and traditional methods by 12 per cent. By far the most commonly used method is female sterilization, which has been adopted by 27 per cent of currently married women. Male sterilization has been used by 4 per cent of couples. Modern temporary methods such as IUDs, pills, and condoms have each been used by only 5-7 per cent. The pattern of use suggests very little switching among the modern temporary methods. Less than 4 per cent of women have ever used more than one spacing method. As expected, ever use of contraceptive methods is higher in urban than in rural areas (59 per cent compared with 43 per cent of currently married women; see Figure 6.2). This is true for every contraceptive method except male sterilization, but the difference is particularly large for modern temporary methods. The proportion of women who have ever used a modern temporary method is almost three times as high in urban areas (27 per cent) as in rural areas (10 per cent). The use of more than one modern temporary method is also higher in urban areas than in rural areas. Ever use of traditional methods is also somewhat higher in urban areas (15 per cent) than in rural areas (10 per cent).

In terms of differences by age, experience with having used contraception rises through age 35-39 and gradually decreases thereafter. Contraceptive use rates are highest in the age group 30-39, where knowledge is also reported to be highest. A very low use rate, even for modern temporary methods, is observed among younger married women age less than 20. Only 2 and 6 per cent of women age 13-14 and 15-19, respectively, reported ever use of any modern temporary method. The use of traditional methods is also low in these two age groups, although it is higher than the use of modern temporary methods. Male sterilization is the only method that increases steadily throughout the age range. The relatively large proportion of male sterilizations in the older age groups undoubtedly reflects the large number of vasectomies that were performed 15-20 years before the survey.

The age pattern of ever use of modern methods of family planning is similar for urban and rural women, peaking in the 35-39 age group. At every age, however, the level of ever use is higher for urban than for rural women.

Current Use of Family Planning Methods

Current contraceptive prevalence in India is moderate with 41 per cent of currently married women age 13-49 practicing family planning; 36 per cent use modern methods (31 per cent using sterilization and 6 per cent using modern temporary methods) and another 4 per cent

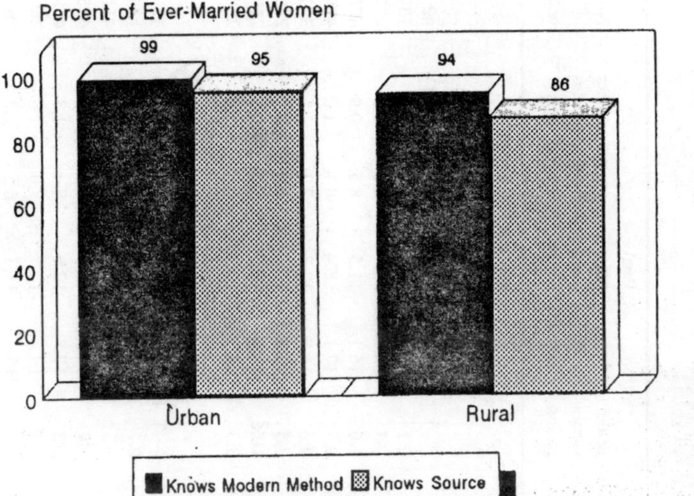

Figure 6.1 Knowledge of Modern Contraceptive Methods and Sources by Residence

use traditional methods (Table 6.5)[2]. Most of the currently married women who have ever used contraception are current users (41 out of 47 per cent). The overall level of contraceptive use is almost the same as the combined level of 42 per cent for all less developed countries excluding China (Population Reference Bureau, 1994). The NFHS estimate of current contraceptive prevalence is somewhat lower than that obtained in the 1988-89 Third All India Survey on Family Planning Practices in India (Operations Research Group, 1990). That survey (which covered currently married women age 15-44 only) found a contraceptive prevalence rate of 45 per cent for India, with 40 per cent using modern methods and 5 per cent using traditional methods. When the NFHS sample is restricted by age to match the All India Survey's sample, the prevalence rate is 40 per cent, with 36 per cent using modern methods. The per centage of couples sterilized is almost identical in the two surveys (between 30 and 31 per cent). The estimates in the two surveys are also close in the case of pills (around 1 per cent) and IUDs (2 per cent). Therefore, the difference between the overall contraceptive prevalence rates estimated in the NFHS and the Third All India Survey is largely in the reported use of condoms, which was 5 per cent in the Third All India Survey and less than 3 per cent in the NFHS. The NFHS sterilization figures are also very close to the unpublished official statistics for 1993

Table 6.4: Ever use of Contraception

Percentage of ever-married and currently married women who have ever used any contraceptive method, by specific method and age, according to residence, India, 1992-93

State	Any method	Any modern method	Any modern Temporary method	Pill	IUO	Injection	Condom	Female sterilization	Male sterilization	Any trad. method	Periodic-abstinence	With drawal	Other methods	Number of women
URBAN														
Ever-married women														
13-14	(11.2)	(—)	(—)	(—)	(—)	(—)	(—)	(—)	(—)	(11.2)	(11.2)	(—)	(—)	42
15-19	14.9	11.9	10.9	3.7	2.7	0.1	5.8	1.2	0.1	4.7	3.1	3.2	0.2	1376
20-24	36.1	31.7	23.6	7.3	9.2	0.2	12.1	9.5	0.3	8.8	6.0	4.5	0.5	4229
25-29	60.6	54.8	33.2	10.1	13.8	0.3	18.0	26.2	1.0	16.1	11.5	8.5	0.9	4705
30-34	70.3	64.7	32.3	10.4	14.3	0.4	17.9	38.8	2.3	17.1	1Z.4	8.1	1.2	4291
35-39	73.8	68.1	26.5	9.3	10.6	0.2	14.3	46.7	4.6	16.8	12.3	7.7	1.5	3715
40-44	66.7	60.8	18.2	7.3	6.1	0.3	9.5	41.9	7.5	14.4	10.6	6.0	1.1	2899
45-49	59.5	52.9	15.8	5.9	4.1	0.2	9.1	32.1	10.6	15.3	11.8	7.0	0.9	2197
Total	57.9	52.5	25.4	8.4	10.0	0.3	13.7	29.7	3.3	14.1	10.2	6.8	1.0	23455
Currently married women														
13-14	(11.2)	(—)	(—)	(—)	(—)	(—)	(—)	(—)	(—)	(11.2)	(11.2)	(—)	(—)	42
15-19	15.1	12.1	11.2	3.8	2.8	0.1	5.9	1.1	0.1	4.8	3.2	3.2	0.2	1339
20-24	36.6	32.1	24.2	7.4	9.5	0.2	12.3	9.5	0.3	9.0	6.2	4.6	0.5	4116
25-29	61.7	55.8	34.1	10.4	14.2	0.3	18.5	26.5	1.0	16.2	11.6	8.6	0.9	4553
30-34	72.3	66.5	33.5	10.8	14.8	0.4	18.5	40.0	2.2	17.8	12.9	8.4	1.3	4082
35-39	75.7	70.0	27.4	9.7	10.9	0.2	14.9	47.9	4.7	17.3	12.7	8.0	1.6	3493
40-44	70.1	64.0	19.4	7.7	6.6	0.3	10.0	44.3	7.7	15.4	11.3	6.5	1.2	2603

45-49	63.4	56.4	17.2	6.5	4.6	0.1	9.7	34.1	11.1	16.4	12.7	7.3	1.0	1849
Total	59.4	53.9	26.5	8.7	10.5	0.3	14.3	30.4	3.3	14.6	10.6	7.0	1.0	22077
							RURAL							
							Ever- married women							
13-14	6.5	2.0	2.0	0.6	—	—	1.4	—	—	4.5	3.2	3.4	—	311
15-19	11.0	5.7	4.4	1.9	0.7	0.1	2.3	1.3	—	6.5	4.8	3.4	0.1	7719
20-24	26.4	20.6	10.4	4.4	3.0	0.2	5.1	10.8	0.4	9.4	7.1	4.7	0.3	13755
25-29	44.7	39.2	12.6	5.2	4.6	0.1	5.8	28.3	1.3	11.2	8.5	5.4	0.7	12735
30-34	56.6	51.3	12.3	5.0	4.4	0.2	5.7	40.2	3.1	12.1	9.3	5.3	1.3	10369
35-39	58.9	53.8	9.8	4.3	3.2	0.3	4.4	41.6	6.1	12.2	9.4	5.1	1.0	8746
40-44	54.5	49.2	7.3	2.8	2.1	0.4	3.6	35.9	9.3	10.8	8.5	4.2	1.0	6850
45-49	45.4	40.8	4.6	1.7	1.5	0.1	2.0	27.4	10.9	8.5	6.4	3.4	0.8	5838
Total	41.6	36.2	9.5	3.9	3.0	0.2	4.5	25.7	3.5	10.2	7.8	4.7	0.7	66322
							Currently married women							
13-14	6.5	2.0	2.0	0.6	—	—	1.4	—	—	4.5	3.2	3.5	—	309
15-19	11.2	5.7	4.5	1.9	0.7	0.1	2.4	1.3	—	6.6	4.9	3.5	0.1	7558
20-24	26.7	20.8	10.6	4.5	3.1	0.2	5.2	10.8	0.4	9.5	7.2	4.8	0.3	13388
25-29	45.7	40.1	13.0	5.4	4.7	0.2	6.0	28.8	1.3	11.4	8.7	5.5	0.7	12254
30-34	57.9	52.6	12.6	5.2	4.5	0.2	5.8	41.3	3.1	12.3	9.4	5.4	1.3	9818
35-39	61.0	55.8	10.3	4.5	3.4	0.3	4.6	43.1	6.2	12.6	9.6	5.4	1.1	8104
40-44	57.3	52.1	7.8	3.1	2.2	0.4	3.8	38.0	9.7	11.1	8.8	4.5	1.0	6122
45-49	48.3	43.7	5.1	2.0	1.7	0.1	2.2	29.3	11.6	8.8	6.6	3.6	0.9	5047
Total	42.5	37.1	9.9	4.1	3.2	0.2	4.6	26.3	3.5	10.4	8.0	4.8	0.7	62601
							TOTAL							
							Ever- married women							
13-14	7.1	1.8	1.8	0.5	—	—	1.3	—	—	5.3	4.1	3.0	—	352
15-19	11.6	6.6	5.4	2.2	1.0	0.1	2.8	1.3	0.1	6.2	4.6	3.4	0.1	9095
20-24	28.6	23.2	13.5	5.1	4.5	0.2	6.8	10.5	0.4	9.2	6.8	4.7	0.4	17983

1	2	3	4	5	6	7	8	9	10	11	12	13	14	15
25-29	49.0	43.4	18.2	6.5	7.0	0.2	9.1	27.7	1.2	12.5	9.3	6.2	0.8	17441
30-34	60.6	55.2	18.2	6.6	7.3	0.2	9.3	39.8	2.9	13.6	10.2	6.1	1.2	14660
35-39	63.3	58.1	14.8	5.8	5.4	0.2	7.4	43.1	5.7	13.6	10.3	5.9	1.2	12461
40-44	58.1	52.6	10.5	4.2	3.3	0.3	5.4	37.7	8.7	11.8	9.1	4.8	1.0	9748
45-49	49.2	44.1	7.7	2.9	2.2	0.1	3.9	28.7	10.8	10.3	7.9	4.3	0.9	8036
Total	45.9	40.5	13.7	5.1	4.9	0.2	6.9	26.8	3.5	11.2	8.5	5.2	0.8	89 777
Currently married women														
13-14	7.1	1.8	1.8	0.5	—	—	1.3	—	—	5.3	4.1	3.0	—	351
15-19	11.8	6.7	5.5	2.2	1.0	0.1	2.9	1.3	0.1	6.3	4.7	3.4	0.1	8897
20-24	29.0	23.5	13.8	5.2	4.6	0.2	6.9	10.5	0.4	9.4	7.0	4.8	0.4	17504
25-29	50.0	44.3	18.7	6.7	7.3	0.2	9.4	28.2	1.2	12.7	9.5	6.3	0.8	16807
30-34	62.2	56.7	18.8	6.8	7.5	0.2	9.5	40.9	2.8	13.9	10.4	6.3	1.3	13900
35-39	65.4	60.1	15.5	6.1	5.6	0.3	7.7	44.6	5.7	14.0	10.6	6.2	1.3	11596
40-44	61.1	55.6	11.2	4.5	3.5	0.4	5.7	39.9	9.1	12.4	9.5	5.1	1.1	8725
45-49	52.4	47.1	8.3	3.2	2.4	0.1	4.2	30.6	11.5	10.8	8.2	4.6	0.9	6896
Total	46.9	41.5	14.2	5.3	5.1	0.2	7.1	27.3	3.5	11.5	8.6	5.4	0.8	84678

( ) Based on 25-49 unweighted cases.

— Less than 0.05 per cent.

(Evaluation and Information Division, Department of Family Welfare, Ministry of Health and Family Welfare), according to which 30 per cent of couples in the country are protected through sterilization compared with 31 per cent in the NFHS.

Table 6.5 shows that female sterilization is the most popular contraceptive method in India. Twenty-seven per cent of currently married women are sterilized and female sterilization alone accounts for 67 per cent of current contraceptive prevalence. Another 3 per cent of currently married women report that their husbands are sterilized, and 2 per cent each report the use of IUDs and condoms. The pill is used by only 1 per cent of currently married women. The preponderance of terminal methods is commensurate with the emphasis on sterilization in the Indian family planning programme.

Contraceptive prevalence is 38 per cent higher in urban than in rural areas (51 per cent compared with 37 per cent), with urban use higher for every single method of family planning, except male sterilization. In rural areas, however, male and female sterilization together account for a higher proportion of total contraceptive use among women age 15-49 (81 per cent) than they do in urban areas (66 per cent). As expected, the use of modern temporary methods is higher in urban areas (12 per cent) than rural areas (3 per cent).

The level of contraceptive use varies with the age of women, increasing from 5 per cent for currently married women age 13-14 to a high of 61 per cent for women age 35-39, and decreasing thereafter. In the age groups with the highest fertility (20-24 and 25-29), contraceptive prevalence rates are 21 and 42 per cent, respectively. Among modern methods, female sterilization is the most widely used method above age 20, and its use peaks in the age group 35-39 (at 45 per cent). The use rate of most of the modern methods, especially female sterilization, shows an expected curvilinear relationship with age. The temporary methods (pills, IUDs, injections, condoms, periodic abstinence and withdrawal) are each consistently used by less than 4 per cent of couples at all ages. The low use rate of any method at early ages and the lack of use of temporary methods suggest that very little attempt is being made by women to space their children. The age pattern of the current use of contraception is similar for urban and rural women, peaking in the age group 35-39. At every age, however, current use is higher for urban than for rural women.

Socioeconomic Differentials in Current Use of Family Planning

Table 6.6 and Figure 6.3 show differences in current contraceptive use by background characteristics. Education has a positive rela-

Table 6.5: Current use of contraception

Per cent distribution of currently married women by contraceptive method currently used, according to age and residence, India, 1992-93

Age	Any meth-od	Any modern method	Any modern Temporary method	Pill	IUD	Injection	Condom	Female sterili-zation	Male sterili-zation	Any trade method	Peri-odic-alasati nence	drawal	Other meth-ods	Not using any method	Total percent	Number of women
								URBAN								
13-14	(10.6)	(—)	(—)	(—)	(—)	(—)	(—)	(—)	(—)	(10.6)	(10.6)	(—)	(—)	(89.4)	100.0	42
15-19	9.8	7.7	6.6	1.7	1.7	—	3.2	1.1	0.1	2.1	0.5	1.4	0.2	90.2	100.0	1339
20-24	26.7	23.0	13.2	2.2	4.6	—	6.4	9.5	0.3	3.7	2.5	1.0	0.1	73.3	100.0	4116
25-29	51.2	44.9	17.4	3.1	6.2	—	8.1	26.5	1.0	6.3	3.6	2.7	0.1	48.8	100.0	4553
30-34	64.2	57.3	15.2	2.2	5.3	0.1	7.5	40.0	2.2	6.9	4.0	2.6	0.3	35.8	100.0	4082
35-39	70.5	62.5	9.9	1.5	3.3	—	5.1	47.9	4.7	8.0	5.0	2.5	0.5	29.5	100.0	3493
40-44	63.5	57.5	5.5	0.8	1.1	—	3.6	44.3	7.6	6.1	3.5	2.3	0.2	36.5	100.0	2603
45-49	51.8	47.4	2.2	0.5	0.4	—	1.4	34.1	11.0	4.5	3.2	0.9	0.3	48.2	100.0	1849
15-44	51.0	45.2	12.6	2.1	4.2	—	6.2	30.1	2.5	5.9	3.5	2.2	0.2	49.0	100.0	20186
15-49	51.1	45.3	11.7	1.9	3.9	—	5.8	30.4	3.2	5.8	3.5	2.1	0.2	48.9	100.0	22035
13-49	51.0	45.3	11.7	1.9	3.9	—	5.8	30.4	3.2	5.8	3.5	2.1	0.2	49.0	100.0	22077
								RURAL								
13-14	3.9	1.0	1.0	0.4	—	—	0.6	—	—	3.0	1.8	1.2	—	96.1	100.0	309
15-19	6.6	3.4	2.0	0.6	0.4	—	0.9	1.3	—	3.3	2.1	1.2	0.1	93.4	100.0	7558
20-24	19.3	15.6	4.3	1.4	1.4	—	1.5	10.8	0.4	3.7	2.3	1.4	—	80.7	100.0	13388
25-29	39.1	35.1	5.1	1.4	1.9	—	1.7	28.8	1.3	4.0	2.4	1.3	0.2	60.9	100.0	12254
30-34	52.4	48.3	3.8	0.9	1.4	—	1.5	41.3	3.1	4.1	2.6	1.1	0.4	47.6	100.0	9818
35-39	56.9	52.3	3.0	0.8	1.2	0.1	1.0	43.1	6.2	4.6	2.9	1.4	0.3	43.1	100.0	8104
40-44	53.2	49.3	1.6	0.2	0.5	0.1	0.7	38.0	9.7	3.9	2.5	1.0	0.4	46.8	100.0	6122
45-49	43.6	41.8	0.9	0.2	0.3	—	0.4	29.3	11.6	1.8	0.9	0.6	0.2	56.4	100.0	5047

15-44	36.5	32.6	3.6	1.0	1.2	—	1.3	26.1	2.8	3.9	2.5	1.2	0.2	63.5	100.0	57244
15-49	37.1	33.3	3.4	0.9	1.2	—	1.2	26.4	3.5	3.8	2.3	1.2	0.2	62.9	100.0	62291
13-49	36.9	33.1	3.4	0.9	1.2	—	1.2	26.3	3.5	3.8	2.3	1.2	0.2	63.1	100.0	62601
								TOTAL								
13-14	4.7	0.8	0.8	0.3	—	—	0.5	—	—	3.9	2.8	1.0	—	95.3	100.0	351
15-19	7.1	4.0	2.7	0.8	0.6	—	1.2	1.3	0.1	3.1	1.8	1.2	0.1	92.9	100.0	8897
20-24	21.0	17.3	6.4	1.6	2.1	—	2.7	10.5	0.4	3.7	2.3	1.3	0.1	D.0	100.0	17504
25-29	42.4	37.8	8.4	1.9	3.1	—	3.5	28.2	1.2	4.6	2.7	1.7	0.2	57.6	100.0	16807
30-34	55.9	50.9	7.2	1.3	2.6	—	3.2	40.9	2.8	4.9	3.0	1.5	0.4	44.1	100.0	13900
35-39	61.0	55.4	5.1	1.0	1.8	—	2.2	44.6	5.7	5.6	3.5	1.7	0.4	39.0	100.0	11596
40-44	56.3	51.7	2.7	0.4	0.7	0.1	1.6	39.9	9.1	4.5	2.8	1.4	0.3	43.7	100.0	8725
45-49	45.8	43.3	1.3	0.3	0.3	—	0.7	30.6	11.4	2.5	1.5	0.7	0.3	54.2	100.0	6896
15-44	40.3	35.8	5.9	1.3	2.0	—	2.6	27.2	2.7	4.4	2.7	1.5	0.2	59.7	100.0	77430
15-49	40.7	36.5	5.6	1.2	1.9	—	2.4	27.4	3.5	4.3	2.6	1.4	0.2	59.3	100.0	84326
13-49	40.6	36.3	5.5	1.2	1.9	—	2.4	27.3	3.4	4.3	2.6	1.4	0.2	59.4	100.0	84678

( ) Based on 25-49 unweighted cases.

— Less than 0.05 per cent.

Table 6.6 Current use by background characteristics

Percent distribution of currently married women by contraceptive method currently used, according to selected background characteristics, India, 1992-93

Age	Any meth od	Any modern method	Any modern Temporary method	Pill	IUD	Injection	Condom	Female sterili-zation	Male sterili-zation	Any trad-mathod	Peri-odic-absti-nence	With drawal	Other meth-ods	Not using any method	Tctal per cent	Number of women
Residence																
Urban	51.0	45.3	11.7	1.9	3.9	—	5.8	30.4	3.2	5.8	3.5	2.1	0.2	49.0	100.0	22077
Rural	36.9	33.1	3.4	0.9	1.2	—	1.2	26.3	3.5	3.8	2.3	1.2	0.2	63.1	100.0	62601
Education																
Illiterate	33.9	31.5	2.1	0.6	0.6	—	0.8	25.7	3.7	2.4	1.6	0.6	0.2	66.1	100.0	53045
Literate, <middle	50.4	44.8	6.1	1.7	2.2	—	2.2	35.1	3.7	5.5	3.2	2.1	0.2	49.6	100.0	15476
Middle school complete	50.8	42.4	9.5	2.3	3.3	—	3.8	30.1	2.8	8.5	4.9	3.4	0.1	49.2	100.0	6280
High school and above	54.7	45.0	20.9	2.8	7.3	—	10.7	22.0	2.1	9.7	5.9	3.4	0.3	45.3	100.0	9879
Religion																
Hindu	41.6	37.7	5.1	1.0	1.7	—	2.2	29.0	3.7	3.9	2.4	1.3	0.2	58.4	100.0	69635
Muslim	27.7	22.0	6.1	1.9	1.7	—	2.4	14.4	1.6	5.7	3.7	1.6	0.4	72.3	100.0	10082
Christian	48.3	40.3	6.5	1.2	2.5	—	2.8	30.2	3.6	8.0	5.2	2.2	0.6	51.7	100.0	1960
Sikh	57.6	50.0	17.0	2.5	6.4	—	8.1	30.3	2.6	7.6	4.2	3.3	—	42.4	100.0	1606
Jain	62.6	58.3	22.3	2.1	7.9	—	12.3	34.3	1.7	4.2	3.3	0.9	—	37.4	100.0	418
Buddhist	50.4	47.9	5.7	1.9	2.8	—	1.0	30.3	11.9	2.5	1.9	0.6	—	49.6	100.0	665
Other	37.4	33.3	4.2	1.0	1.4	—	1.8	23.8	5.3	4.1	3.1	0.6	0.4	62.6	100.0	312

Caste/tribe																	
Scheduled caste	34.5	31.7	2.8	0.7	0.8	—	1.3	25.6	3.2	2.8	1.9	0.8	0.2	65.5	100.0	10350
Scheduled tribe	33.0	30.8	2.0	0.7	0.5	—	0.7	23.2	5.6	2.2	1.2	0.6	0.4	67.0	100.0	7422
Other	42.4	37.6	6.4	1.3	2.2	—	2.8	28.0	3.2	4.7	2.9	1.6	0.2	57.6	100.0	66906
Number and sex of living children																
None	4.2	2.1	1.4	0.3	0.1	—	1.1	0.3	0.4	2.1	1.2	0.8	—	95.8	100.0	11265
1 child	19.3	12.8	8.5	1.6	3.2	—	3.6	3.1	1.2	6.5	3.8	2.5	0.2	80.7	100.0	13843
1 son	20.9	14.1	9.2	1.8	3.7	0.1	3.7	3.5	1.4	6.9	4.0	2.7	0.2	79.1	100.0	7271
No sons	17.4	11.4	7.8	1.5	2.7	—	3.6	2.6	1.0	6.0	3.6	2.3	0.1	82.6	100.0	6572
2 children	46.1	40.2	9.5	1.7	3.6	—	4.2	27.1	3.6	5.9	3.7	2.0	0.2	53.9	100.0	17695
2 sons	55.0	50.0	9.0	1.6	3.7	—	3.6	37.0	4.0	5.1	3.1	1.9	0.1	45.0	100.0	5233
1 son	46.4	40.2	10.0	1.9	3.6	0.1	4.5	26.3	3.8	6.2	3.9	2.0	0.2	53.6	100.0	9134
No sons	31.5	24.9	8.9	1.4	3.4	—	4.1	13.4	2.5	6.6	4.2	2.3	0.2	68.5	100.0	3328
3 children	58.9	55.4	4.8	1.1	1.5	—	2.1	45.3	5.3	3.5	2.2	1.1	0.2	41.1	100.0	17204
3 sons	64.9	62.4	3.1	0.9	0.8	—	1.4	52.3	7.0	2.5	1.6	0.8	0.2	35.1	100.0	2342
2 sons	68.0	65.1	4.1	1.1	1.3	—	1.8	54.9	6.0	2.9	1.8	1.0	0.2	32.0	100.0	7662
1 son	51.2	47.1	6.0	1.1	2.2	—	2.7	36.4	4.7	4.1	2.5	1.3	0.3	48.8	100.0	5778
No sons	31.7	25.9	6.1	2.1	1.6	—	2.5	18.0	1.8	5.7	4.2	1.3	0.3	68.3	100.0	1422
4+ children	52.4	49.0	3.4	1.0	1.0	0.1	1.3	40.9	4.6	3.4	2.1	0.9	0.4	47.6	100.0	24672
2+ sons	53.8	50.5	3.0	0.9	0.8	0.1	1.2	42.8	4.7	3.3	2.0	0.9	0.5	46.2	100.0	19408
1 son	44.5	45.6	5.1	1.6	1.5	0.1	1.9	36.1	4.3	3.9	2.6	1.1	0.3	50.5	100.0	4471
No sons	34.8	30.9	4.4	0.8	1.4	0.2	2.0	22.5	4.1	3.9	2.6	1.3	—	65.2	100.0	794
Total	40.6	36.3	5.5	1.2	1.9	—	2.4	27.3	3.4	4.3	2.6	1.4	0.2	59.4	100.0	84678

— Less than 0.05 per cent.

tionship to current use, although the differences are most evident between illiterate women and women with the lowest level of education (literate but primary school not completed). Further increases in the contraceptive use rate with education are marginal. A little more than one-third of illiterate women currently use a family planning method, compared to 51-55 per cent of literate women. A strong positive relationship between education and the level of current use is seen for spacing methods, both for modern and traditional methods. The use of sterilization, however, decreases with an increase in education among literate women, although female sterilization is also lower among illiterate women than among women with less than a high school education. Since female sterilization is the most dominant method, this curvilinear relationship tends to weaken the otherwise strong positive relationship between the level of education and the current use of any method. It should also be noted that women with the highest levels of education come disproportionately from the younger age groups, where the use of contraception is generally lower.

Religious differences in the use of contraception are even more substantial than the differences by education. The prevalence rate is highest among Jains (63 per cent) and lowest among Muslims (28 per cent). Contraceptive prevalence is also higher among Sikhs (58 per cent), Buddhists (50 per cent), and Christians (48 per cent) than among Hindus (42 per cent). The use of modern temporary methods is particularly high among Jains and Sikhs. Twenty-two per cent of pains and 17 per cent of Sikhs are using a modern temporary method compared to only 4-7 per cent among other religious groups. The prevalence of female sterilization does not differ much among most religious groups, except for the fact that it is very low among Muslims and the small proportion of women belonging to "other" religious groups. The proportion of women and men who have been sterilized is twice as high for Hindus as for Muslims. Religious differentials in contraceptive use may be partly an artifact of the relationship between the level of education and contraceptive use. That is, a portion of these differentials may disappear once the level of education of women is controlled. Further discussion on this issue is presented later in this chapter.

Caste/tribe is also related to current use of contraception, although not as strongly as religion or parity. The practice of family planning is lower among scheduled caste and scheduled tribe women (33-35 per cent) than among non-SC/ST women (42 per cent). Between 83 and 87 per cent of current use among scheduled caste and scheduled tribe women consists of sterilization, a figure that is 74 per cent among non-SC/ST women.

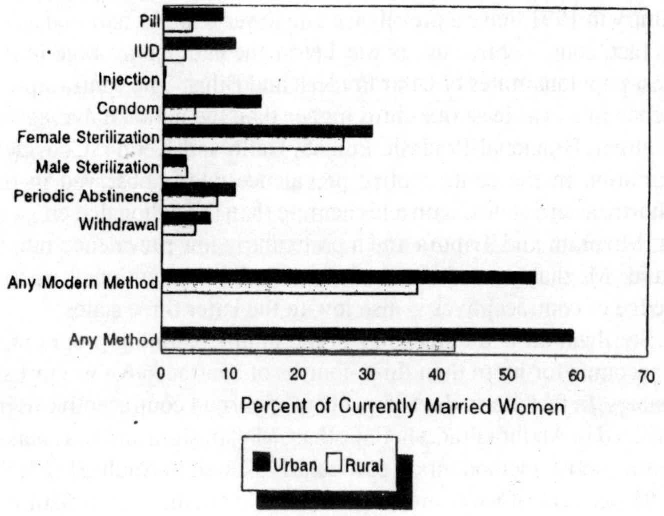

Figure 6.2 Ever Use of Contraception by Residence

Table 6.6 also shows differences in current use by the number and sex of living children. A curvilinear relationship exists between the number of living children a woman has and her current practice of contraception. Current use of any modern method increases steadily from only 2 per cent for women with no living children to 13 per cent for women with one child, 40 per cent with two children, and 55 per cent with three children, before declining to 49 per cent among women with four or more children. A similar trend is evident for sterilized women. The data on the prevalence rate by the sex composition of living children indicate the existence of son preference; at each parity, the current use of family planning is lowest for women having no sons and highest for women who have two or more sons. The contraceptive prevalence rate is highest (between 64 and 68 per cent) among women who have exactly three sons or two sons and one daughter. As expected, sterilization is a particularly unpopular method for women who do not have any sons.

Table 6.7 and Figure 6.4 show variations in the current use of contraception by state. Among the major states, the current use of any method varies from a low of 20 per cent in Uttar Pradesh to a high of 63 per cent in Kerala. Uttar Pradesh, Bihar, Rajasthan, Orissa and Madhya

Pradesh, which together accounted for 43 per cent of the population of the country in 1991, have a prevalence rate lower than the national average. In fact, contraceptive use is way below the national average in the two most populous states of Uttar Pradesh and Bihar. The contraceptive prevalence rate is at least one-third higher than the national average in West Bengal, Himachal Pradesh, Punjab, Delhi and Kerala. Considerable variation in the contraceptive prevalence rate is observed in the seven northeastern states, with a higher rate than the national average in Assam, Mizoram and Tripura and a particularly low prevalence rate in Nagaland, Meghalaya and Arunachal Pradesh. As mentioned earlier, knowledge of contraceptives is also low in the latter three states.

Sterilization is the mainstay of the family planning programme and it accounts for more than three-fourths of contraceptive use in half of the states. In fact, more than 85 per cent of current contraceptive users are sterilized in Andhra Pradesh, Rajasthan, Maharashtra and Karnataka. The contraceptive method mix is particularly skewed in Andhra Pradesh, where 95 per cent of users are sterilized. Male sterilization constitutes 11 per cent of total sterilizations in India. The use of male sterilization is noticeably high in Himachal Pradesh, where this method is used by 13 per cent of couples. Assam, West Bengal, Punjab and Uttar Pradesh are the only major states where the relative contribution of methods other than sterilization is large.

The use of modern temporary methods is low in all states except in Delhi, where 31 per cent of currently married women use a modern temporary method. The use rate for any modern temporary method ranges from 10-17 per cent in Jammu, Manipur and Punjab. In the remaining states, less than 10 per cent of currently married women use a modern temporary method. The contribution of modern temporary methods to total contraceptive use is relatively high in Delhi (52 per cent), Punjab (29 per cent) and Uttar Pradesh (28 per cent).

Traditional methods of family planning, mostly periodic abstinence, are used by only 4 per cent of Indian women, ranging from a low of less than 1 per cent in several states to a high of 28 per cent in Tripura. Among the major states, West Bengal and Assam are characterized by an unusually high prevalence of traditional methods, which constitute 35 per cent and 54 per cent of total contraceptive prevalence, respectively. In Tripura, which borders on Assam, nearly half of all contraceptive users rely on traditional methods.

There are considerable urban-rural differentials in the use of contraception in almost all states. Maharashtra is the only state where the prevalence rate is slightly higher in rural areas (54 per cent) than in urban areas (53 per cent). The urban-rural differentials are also quite small in Tamil Nadu and several other low fertility states. The gap between the urban and rural rates is substantial in Bihar, Uttar Pradesh, and several small northeastern states, where the contraceptive prevalence rate is approximately twice as high in urban areas as in rural areas.

The patterns of contraceptive use by age for the states are shown in Table 6.8. Although the extent of contraceptive use varies considerably across the states, the age pattern of use is more or less invariant. In all states except Haryana, Manipur, Nagaland, Himachal Pradesh, Tamil Nadu and Andhra Pradesh, the use rate reaches a maximum at age 35-39. In Haryana and Manipur, the peak is attained at age 40-44, whereas in the other four states the peak is at age 30-34. In Kerala, Punjab and Himachal Pradesh, at least 80 per cent of women age 35-39 are using contraception. In Uttar Pradesh, Bihar, Rajasthan and some of the small northeastern states, where the overall practice of family planning is low, the use of contraception in the early reproductive ages of 15-24 is negligible (less than 10 per cent). West Bengal, Delhi and Tripura are the only states where the contraceptive use rate at age 20-24 is higher than 40 per cent. In addition to these states, the contraceptive prevalence rate at age 25-29 is also high (more than 50 per cent) in Himachal Pradesh, Haryana, Punjab, Maharashtra and the four southern states.

The pattern of contraceptive use by the number and sex of living children for the states is presented in Table 6.9. West Bengal, Delhi and Tripura stand out as having relatively high levels of use (more than 40 per cent) among women with one child. The early use of contraception is consistent with the fact that spacing methods are particularly popular in these states. More than 60 per cent of two-child couples are using family planning in these three states, as well as in Himachal Pradesh, Punjab and Kerala. The table reveals a strong association between the sex composition of children and the use of contraception. For a given number of living children, women with more sons are generally more likely to be using contraception. The differentials are quite small for women with one living child. For women with two living children, son preference is observed in every state except Nagaland and Meghalaya, although a slight preference for a balanced sex composition exists together with son preference in Delhi, Kerala and several small northeastern states. At parity three, son preference persists, but a desire to have at least one daughter emerges in half of the states. Overall, son preference is evident in every state. Son preference is extremely high in Rajasthan, Gujarat, Haryana, Madhya Pradesh, Bihar and Himachal Pradesh. Son preference is relatively low (but still pronounced) in the southern states

Table 6.7: Current use by state

Percent distribution of currently married women age 13-49 by contraceptive method currently used, according to state and residence, India, 1992-93

State	Any meth od	Any modern method	Any modern Temporary method	Pill	IUO	Injection	Condom	Female sterili- zation	Male sterili- zation	Any trad mathod	Peri- odic- absti nence	with drawal	Other meth- ods	Not using andy method	Total percent
1	2	3	4	5	6	7	8	9	10	11	12	13	14	15	16
							URBAN								
India	51.0	45.3	11.7	1.9	3.9	—	5.8	30.4	3.2	5.8	3.5	2.1	0.Z	49.0	100.0
North															
Delhi	60.7	54.9	31.5	3.0	8.1	0.1	20.3	20.2	3.1	5.8	3.2	2.5	0.1	39.3	100.0
Haryana	58.0	48.7	20.2	1.5	5.4	—	13.3	23.5	5.0	9.3	3.0	6.1	0.2	42.0	100.0
Himachal Pradesh	70.4	63.0	24.4	1.2	8.9	—	14.3	29.1	9.6	7.4	2.4	4.9	0.1	29.6	100.0
Jammu Region of J & K	64.4	50.1	22.5	2.5	7.0	—	13.1	22.5	5.0	14.3	3.9	9.9	0.4	35.6	100.0
Punjab	62.8	54.3	23.9	1.8	7.8	—	14.4	27.6	2.8	8.5	4.3	4.0	0.3	37.3	100.0
Rajasthan	47.1	46.8	8.6	0.8	2.5	0.1	5.1	34.9	3.4	0.3	0.1	0.2	—	52.9	100.0
Central															
Madhya Pradesh	47.7	46.2	11.6	1.2	3.6	—	6.8	29.9	4.7	1.5	1.0	0.2	0.2	52.3	100.0
Uttar Pradesh	32.0	29.6	13.7	1.5	3.4	—	8.8	13.6	2.2	2.4	1.6	0.6	0.2	68.0	100.0
East															
Bihar	42.5	39.2	8.5	2.3	1.6	0.2	4.5	27.4	3.3	3.3	1.7	1.1	0.5	57.5	100.0
Orissa	47.4	45.1	7.9	2.5	3.2	—	2.2	33.1	4.1	2.3	1.2	0.7	0.4	52.6	100.0
West Bengal	61.8	36.5	11.1	5.2	1.6	—	4.3	23.3	2.1	25.3	12.8	11.8	0.7	38.2	100.0

Northeast															
Arunachal Pradesh	39.5	29.0	13.7	4.0	5.6	—	4.0	14.5	0.8	10.5	8.9	1.6	—	60.5	100.0
Assam	62.3	33.6	10.9	3.9	1.6	—	5.5	21.4	1.3	28.7	17.2	11.0	0.5	37.7	100.0
Manipur	44.3	31.6	17.2	3.4	12.0	—	1.7	11.0	3.4	12.7	12.0	0.7	—	55.7	100.0
Meghalaya	31.9	27.7	7.9	3.7	3.7	—	0.5	19.4	0.5	4.2	2.1	2.1		68.1	100.0
Mizoram	57.1	55.8	9.5	3.6	4.5	—	1.4	46.0	0.2	1.4	0.9	0.5	—	42.9	100.0
Nagaland	20.6	20.6	8.3	3.2	3.2	—	1.8	11.9	0.5	—	—	—	—	79.4	100.0
Tripura	71.1	39.3	13.9	9.5	2.0	—	2.5	23.4	2.0	31.8	15.4	15.9	0.5	28.9	100.0
West															
Goa	51.2	36.7	9.3	0.9	3.0	—	5.4	26.0	1.4	14.5	11.3	3.1	0.1	48.8	100.0
Gujarat	52.7	49.0	11.0	1.7	5.5	0.1	3.7	34.8	3.3	3.7	2.8	0.9	—	47.3	100.0
Maharashtra	52.9	50.8	11.3	2.3	4.6		4.4	36.7	2.8	2.2	2.0	0.1	0.1	47.1	100.0
South															
Andhra Pradesh	56.6	55.6	4.3	1.1	1.0	—	2.1	44.1	7.2	1.0	0.8	—	0.2	43.4	100.0
Karnataka	52.0	49.1	8.7	0.7	5.0	—	2.9	39.4	1.0	2.9	2.6	0.2	0.1	48.0	100.0
Kerala	68.2	57.3	6.9	0.6	2.3	—	3.9	42.6	7.8	10.9	7.9	3.0	—	31.8	100.0
Tamil Nadu	50.9	44.5	9.9	0.9	6.1	—	3.0	33.3	1.4	6.3	4.3	1.6	0.5	49.1	100.0
							RURAL								
India	36.9	33.1	3.4	0.9	1.2	—	1.2	26.3	3.5	3.8	2.3	1.2	0.2	63.1	100.0
North															
Delhi	55.3	50.6	28.4	1.6	4.3	—	22.6	17.9	4.3	4.7	2.3	1.9	0.4	44.7	100.0
Haryana	46.7	42.8	5.8	1.1	2.4	0.1	2.3	32.0	5.0	3.9	2.0	1.9	—	53.3	100 0
Himachal Pradesh	57.1	53.4	6.9	0.5	2.0	0.1	4.3	33.0	13.6	3.6	1.6	1.9	0.1	42.9	100 0
Jammu Region of J & K	46.2	37.5	7.3	1.1	1.9	—	4.4	25.9	4.2	8.8	3.3	5.4	—	53.8	100.0
Punjab	57.2	50.2	14.8	2.3	5.7	—	6.8	33.0	2.4	7.0	4.5	2.5	—	42.8	100.0
Rajasthan	28.2	27.1	2.0	0.4	0.9	—	0.6	23.0	2.1	1.0	0.5	0.4	0.1	71.8	100.0

1	2	3	4	5	6	7	8	9	10	11	12	13	14	15	16
Central															
Madhya Pradesh	33.4	32.5	1.8	0.5	0.4	—	0.9	25.4	5.3	0.9	0.6	—	0.3	66.6	100.0
Uttar Pradesh	16.7	15.8	3.4	0.9	0.6	0.2	1.8	11.2	1.2	1.0	0.7	0.1	0.1	83.3	100.0
East															
Bihar	19.8	18.5	2.0	0.9	0.4	—	0.7	15.6	1.0	1.2	0.8	0.4	—	80.2	100.0
Orissa	34.2	32.7	2.1	0.6	1.2	—	0.3	27.3	3.3	1.5	0.9	0.2	0.5	65.8	100.0
West Bengal	55.7	37.6	5.0	2.9	1.1	0.1	0.9	27.4	5.1	18.2	10.8	6.9	0.5	44.3	100.0
Northeast															
Arunachal Pradesh	20.8	17.6	7.7	3.1	4.4	0.1	0.1	9.6	0.3	3.2	3.0	0.3	—	79.2	100.0
Assam	40.1	18.0	4.7	2.7	0.8	—	1.2	10.8	2.5	22.1	15.5	5.7	1.0	59.9	100.0
Manipur	30.3	20.5	7.0	1.8	4.2	—	1.0	10.8	2.7	9.8	9.0	0.8	—	69.7	100.0
Meghalaya	18.0	12.1	4.4	2.1	1.8	—	0.5	7.0	0.6	5.9	1.0	0.2	4.7	82.0	100.0
Mizoram	50.5	50.1	7.1	1.5	5.6	—	—	43.0	—	0.4	0.4	—	—	49.5	100.0
Nagaland	10.9	10.9	6.1	1.9	1.7	0.2	2.2	4.8	—	—	—	—	—	89.1	100.0
Tripura	52.4	25.9	8.4	5.6	1.4	—	1.4	15.1	2.5	26.4	17.0	9.1	0.4	47.6	100.0
West															
Goa	44.4	39.0	5.4	0.5	2.4	—	2.5	33.0	0.6	5.3	3.7	1.6	—	55.6	100.0
Gujarat	47.5	45.7	3.2	0.7	1.7	—	0.8	38.9	3.7	1.7	1.1	0.6	—	52.5	100.0
Maharashtra	54.3	53.8	2.9	0.7	1.1		1.2	42.3	8.5	0.5	0.4	—	0.1	45.7	100.0
South															
Andhra Pradesh	43.6	43.3	0.9	0.2	0.4	—	0.2	36.0	6.4	0.3	0.1	—	0.2	56.4	100.0
Karnataka	47.7	46.4	2.9	0.3	2.3	—	0.3	41.7	1.8	1.2	1.0	0.1	0.1	52.3	100.0
Kerala	61.4	53.2	5.8	0.4	2.9		2.5	41.5	6.0	8.1	5.2	2.8	0.1	38.6	100.0

Tamil Nadu	49.2	45.5	3.4	0.4	2.2	—	0.8	39.9	2.3	3.7	1.7	1.3	0.7	50.8	100.0
							TOTAL								
India	40.6	36.3	5.5	1.2	1.9	—	2.4	27.3	3.4	4.3	2.6	1.4	0.2	59.4	100.0
North															
Delhi	60.3	54.6	31.3	2.9	7.8	0.1	20.5	20.0	3.2	5.7	3.1	2.5	0.2	39.7	100.0
Haryana	49.7	44.3	9.6	1.2	3.2	—	5.2	29.7	5.0	5.3	2.2	3.0	0.1	50.3	100.0
Himachal Pradesh	58.4	54.4	8.6	0.5	2.7	—	5.3	32.6	13.2	4.0	1.7	2.2	0.1	41.6	100.0
Jammu Region of J& K	49.4	39.7	10.0	1.3	2.8	—	5.9	25.3	4.4	9.7	3.4	6.2	0.1	50.6	100.0
Punjab	58.7	51.3	17.3	2.2	6.3	—	8.9	31.5	2.5	7.4	4.4	2.9	0.1	41.3	100.0
Rajasthan	31.8	30.9	3.3	0.5	1.2	0.1	1.5	25.3	2.4	0.9	0.4	0.4	0.1	68.2	100.0
Central															
Madhya Pradesh	36.5	35.5	4.0	0.7	1.1	—	2.2	26.4	5.1	1.0	0.7	0.1	0.3	63.5	100.0
Uttar Pradesh	19.8	18.5	5.5	1.0	1.1	0.1	3.2	11.7	1.4	1.3	0.9	0.2	0.1	80.2	100.0
East															
Bihar	23.1	21.6	2.9	1.1	0.5	—	1.3	17.3	1.3	1.5	0.9	0.5	0.1	76.9	100.0
Orissa	36.3	34.6	3.0	0.9	1.5	—	0.6	28.2	3.4	1.6	0.9	0.3	0.5	63.7	100.0
West Bengal	57.4	37.3	6.7	3.5	1.3	0.1	1.9	26.3	4.3	20.1	11.3	8.3	0.5	42.6	100.0
Northeast															
Arunachal Pradesh	23.6	19.3	8.6	3.2	4.6	0.1	0.7	10.3	0.4	4.3	3.8	0.5	—	76.4	100.0
Assam	42.8	19.8	5.4	2.8	0.9	—	1.7	12.1	2.3	22.9	15.7	6.3	0.9	57.2	100.0
Manipur	34.9	24.1	10.3	2.4	6.7	—	1.2	10.9	2.9	10.8	10.0	0.8	—	65.1	100 0
Meghalaya	20.7	15.1	5.1	2.4	2.2	—	0.5	9.4	0.6	5.6	1.2	0.6	3.8	79.3	100 0
Mizoram	53.8	52.9	8.3	2.5	5.1	—	0.7	44.5	0.1	0.9	0.7	0.2	—	46.2	100.0
Nagaland	13.0	13.0	6.5	2.1	2.0	0.2	2.1	6.3	0.1	—	—	—	—	87.0	100.0

1	2	3	4	5	6	7	8	9	10	11	12	13	14	15	16
Tripura	56.1	28.6	9.5	6.4	1.5	—	1.6	16.7	2.4	27.5	16.7	10.5	0.4	43.9	100.0
West															
Goa	47.8	37.9	7.3	0.7	2.7	—	3.9	29.5	1.0	9.9	7.5	2.4	0.1	52.2	100.0
Gujarat	49.3	46.9	5.9	1.0	3.0	—	0.1	1.8	37.5	3.5	2.4	1.7	0.7	50.7	100.0
Maharashtra	53.7	52.5	6.4	1.4	2.5	—	2.5	40.0	6.2	1.2	1.1	0.1	0.1	46.3	100.0
South															
Andhra Pradesh	47.0	46.5	1.8	0.5	0.6	—	0.7	38.1	6.6	0.5	0.3	—	0.2	53.0	100.0
Karnataka	49.1	47.3	4.8	0.4	3.2	—	1.2	41.0	1.5	1.8	1.5	0.1	0.1	50.9	100.0
Kerala	63.3	54.4	6.1	0.5	2.7	—	2.9	41.8	6.5	8.9	6.0	2.9	0.1	36.7	100.0
Tamil Nadu	49.8	45.2	5.7	0.6	3.5	—	1.6	37.5	2.0	4.6	2.6	1.4	0.6	50.2	100.0

— Less than 0.05 per cent.

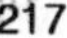

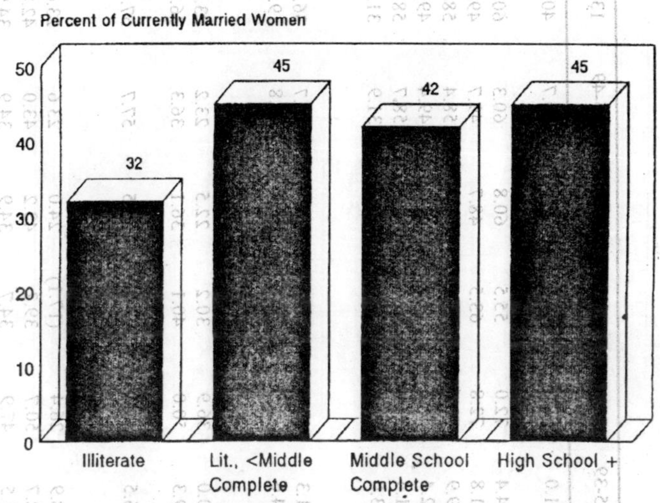

Figure 6.3 Current Use of Modern Contraceptive Methods by Education

(except in Karnataka) and in Goa, West Bengal, Delhi and parts of the northeast. The contraceptive prevalence rate is highest for women with three sons and no daughter in most major states except Madhya Pradesh, Bihar, Orissa, Assam and Southern states where the prevalence rate is highest for women with 2 sons and 1 daughter.

The gap in the contraceptive prevalence rate between illiterate and literate women is conspicuous in Uttar Pradesh, Bihar and Rajasthan (Table 6.10). Contraceptive use differentials by literacy are also large in West Bengal and Assam, where the use of spacing methods is prominent. In Uttar Pradesh, only 16 per cent of illiterate women use family planning compared with 40 per cent of women who have completed high school. In general, the use of family planning is higher among literate than illiterate women, but literacy is not strongly related to the use of family planning in Himachal Pradesh, Maharashtra, Goa, Kerala and Tamil Nadu, all of which have relatively high average levels of education.

Table 6.10 also shows that in all states except Madhya Pradesh, the contraceptive prevalence rate is higher among Hindus than Muslims. However, the gap in the contraceptive prevalence rate between the two religious groups is marginal in Andhra Pradesh, Tamil Nadu, and Goa. In general, the practice of family planning is relatively low among

Table 6.8: Current use by

Percentage of currently married women age 13-49 who are currently using any contraceptive method, according to state and age, India, 1992-93

State	Current age										
	13-14	15-19	20-24	25-29	30-34	35-39	40-44	45-49	15- 44	15-49	13-49
India	4.7	7.1	21.0	42.4	55.9	61.0	56.3	45.8	40.3	40.7	40.6
North											
Delhi	*	14.7	42.1	61.0	74.3	74.4	72.0	55.5	60.8	60.3	60.3
Haryana	*	8.2	25.9	53.8	68.2	71.8	72.8	63.5	48.7	49.7	49.7
Himachal Pradesh	NC	9.1	24.2	63.8	81.2	79.9	73 .5	57.9	58.4	58.4	58.4
Jammu Region of J & K	*	6.2	22.9	42.8	65.4	72.4	68.8	59.5	48.5	49.4	49.4
Punjab	*	10.7	28.0	55.3	73 .6	81.4	73.6	57.6	58.8	58.7	58.7
Rajasthan	*	2.1	9.1	28.6	43.9	53.0	52.2	46.0	30.6	31.9	31.8
Central											
Madhya Pradesh	(—)	3.8	12.8	35.0	57.6	61.3	61.0	53.2	35.5	36.7	36.5
Uttar Pradesh	(—)	2.6	7.4	17.4	27.7	34.6	32.5	26.1	19.2	19.8	19.8
East											
Bihar	(—)	2.7	7.8	23.5	35.8	40.0	36.9	30.2	22.5	23.2	23.1
Orissa	*	1.8	16.3	33.5	53.6	59.3	50.0	40.1	36.1	36.3	36.3
West Bengal	(20.6)	27.2	44.9	63.9	72.3	76.5	66.3	47.9	58.5	57.7	57.4
Northeast											
Arunachal Pradesh	*	9.0	11.6	26.9	31.6	38.9	26.4	(17.1)	24.0	23 6	23.6
Assam	*	18.1	31.4	41.0	54.6	62.7	50.7	39.2	43.2	43.0	42.8
Manipur	NC	*	17.4	27.6	42.2	45.5	47.9	34.7	34.9	34.9	34.9

Meghalaya	*	3.5	9.1	19.6	31.8	32.5	28.6	22.4	20.5	20.7	20.7
Mizoram	NC	(5.9)	22.0	37.6	65.1	76.1	73.1	63.6	51.9	53.8	53.8
Nagaland	NC	(5.0)	4.0	9.2	23.1	22.2	16.1	10.7	13.4	13.0	13.0
Tripura	*	26.4	40.0	60.9	70.8	74.7	61.3	42.0	57.8	56.4	56.1
West											
Goa	*	(18.8)	21.4	38.1	51.8	59.0	57.3	49.8	47.5	47.8	47.8
Gujarat	*	3.2	18.1	42.4	63.8	76.9	73.9	64.3	47.8	49.3	49.3
Maharashtra	(—)	9.1	29.5	59.2	72.4	76.8	71.0	67.4	53.0	54.1	53.7
South											
Andhra Pradesh	(—)	4.5	31.6	57.5	70.4	65.3	62.3	54.3	46.9	47.4	47.0
Karnataka	(4.0)	4.3	31.8	59.4	67.2	69.7	62.0	48.4	49.5	49.4	49.1
Kerala	*	13.0	28.5	61.0	75.5	83.1	77.4	68.1	62.8	63.3	63.3
Tamil Nadu	*	10.6	29.2	55.1	66.9	66.4	58.3	41.7	50.6	49.8	49.8

NC: Not calculated because there are no currently married women age 13-14.
( ) Based on 25-49 unweighted cases.
* Percentage not shown; based on fewer than 25 unweighted cases.
—Less than 0.05 per cent.

Table 6.9: Current use by state and number and sex of living children

Percentage of currenty married women age 13-49 who are currently using any contraceptive method, by state and number and sex of living children, India, 1992-93

Number and sex of living children

State	None	1 child	1 son	No son	2 child	2 sons	1 son	No sons	3 child	3 son	2 sons	1 son	No sons	4+ child	2+ sons	1 son	No sons
India	4.2	19.3	20.9	17.4	46.1	55.0	46.4	31.5	58.9	64.9	68.0	51.2	31.7	52.4	53.8	49.5	34.8
North																	
Delhi	13.1	47.6	48.5	46.4	70.8	69.3	75.4	57.6	71.4	76.6	73 .9	71.3	53.7	67.9	68.7	67.7	*
Haryana	3.4	19.8	20.6	18.8	48.1	65.3	42.6	26.0	70.6	84.9	81.9	51.3	(12.8)	67.1	71.0	55.8	*
Himachal Pradesh	6.8	20.1	22.5	16.8	64.6	77.9	63.1	31.6	76.4	99.4	87.0	66.2	(19.4)	75.3	79.5	68.0	*
Jammu Region of																	
J & K	3.9	23.3	24.3	22.1	49.9	55.3	53.2	30.8	67.9	76.8	75.3	57.1	(43.4)	65.0	69.3	44.4	*
Punjab	2.3	28.9	31.2	26.3	61.1	70.2	61.5	34.8	74.1	85.7	82.3	65.9	(29.8)	76.1	80.9	61.8	*
Rajasthan	1.9	6.9	6.9	7.0	27.6	34.2	30.6	5.8	47.2	63.9	57.4	27.2	12.0 4	9.3	52.2	36.4	(26.5)
Central																	
Madhya Pradesh	2.2	9.3	9.1	9.6	35.2	52.6	32.2	16.2	54.9	57.3	70.4	39.3	16.4	57.6	60.9	48.2	33.3
Uttar Pradesh	1.8	7.8	9.2	6.3	18.6	26.9	17.1	9.7	28.1	35.6	35.3	19.0	14.8	28.5	30.4	21.2	10.8
East																	
Bihar	1.7	7.9	7.8	8.0	24.7	34.5	23.1	14.7	34.3	38.0	46.9	24.7	4.0 3	3.4	36.3	23.9	8.9
Orissa	2.7	12.1	14.0	9.9	39.9	51.8	40.0	20.0	51.7	60.2	61.5	43.3	21.5 54.3		55.8	51.0	(42.7)
West Bengal	19.8	49.5	53.9	44.8	66.4	74.8	67.0	52.7	74.2	82.3	78.0	72.0	53.2 62.0		61.4	66.7	(47.3)
Northeast																	
Arunachal Pradesh	4.1	14.2	19.8	5.9	25.0	(26.2)	29.2	(15.8)	25.5	(30.8)	33.3	19.2	*	34.5	37.0	*	*
Assam	18.0	28.4	32.8	23.9	46.4	54.4	46.6	35.0	51.4	51.8	59.2	48.0	27.8	49.6	50.5	46.6	(42.9)
Manipur	4.8	20.3	26.6	15.2	35.0	(43.6)	35.6	(20.0)	46.9	*	51.4	41.3	*	42.2	43.2	37.5	*

State																	
Meghalaya	4.0	13.5	14.3	12.5	23.5	20.8	24.7	(24.4)	32.1	*	39.7	27.0	*	23.4	22.5	(30.6)	*
Mizoram	0.9	25.2	33.3	14.0	48.9	(61.1)	43.5	(47.1)	67.0	(71.9)	67.5	71.9	*	74.3	75.7	70.9	*
Nagaland	2.4	7.3	6.4	9.0	9.6	(8.5)	10.6	(8.7)	17.5	*	17.1	21.6	*	17.3	18.0	14.0	*
Tripura	15.7	45.1	49.5	40.2	60.8	61.4	64.6	(48.7)	71.4	*	67.4	77.0	*	62.5	59.7	78.4	*
West																	
Goa	4.6	27.1	26.9	27.2	48.6	52.0	48.9	43.2	63.0	63.0	70.3	58.2	46.3	66.6	68.7	62.8	(44.4)
Gujarat	3.3	18.2	23.3	11.7	55.6	70.0	54.7	26.2	67.7	84.0	81.6	53.3	18.3	68.6	n.9	56.5	(11.1)
Maharashtra	3.1	22.8	27.3	17.8	50.3	65.9	48.1	27.9	74.8	86.0	84.7	63.9	30.8	76.0	79.7	69.5	(48.6)
South																	
Andhra Pradesh	1.6	15.2	16.2	14.2	53.2	55.5	54.9	45.7	73.5	76.9	79.9	70.8	51.7	69.9	70.4	70.7	t59.1)
Karnataka	2.2	18.5	19.4	17.5	54.9	67.3	54.6	35.0	72.3	76.0	79.8	69.9	38.9	63.5	64.5	62.6	47.4)
Kerala	8.5	37.1	38.1	36.0	78.1	78.2	80.1	n.1	83.1	85.3	86.5	81.8	74.3	68.9	67.1	77.4	(65.5)
Tamil Nadu	3.3	24.4	24.9	23.9	59.5	62.5	61.9	49.0	72.6	74.2	80.4	70.4	50.6	64.6	64.1	68.0	(59.5)

( ) Based on 25-49 unweighted cases.
* Percentage not shown; based on fewer than 25 unweighted cases.

Table 6.10: Current use by state and background characteristics

Percentage of currently married women age 13-49 who are currently using any contraceptive method, by state and selected background characteristics, India, 1992-93

	Education				Religion							Caste/tribe		
State	Illi-literate	Lit., <middle	Middle complete	High school & above	Hindu	Muslim	Christian	Sikh	Jain	Buddhist	other	Scheduled caste	Scheduled tribe	other
India	33.9	50.4	50.8	54.7	41.6	27.7	48.3	57.6 6	2.6	50.4	37.4	34.5	33.0	42.4
North														
Delhi	50.2	60.8	65.8	68.4	61.2	47.4	(68.0)	65.8	(73.5)	*	*	58.8	61.5	60.4
Haryana	47.8	50.7	52.6	55.4	51.3	13.8	*	47.2	*	*	*	43.5	NC	51.9
Himachal Pradesh	58.0	59.4	55.4	59.6	58.8	(41.4)	*	(72.9)	NC	*	*	56.6	39 5	60 1
Jammu Region of J & K	45.7	47.8	49.7	61.1	51.8	34.3	*	61.8	*	NC	*	43.4	*	51 9
Punjab	56.7	61.0	58.0	62.4	59.9	(40.6)	(34.8)	59.0	*	NC	*	57.2	NC	59.3
Rajasthan	29.2	42.5	43.5	46.9	32.3	18.4	*	41.5	(61.3)	*	*	28.5	23.9	35.1
Central														
Madhya Pradesh	33.6	43.4	42.7	49.6	36.1	38.6	(33.1)	*	(64.4)	*	*	33.2	30.2	39.4
Uttar Pradesh	15.5	28.4	29.5	40.4	21.2	10.5	*	*	(55.7)	*	*	15.1	12.0	20.9
East														
Bihar	17.6	39.2	42.4	45.7	26.0	7.5	(19.6)	*	*	(22.9)	(22.6)	14.7	16.4	24.7
Orissa	33.8	40.5	33.8	47.5	36.5	16.1	45.6	39.7	*	NC	*	33.7	30.0	38.5
West Bengal	49.1	61.6	66.9	75.1	61.4	43.0	*	NC	*	*	(41.3)	54.5	44.8	58.4

Northeast														
Arunachal Pradesh	19.9	26.4	27.5	46.9	35.5	*	23.7	*	NC	29.7	10.9	NC	18.4	41.3
Assam	32.1	51.7	63.7	69.3	48.3	32.3	19.1	*	*	NC	NC	52.9	31.4	44.5
Manipur	30.4	35.3	40.8	41.0	39.9	25.0	22.8	*	*	NC	(45.7)	NC	22.6	39.2
Meghalaya	17.0	20.1	30.8	32.0	45.7	(28.0)	18.7	NC	NC	*	11.2	*	17.9	42.3
Mizoram	35.4	58.5	49.4	51.5	*	*	54.1	NC	*	*	NC	NC	54.1	40.0
Nagaland	6.6	16.0	17.8	20.8	12.1	*	13.1	NC	*	NC	*	NC	12.9	14.0
Tripura	45.0	61.0	66.9	67.8	58.6	28.6	*	NC	NC	(44.0)	NC	*	51.0	56.8
West														
Goa	46.6	49.4	41.3	49.8	52.3	48.3	36.1	*	*	*	*	45.1	41.5	48.0
Gujarat	46.3	51.2	53.9	54.8	50.3	35.0	*	*	(68.3)	*	*	53.5	47.3	49.4
Maharashtra	54.1	53.2	45.4	58.0	56.6	36.1	(41.4)	*	59.7	52.0	(70.4)	55.1	49.2	54.2
South														
Andhra Pradesh	43.5	55.8	55.3	52.2	47.0	44.7	52.3	*	*	*	*	35.9	36.5	49.7
Karnataka	45.5	53.3	52.8	56.9	50.6	36.8	47.6	*	(61.8)	NC	*	45.1	45.7	49.9
Kerala	66.7	64.1	60.5	62.9	72.5	37.8	71.7	*	*	NC	*	76.7	75.0	62.5
Tamil Nadu	47.5	51.7	52.6	52.3	50.2	45.8	48.8	NC	*	NC	*	45.0	*	51.0

NC: Not calculated because there are no cases on which to base a percentage.
( ) Based on 25-49 unweighted cases
* Percentage not shown; based on fewer than 25 unweighted cases

women from both scheduled castes and scheduled tribes. In Assam, Gujarat, Maharashtra and Kerala, the prevalence rate is higher among scheduled caste women than women from either of the other two caste/ tribe groups. Similarly, in Delhi, the practice of contraception is highest among scheduled tribe women.

The religious differentials in the contraceptive use rate can be understood better from Table 6.11, which provides these rates by religious composition as well as level of education of women. The contraceptive prevalence rate is lowest among Muslims and highest among Sikhs for each educational category of women. With more education, the religious differentials in the use rate tend to narrow. For women with at least a high school education, the contraceptive prevalence rate ranges from a low level of 45 per cent among Muslims to a high of 62 per cent among Sikhs. For illiterates, the variation is from a low of 22 per cent among Muslims to a high of 56 per cent among Sikhs. The use of any modern temporary method is, however, higher among Muslims than among Hindus in each educational category. The analysis suggests that educational differentials among different religious groups partly explain the religious differences in contraceptive use; however, the religious differentials persist even after controlling for education.

Number of Children at First Use of Contraception

In order to examine the timing of initial family planning use, the NFHS included a question on how many living children women had when they first used a method. The distribution of ever-married women according to the number of living children at first contraceptive use is shown in Table 6.12. Overall, only 7 per cent of contraceptors (3 per cent of all ever-married women) initiated the use of contraception before having any children, and another 19 per cent started after the first child. As mentioned earlier, use of spacing methods is minimal and there is hardly any effort to space the first child. However, although early use of contraception is rare, the majority of those who ever used family planning (68 per cent) initiated use when they had fewer than four living children. This pattern of first acceptance at relatively low parities means that family planning has a larger demographic impact than it would if contraceptive use were initiated later.

Table 6.12 suggests that there has been a shift over time toward initiating contraceptive use at lower parities. In the older cohorts, the average parity at which women who ever used contraception first did so was considerably higher than the parity at which ever users in the younger cohorts first used. For example, 30 per cent of ever users age 25-29

Table 6.11: Current use by religion and education
Percentage of currently married women age 13-49 currently using any method, any modern method, and any modern temporary method of contraception, by religion and education, India, 1992-93

Religion	Any method				Any modern method				Any modern temporary method			
	Illit-erate	Literate, < middle school	Middle school complete	High school and above	Illit-erate	Literate, < middle school	Middle school complete	High school and above	Illit-erate	Literate, < middle school	Middle school complete	High school and above
Hindu	35.1	52.2	51.7	55.2	33.1	47.3	43.5	45.5	1.8	5.3	8.8	20.3
Muslim	21.8	37.2	40.5	44.9	17.3	29.0	31.4	38.9	3.1	8.0	13.6	24.6
Christian	36.4	55.6	55.0	52.0	32.1	50.1	44.0	39.2	2.1	4.2	7.2	13.4
Sikh	55.9	57.4	57.0	61.9	50.6	49.3	45.8	50.6	8.3	20.7	20.2	34.1
Other	43.1	56.7	50.2	57.3	42.4	51.7	45.2	50.3	2.0	8.6	12.1	30.0

began their first use when they had fewer than two living children, whereas only 12 per cent of ever users age 45-49 initiated the use of contraception at such an early stage in the family building process. The average parity at which urban women initiate contraceptive use also is slightly lower than the average parity at which rural women initiate use, but the difference is small, despite the very substantial urban-rural difference in total contraceptive prevalence.

Problems in the Current Use of Family Planning

Table 6.13 deals with the problems faced by women while using the pill, IUD, and sterilization. Most women using these methods did not report any problems. For pill and IUD users, however, the extent of problems may be underestimated because women who had serious problems with these methods may have already discontinued use. Among the specific problems listed in the case of pill users, headache is most common (6 per cent of users) followed by dizziness and body ache (each was mentioned by 4 per cent of users). In the case of the IUD, the major problems are excessive bleeding (8 per cent) and backache (7 per cent). The proportion of women complaining of a problem is higher in the case of female sterilization, the most commonly used method. The major causes of discomfort reported in this case are pain or backache (15 per cent) and weakness or inability to work (10 per cent). The same problems were most commonly mentioned in the case of male sterilization. Sepsis was mentioned in a few cases, as was the failure of the operation, but even fewer women mentioned the loss of sexual power as a result of female or male sterilization.

Family Planning Services

The NFHS included some questions designed to elicit information on the extent of followup services provided by health workers to the users of various contraceptive methods, either at home or outside the home. Such data can provide useful information about the mechanisms to encourage continuity in use, which is an important element in the framework for assessing the quality of care provided by the family welfare programme (Bruce, 1990). In a recent study conducted in India, it was found that home visits by health workers can be an important factor affecting the utilization of government family welfare services (Verma *et al.*, 1994).

Table 6.12: Number of living children at first use
Per cent distribution of ever-married women by number of living children at the time of first use of contraception, according to current age and residence, India, 1992-93

Current age	Never used	Number of living children at the time of first use 0	1	2	3	4+	Missing	Total per cent	Number of women
				URBAN					
13-14	(88.8)	(10.6)	(0.6)	(—)	(—)	(—)	(—)	100.0	42
15-19	85.1	5.5	7.4	1.4	0.3	0.2	0.2	100.0	1376
20-24	63.9	6.7	15.7	8.4	4.0	1.2	0.2	100.0	4229
25-29	39.4	6.0	19.3	15.9	11.5	7.7	0.1	100.0	4705
30-34	29.7	3.8	16.7	16.9	16.5	16.1	0.2	100.0	4291
35-39	26.2	3.4	12.5	14.8	17.1	25.9	—	100.0	3715
40-44	33.3	2.2	9.4	11.3	15.0	28.7	0.1	100.0	2899
45-49	40.5	1.9	8.3	9.2	12.4	27.5	0.3	100.0	2197
Total	42.1	4.4	14.1	12.5	11.8	15.0	0.2	100.0	23455
				RURAL					
13-14	93.5	5.6	0.9	—	—	—	—	100.0	311
15-19	89.0	5.5	3.9	1.3	0.3	—	0.1	100.0	7719
20-24	73 .6	4.0	8.9	7.4	4.6	1.3	0.1	100.0	13755
25-29	55.3	2.4	8.4	12.0	13.5	8.2	0.1	100.0	12 735
30-34	43.4	1.7	7.6	10.7	16.5	20.0	0.1	100.0	10369
35-39	41.1	1.5	6.1	9.4	15.6	26.3	0.1	100.0	8746
40-44	45.5	1.4	4.9	6.5	11.5	30.1	0.1	100.0	6850
45-49	54.6	0.6	3.4	4.5	8.0	28.6	0.2	100.0	5838
Total	58.4	2.6	6.7	8.0	10.1	14.1	0.1	100.0	66322
				TOTAL					
13-14	92.9	6.2	0.9	—	—	—	—	100.0	352
15-19	88.4	5.5	4.4	1.3	0.3	—	0.1	100.0	9095
20-24	71.3	4.6	10.5	7.6	4.5	1.3	0.1	100.0	17983
25-29	51.0	3.4	11.4	13.1	13.0	8.1	0.1	100.0	17441
30-34	39.4	2.4	10.3	12.5	16.5	18.8	0.1	100.0	14660
35-39	36.7	2.1	8.0	11.0	16.0	26.2	0.1	100.0	12461
40-44	41.9	1.6	6.2	8.0	12.5	29.7	0.1	100.0	9748
45-49	50.8	1.0	4.8	5.8	9.2	28.3	0.2	100.0	8036
Total	54.1	3.1	8.7	9.1	10.5	14.3	0.1	100.0	89 w

( ) Based on 25-49 unweighted cases.
— Less than 0.05 per cent.

Table 6.13: Problems with current method

Percentage of current users of the pill, copper T/IUD, and female/male sterilization who have had problems in using the method, India, 1992-93

Problem	Method	
	Pill	
No problems	80.0	
Cramps	0.8	
Dizziness	3.8	
Body ache	3.8	
Spotting/bleeding	2.4	
White discharge	1.5	
Headache	5.9	
Other	5.8	
Number of pill users	1013	
	Copper T/IUD	
No problems	81.1	
Backache	6.5	
Irregular periods	2.6	
Excessive bleeding	7.8	
Weakness/inability to work	3.0	
Other	3.4	
Number of IUD users	1589	
	Female sterilization	**Male sterilization**
No problems	76.7	84.9
Fever	1.7	1.0
Pain/backache	14.6	7.3
Seps is	2.0	1.8
Weakness/inability to Work	9.5	6.1
Failure/woman got pregnant	0.6	1.2
Loss of sexual power	0.3	0.6
Other	3.0	0.8
Number sterilized	23136	2916

Note: Percentages may sum to more than 100.0 because multiple problems could be recorded.

The follow-up care provided by the family welfare programme needs improvement. Only 15 per cent of IUD and pill users reported having received a follow-up visit at home, and for the most popular method (sterilization), follow-up care was received by 30 per cent of users (Table 6.14). There are wide interstate variations in the extent of follow-up home care provided by the programme. Only in Karnataka and Orissa did more than 50 per cent of sterilized women or their sterilized husbands receive follow-up care services at home. Even in Kerala and Maharashtra, where the programme has been performing well, health workers are generally not providing follow-up home visits. Only one-fifth of sterilized couples in Maharashtra and less than one-fifth (18 per cent) of sterilized couples in Kerala reported a follow-up home visit.

A larger proportion of acceptors, however, went outside the home for a follow-up consultation with medical or health personnel. Sixty per cent of IUD users, 49 per cent of pill users and 43 per cent of sterilization acceptors made such a visit. It appears that women using spacing methods had a substantial need for counselling regarding side effects and other methodrelated problems, and follow-up home care was particularly lacking in such cases. For example, 79 per cent of IUD users in Maharashtra went outside the home for a consultation with a medical or a health person. Only 18 per cent of the IUD users in Maharashtra were given the required follow-up home visits by health workers.

The quality of care and services offered by the programme was further assessed by asking sterilized women about the quality of care they received during and just after the operation, as well as the quality of follow-up home care if they were visited by a health worker. A majority of sterilized women (53 per cent) rated the operative and postoperative care as either very good or excellent (Table 6.15). More than 60 per cent of women rated the care as either very good or excellent in Gujarat (79 per cent), Karnataka (72 per cent), Mizoram (72 per cent), Goa (66 per cent), Maharashtra (66 per cent), Tripura (64 per cent), Tamil Nadu (63 per cent) and Manipur (61 per cent).

Ratings of the quality of follow-up home care received after the operation are similar to ratings given to the care during and just after the operation. Only 4 per cent thought the followup care was not so good or very bad. Not only was the extent of follow-up services very high in Karnataka, but a large majority of women in that state (70 per cent) also rated the services as very good or excellent. In Orissa, on the other hand, where the extent of follow-up visits was also relatively good, the majority of women (55 per cent) rated the service as "alright". In Gujarat and Maharashtra, where the extent of follow-up care was relatively low, a large majority of women rated the services as very good or excellent.

Duration of Contraceptive Use

In the NFHS, the duration of continuous use of a method was ascertained from each current user of family planning. Table 6.16 shows that the mean duration of continuous use of any method of family planning is 77 months, or 6.4 years. On average, female sterilizations took

Table 6.14: Follow-up from a health worker.

Percentage of currently married women age 13-49 currently using the pill, IUD or sterilization who had a follow-up visit from a health worker, by place of visit and state, India, 1992-93

State	Follow-up at home			Follow-up outside home			Follow-up of any type		
	Pill	IUD	Steril-ization	Pill	IUD	Steril-ization	Pill	IUD	Steril ization
India	15.0	14.7	30.1	48.8	60.4	43.4	54.6	65.3	61.9
North									
Delhi	3.1	1.9	10.8	51.0	67.2	60.3	53.1	68.3	66.1
Haryana	(15.6)	3.9	44.5	(52.2)	59.0	50.5	(58.9)	61.2	81.1
Himachal Pradesh	*	2.1	34.4	*	65.7	50.8	*	67.8	72.5
Jammu Region of J & K	(—)	3.1	12.9	(43.2)	66.7	69.4	(43.2)	68.4	76.6
Punjab	3.2	4.4	35.0	38.7	71.3	53.1	40.3	73.5	75.4
Rajasthan	(24.0)	22.2	24.3	(44.0)	54.0	41.4	(48.0)	61.9	53.8
Central									
Madhya Pradesh	(25.3)	16.9	32.0	(69.3)	71.8	42.3	(79.5)	77.1	60.0
Uttar Pradesh	21.6	5.8	28.4	45.0	56.9	36.5	57.0	59.3	53.8
East									
Bihar	3.0	(8.6)	16.8	31.3	(49.6)	37.2	31.9	(55.8)	48.1
Orissa	(11.5)	25.3	52.7	(29.4)	58.9	36.1	(32.7)	72.1	71.8
West Bengal	7.2	(13.2)	17.8	49.8	(49.4)	50.3	53.2	(55.2)	60.2
Northeast									
Arunachal Pradesh	(7.4)	(5.3)	4.5	(74.1)	(63.2)	67.4	(74.1)	(65.8)	70.8

Assam	9.5	(1.3)	11.3	40.5	(58.3)	57.2	44.1	(59.6)	64.0
Manipur	*	—	4.9	*	45.0	53.7	*	45.0	53.7
Meghalaya	*	*	6.0	*	*	67.0	*	*	67.0
Mizoram	*	(17.4)	10.4	*	(78.3)	18.8	*	(82.6)	25.7
Nagaland	*	*	12.1	*	*	56.1	*	*	56.1
Tripura	1.6	*	7.8	50.0	*	66.1	51.6	*	69.3
West									
Goa	*	21.5	22.2	*	65.8	73.5	*	77.2	79.5
Gujarat	(37.8)	13.8	38.4	(35.1)	53.2	32.9	(54.1)	56.0	63.7
Maharashtra	32.7	17.7	20.1	78.8	79.2	45.5	78.8	81.3	57.9
South									
Andhra Pradesh	*	*	37.6	*	*	50.8	*	*	71 4
Karnataka	*	33.8	53.7	*	59.2	46.7	*	66.2	75 5
Kerala	*	28.7	17.9	*	35.2	31.5	*	51.9	43.6
Tamil Nadu	*	13.2	32.2	*	50.4	40.3	*	57.4	63.0

( ) Based on 25-49 unweighted cases.
* Percentage not shown; based on fewer than 25 unweighted cases.
— Less than 0.05 per cent.

Table 6.15: Quality of care during sterilization and follow-up after sterilization
Per cent distribution of sterilization acceptors by reported quality of care during sterilization and at the time of follow-up visit by state, India, 1992-93

State	Care during sterilization							Follow-up care[1]						
	Excel-lent	Very good	Al-right	Not so good	Very bad	DK/ missing	Total per cent	Excel-lent	Very good	Al-right	Not so good	Very bad	DK/ missing	Total per cent
India	10.0	42.6	39.2	5.6	1.5	1.1	100.0	8.5	47.6	40.0	3.2	0.5	0.3	100.0
North														
Delhi	16.4	35.5	41.2	3.6	1.2	2.2	100.0	15.7	42.2	39.8	2.4	—	—	100.0
Haryana	3.7	40.6	44.6	7.1	0.4	3.5	100.0	2.8	40.0	53.3	3.9	—	—	100.0
Himachal Pradesh	3.9	30.5	58.7	4.8	1.5	0.7	100.0	6.2	37.2	53.8	1.9	0.6	0.3	100.0
Jammu Region of J & K	4.6	26.1	57.5	7.8	1.3	2.7	100.0	6.5	23.9	66.6	1.7	1.2	—	100.0
Punjab	8.8	30.5	54.4	4.6	0.5	1.2	100.0	7.9	43.0	46.8	2.3	—	—	100.0
Rajasthan	13.3	20.1	52.3	7.4	3.6	3.3	100.0	15.0	25.3	54.1	3.8	0.9	0.9	100.0
Central														
Madhya Pradesh	7.5	29.3	50.1	9.1	3.0	1.1	100.0	7.0	35.6	52.0	4.4	0.8	0.1	100.0
Uttar Pradesh	11.0	37.2	40.5	6.9	2.8	1.6	100.0	14.7	44.9	34.8	3.5	1.0	1.0	100.0
East														
Bihar	4.2	35.9	51.2	7.0	0.8	0.8	100.0	1.5	34.9	57.8	4.6	—	1.3	100.0
Orissa	3.2	30.7	53.7	8.7	1.1	2.6	100.0	3.4	30.4	55.1	9.7	0.9	0.6	100.0
West Bengal	7.6	39.3	40.7	9.5	2.7	0.2	100.0	7.5	47.6	41.1	2.7	1.0	—	100.0
Northeast														
Arunachal Pradesh	4.5	49.4	34.8	9.0	1.1	1.1	100.0	*	*	*	*	*	*	100.0

Assam	2.2	48.7	38.4	5.6	0.6	4.5	100.0	(3.8)	(57.6)	(32.4)	(6.2)	(—)	(—)	100.0
Manipur	1.6	59.3	25.2	9.8	4.1	—	100.0	*	*	*	*	*	*	100.0
Meghalaya	13.0	18.0	60.0	6.0	1.0	2.0	100.0	*	*	*	*	*	*	100.0
Mizoram	22.0	49.5	19.3	8.2	1.0	—	100.0	(23.8)	(45.2)	(26.2)	(4.8)	(—)	(—)	100.0
Nagaland	21.2	13.6	48.5	16.7	—	—	100.0	*	*	*	*	*	*	100.0
Tripura	4.2	59.9	26.0	6.8	—	3.1	100.0	*	*	*	*	*	*	100.0
West														
Goa	10.6	55.8	29.0	3.1	0.9	0.6	100.0	6.6	49.7	38.1	4.6	1.0	—	100.0
Gujarat	8.1	70.4	18.0	2.4	0.5	0.6	100.0	7.6	69.1	22.4	0.9	—	—	100.0
Maharashtra	18.1	47.4	29.4	3.3	1.0	0.7	100.0	10.7	56.5	28.8	2.8	0.6	0.6	100.0
South														
Andhra Pradesh	8.8	41.2	44.1	4.6	1.1	0.3	100.0	8.1	45.0	44.7	1.9	0.3	—	100.0
Karnataka	13.9	58.1	23.6	3.2	0.6	0.6	100.0	10.0	59.6	27.6	2.6	0.2	—	100.0
Kerala	4.9	43.2	45.2	3.8	1.0	1.9	100.0	6.4	37.5	48.8	5.2	1.7	0.3	100.0
Tamil Nadu	12.2	51.0	29.5	5.2	1.4	0.8	100.0	9.7	55.3	33.5	1.3	0.2	—	100.0

DK: Don't know.
( ) Based on 25-49 unweighted cases.
* Percentage not shown; based on 25-49 unweighted cases.
— Less than 0.05 per cent.
[1] For those receiving follow-up home care from a health worker.

place 7 years before the time of the survey and male sterilizations were performed nearly 13 years before the survey. Among the modern temporary methods, the mean duration of use is the highest for condoms (28 months), followed by the IUD (23 months). The shortest mean duration of use for any method is for the pill (17 months). The duration of use for each method increases with the current age of the woman.

Age at Sterilization

Table 6.17 shows the age and time at which couples obtained a sterilization. A total of 26,051 sterilization operations were reported, of which 42 per cent were conducted fewer than 6 years before the survey, another 26 per cent were conducted 6-9 years before the survey and the remaining 32 per cent were conducted 10 or more years before the survey. Sixty-nine per cent of the vasectomy operations (which constitute only 11 per cent of total sterilization operations) were performed more than 10 years before the survey. About three-fourths (73 per cent) of couples had undergone sterilization before the wife was age 30, and there are only a negligible proportion of cases of sterilization being performed when the wife was age 40 and above. The median age of the woman at the time of sterilization is 27 years. There has been a gradual decline in the median age at sterilization, from 27.3 years among those who underwent the operation 8-9 years ago to 26.3 years among those who were sterilized in the last two years. One cannot assess the trend in the median age at sterilization more than 10 years before the survey because the NFHS only interviewed ever-married women age 13-49. This means that, for the period 10 or more years before the survey, there are no women age 40-49 because these women would have been age 50-59 at the time of survey.

The median age of women at the time of sterilization varies from a low of 24.5 years in Andhra Pradesh to a high of 29.7 years in Manipur (Table 6.18). The median age at sterilization is relatively high in the larger North Indian states, such as Uttar Pradesh (29.6 years), Bihar (28.1 years) and Rajasthan (27.7 years) where the current use of contraception is also low. The median age at sterilization is relatively low in Maharashtra and the four southern states, and it has registered a decline, particularly in recent years, in Tamil Nadu and Maharashtra.

Methods Used Before Sterilization

The NFHS did not collect information on the sequence of contraceptive methods used in the past, but some information on method switching is provided by the survey data. Table 6.19 shows the extent to which sterilization users have used other temporary methods before accepting

Table 6.16: Mean duration of use of contraceptive methods

Mean duration of use of contraceptive methods in months, by woman's age, India, 1992-93

Women's current age	Any method	Any modern method	Any modern Temporary method	Pill	IUD	Injection	Condom	Female sterili-zation	Male sterili-zation	Peri-odic-absti nence	With drawal
15-19	6.7	8.8	5.1	7.8	(5.8)	*	6.0	10.0	*	5.3	1.7
20-24	17.3	19.4	9.2	9.1	11.8	*	9.2	24.9	29.2	9.1	4.7
25-29	36.6	39.3	16.2	15.7	18.7	*	17.3	45.1	60.6	15.2	11.3
30-34	63.1	66.5	29.1	22.3	29.7	*	35.2	70.8	97.1	26.8	25.9
35-39	94.9	100.0	42.8	26.9	39.8	*	53.1	101.6	140.9	44.6	38.5
40-44	130.7	137.4	54.6	(46.4)	45.1	*	70.7	134.3	177.3	51.0	51.4
45-49	166.7	173.0	56.3	*	(62.2)	*	71.3	167.2	202.7	57.4	47.3
Total	76.7	82.7	24.5	17.1	23.4	(23.0)	28.1	86.5	152.9	26.8	21.7

( ) Based on 25-49 unweighted cases.
* Mean not shown; based on fewer than 25 unweighted cases.

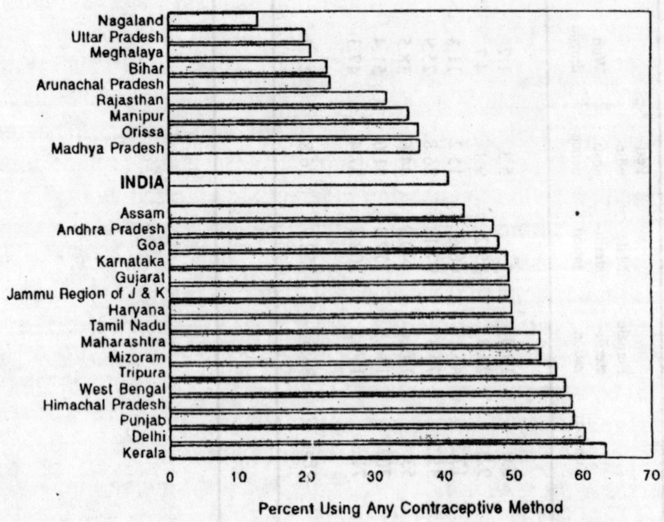

Figure 6.4 Current Use of Any Contraceptive Method by State

the terminal method. For India as a whole, 82 per cent of sterilization users never used any other method of contraception before sterilization. Seven per cent used periodic abstinence previously, 6 per cent used condoms and 4 per cent each used the pill, the IUD or withdrawal. Two-thirds of sterilized couples in Tripura used some temporary method, especially the traditional methods, before accepting sterilization. The extent of prior use of temporary methods before sterilization is also substantial in Assam (54 per cent), Delhi (50 per cent), West Bengal (43 per cent) and Kerala (39 per cent). In Delhi, more of the couples used modern temporary methods (particularly condoms) prior to the sterilization, but couples in the other three states relied more on the use of traditional methods. In Andhra Pradesh, Bihar, Rajasthan, Uttar Pradesh and Orissa, very few of the sterilized couples (less than 12 per cent) had any prior experience with contraceptive use.

6.3 Source of Supply of Contraception

Family planning methods and services in India are provided through a network of government hospitals and urban family welfare centres in urban areas and Primary Health Centres and sub-centres in rural areas. Besides these government outlets, family planning services are also provided by a few private hospitals and clinics as well as by nongovernmental organizations. Sterilization operations and IUD insertions are carried out mostly in government hospitals and Primary Health Centres. Sterilization camps, organized from time to time, also provide sterilization services. Modern spacing methods such as the IUD, the pill and condoms are available through both the government and private sectors.

Tabte 6.17: Timing of sterilization

Per cent distribution of currently married sterilized women and wives of sterilized men by age at the time of sterilization, according to the number of years since the operation, India 1992-93

	Woman's age at the time of operation								
Years since operation	<25	25-29	30-34	35-39	40-44	45-49	Total per cent	Number	Median age[1]
				STERILIZED WOMEN					
<2	38.6	34.8	18.2	6.4	1.5	0.5	100 0	3654	26.3
2-3	39.2	34.5	17.8	6.7	1.6	0.2	100 0	3165	26 2
4-5	37.2	33.8	19.4	6.8	2.7	0.1	100.0	3669	26 4
6-7	35.4	34.0	20.2	8.0	2.3	U	100.0	3497	26.9
8-9	31.1	37.4	20.8	9.8	0.9	U	100.0	2901	27.2
10+	35.0	40.5	20.3	4.2	U	U	100.0	6248	NC
Total	36.1	36.3	19.5	6.6	1.3	0.1	100.0	23136	26.6
				WIVES OF STERILIZED MEN					
<2	33.9	26.2	24.3	9.1	3.5	2.9	100.0	122	27.1
2-3	27.7	34.3	22.4	10.2	4.1	1.3	100.0	124	27.4
4-5	39.6	28.1	15.6	11.4	5.2	—	100 0	205	25 8
6-7	32.9	28.0	25.7	9.5	3.9	U	100 0	222	27 9
8-9	32.5	33.2	21.1	12.1	1.0	U	100.0	221	27.7
10+	38.5	39.9	18.5	3.1	U	U	100.0	2021	NC
Total	37.1	36.8	19.5	5.4	1.1	0.2	100.0	2916	26.7
				STERILIZED COUPLES					
<2	38.5	34.5	18.4	6.4	1.5	0.6	100 0	3776	26.3
2-3	38.8	34.5	17.9	6.8	1.7	0.3	100 0	3289	26 2
4-5	37.3	33.5	19.2	7.0	2.8	0.1	100.0	3873	26 4
6-7	35.3	33.7	20.5	8.1	2.4	U	100.0	3719	27.0
8-9	31.2	37.1	20.8	9.9	0.9	U	100.0	3123	27.3
10+	35.9	40.3	19.9	3.9	U	U	100.0	8269	NC
Totat	36.2	36.4	19.5	6.4	1.3	0.1	100.0	26051	26.6

NC: Not calculated due to censoring. U.: Not available.

— Less than 0.05 per cent.

1 Median ages are Calculated only for persons sterilized at less than 40 years of age to avoid problems of censoring.

Table 6.18: Timing of sterilization by state

Median age of currently married sterilized women or wives of sterilized men at the time of sterilization, by number of years since operation and state, India, 1992-93

State	Years since operation					
	<2	2-3	4-5	6-7	8-9	Total
India	26.3	26.2	26.4	27.0	27.3	26.6
North						
Delhi	29.0	27.6	28.4	28.4	27.7	28.2
Haryana	26.3	26.7	27.4	27.0	28.4	27.3
Himachal Pradesh	26.2	26.5	26.9	27.4	26.4	26.9
Jammu Region of J & K	28.4	27.8	28.2	29.8	29.4	28.6
Punjab	27.4	27.1	28.4	28.4	28.5	27.9
Rajasthan	28.3	27.9	27.2	27.1	28.0	27.7
Central						
Madhya Pradesh	28.0	26.9	26.8	27.5	27.5	27.3
Uttar Pradesh	29.3	29.1	30.2	29.7	29.7	29.6
East						
Bihar	28.1	27.5	27.2	28.3	29.3	28.1
Orissa	27.7	27.2	26.4	26.7	27.1	26.8
West Sengal	25.7	25.2	25.8	26.7	26.1	26.0
Northeast						
Arunachal Pradesh	28.3	28.5	29.5	30.5	24.8	28.0
Assam	28.0	26.6	27.1	27.7	28.3	27.1
Manipur	28.3	29.0	30.0	29.7	31.8	29.7
Meghalaya	29.8	31.8	29.0	28.0	27.0	27.9
Mizoram	28.6	29.5	28.3	28.3	28.9	28.8
Nagaland	31.5	33.0	30.5	29.3	26.8	29.3
Tripura	28.3	27.7	26.0	30.6	29.2	28.1
West						
Goa	28.7	29.3	29.3	28.8	29.4	28.5
Gujarat	27.8	27.7	27.2	27.7	27.6	27.5
Maharashtra	24.7	25.6	24.9	26.5	26.0	25.6
South						
Andhra Pradesh	24.3	23.8	24.2	24.3	25.7	24.5
Karnataka	24.9	25.0	24.6	24.9	25.9	25.2
Kerala	26.6	26.1	27.0	26.8	27.5	26.5
Tamil Nadu	25.0	26.2	26.4	26.4	27.4	26.2

Note: Medians are not shown for persons sterilized 10 or more years before the survey, and median ages are calculated only for persons sterilized at less than 40 years of age to avoid problems of censoring.

Table 6.19: Methods used before sterilization

Per centage of sterilized persons who used specific contraceptive methods before the sterilization by state, India, 1992-93

	Method used before sterilization							
State	None	Pill	IUD	Injection	Condom	Periodic abstinence	Withdrawal	Other
India	81.9	4.2	4.3	0.2	5.5	7.2	3.8	0.6
North								
Delhi	49.7	10.1	17.8	0.5	30.0	11.0	7.0	2.7
Haryana	76.7	3.7	5.0	0.2	9 9	9 0	7.2	0.9
Himachal Pradesh	67.6	4.5	8.2	0.4	13 0	12 6	7 4	1.6
Jammu Resion of J & K	64.7	8.1	5.8	—	15.1	12.7	11 2	0.4
Punjab	73.1	3.7	7.1	0.3	9.6	8 4	5 1	0.4
Rajasthan	91.3	2.5	2.2	0.4	2.5	2 0	1 9	0.1
Central								
Madhya Pradesh	86.7	3.6	2.4	0.3	6.4	3.4	0.9	0.2
Uttar Pradesh	88.9	3.5	3.5	0.1	3.7	3.1	1.0	0.5
East								
Bihar	91.6	2.3	0.8	—	2.9	2.5	1.0	0.2
Orissa	88.2	3.4	3.9	—	1.9	4.3	0.8	0.8
West Bengal	57.3	10.9	2.2	0.6	7.1	27.8	15.9	1.4
Northeast								
Arunachal Pradesh	62.9	19.1	13.5	1.1	5.6	10.1	3.4	1.1
Assam	46.2	13.8	5.8	0.4	5.8	37.2	17.6	2.5
Manipur	70.7	2.4	9.8		2.4	17.1	—	2.4
Meghalaya	77.0	10.0	5.0	—	2.0	4.0	2.0	4.0
Mizoram	85.4	5.7	6.7	0.2	0.7	1.7	1.5	—
Nagaland	86.4	7.6	4.5	7.6	7.6	3 0	4.5	—
Tripura	33.3	22.9	4.7	—	7.3	39 1	24.0	1.6
West								
Goa	84.4	3.3	4.7	—	5.3	5.6	3.1	0.7
Gujarat	86.0	2.5	4.1	0.1	4.0	5.6	1.3	0.2
Maharashtra	86.9	4.7	5.2	0.1	5.6	2.5	0.5	—
South								
Andhra Pradesh	93.0	2.3	2.0	0.3	2.1	1.1	0.2	0.3
Karnataka	83.1	3.2	7.5	0 2	3.4	5 9	0 6	1 1
Kerala	60.6	4.8	8.6	0 2	14.9	18 1	16 4	0 5
Tamil Nadu	81.3	3.1	5.6	0.2	5.1	6.7	4.9	0.8

Note: Percentages may add to more than 100.0 because all prior methods are included
— Less than 0.05 per cent.

In order to assess the relative importance of various sources of contraceptive methods, the NFHS included a question about where current users of contraception obtained their methods. Overall, the public sector, consisting of government/municipal hospitals, Primary Health Centres and other governmental health infrastructure, provide services to 79 per cent of the current users of all modem methods, while the private medical sector, including private hospitals and clinics, private doctors, and pharmacies/drugstores serve 15 per cent of current users (Table 6.20 and Figure 6.5). Only 6 per cent of users obtain their methods from other sources, such as shops, friends or relatives.

The mix of public and private sector sources varies substantially according to the method used. For clinical methods (sterilizations and the IUD), the government is by far the major source of supply - 93 per cent of male sterilizations, 86 per cent of female sterilizations and 63 per cent of IUD insertions were done at a government source. The pill is obtained from both the government sector (31 per cent) and the private medical sector (42 per cent). More than onequarter of pill users obtain the pill from shops, friends and relatives. One-fifth of condom users obtain their supplies from the private medical sector, and another 65 per cent of condom users obtain their supplies from other sources, such as shops, friends or relatives.

With regard to specific sources of contraception, Primary Health Centres and government/municipal hospitals (the main institutions that provide contraceptive services) are the most important sources. Seventy-seven per cent of female sterilization acceptors, 81 per cent of male sterilization acceptors, 56 per cent of IUD users, and 21 per cent of pill users are served by these institutions. Private shops are major sources for condoms (39 per cent of condom users), and they also are the sources for 24 per cent of pill users. Pharmacies and drugstores serve 30 per cent of pill users. Twenty-four per cent of IUD insertions are done at private hospitals or clinics and 12 per cent by private doctors. Seven per cent of female sterilizations and 9 per cent of male sterilizations were done in sterilization camps.

Urban and rural areas differ regarding the sources of contraceptive methods. In rural areas, the public sector is the source of supply for 87 per cent of users, while in urban areas, the public sector is the source of supply for only 62 per cent of all users. In urban areas, private medical sources provide contraception to 26 per cent of users and other non-medical sources to 11 per cent of them; together, they supply 25 per cent of female sterilizations, 48 per cent of the IUD users, and 83 per cent of the pill users. As expected, other (non-medical) sources provided condoms for a sizeable per centage of users (70 per cent) in urban areas. Thus while government sources are important in urban as well as rural areas, their importance is particularly great in rural areas. In rural areas, the predominance of the public sector is particularly evident in the case of female and male sterilizations (91 and 96 per cent, respectively).

Table 6.20: Source of supply of modern contraceptive methods
Per cent distribution of current users of modern contraceptive methods by most recent source of supply, according to specific method and residence, India, 1992-93

Source of supply	Pill	Copper T./ IUD	in-jec-tion	Con-dom	Female sterile ization	Male steril-ization	All modern methods
			URBAN				
Public sector	17.3	52.2	*	7.8	74.6	86.1	62.4
Government/municipal hospital	11.3	44.3	*	5.0	62.5	66.6	51.6
Primary Health Centre	4.1	5.0	*	1.6	7.0	8.7	6.1
Sub-centre	0.3	0.4	*	0.4	0.2	—	0.2
Family planning clinic	0.3	0.8	*	0.3	0.7	2.5	0.8
Public mobile clinic	0.1	0.2	*	0.2	0.1	0.4	0.1
Camp	—	—	*	—	3.6	7.8	3.0
Government paramedic	0.9	0.5	*	0.1	—	—	0.1
Other	0.3	1.1	*	0.2	0.5	0.2	0.5
Private Medical sector	49.9	46.1	*	21.8	24.9	9.8	26.3
Private hospital or clinic	5.0	32.8	*	0.8	22.8	7.3	19.0
Pharmacy/drugstore	35.6	—	*	19.4	—	—	4.0
Private doctor	8.8	13.2	*	1.5	2.0	2.4	3.2
Other	0.5	—	*	0.2	0.1	—	0.1
Other source	32.8	1.7	*	70.3	0.6	4.1	11.2
Shop	30.3	—	*	46.3	—	—	7.2
Husband	—	—	*	19.7	—	—	2.5
Friend/relative	1.9	—	*	0.8	—	—	0.2
Other	0.6	1.7	*	3.5	0.6	4.1	1.3
Total per cent	100.0	100.0	100.0	100.0	100.0	100.0	100.0
Number	425	865	5	1280	6702	715	9992
			RURAL				
Public sector	41.0	74.9	*	27.4	90.8	95.7	87.0
Government/municipal hospital	8.0	31.5	*	7.4	54.2	47.2	49.6
Primary Health Centre	16.3	32.1	*	11.7	26.5	36.2	26.9
Sub-centre	11.5	8.0	*	6.6	0.7	1.5	1.6

{Cont}.....

Family planning clinic	0.9	0.7	*	0.2	0.7	0.7	0.7
Public mobile clinic	0.2	0.2	*	0.1	0.4	0.5	0.4
Camp	—	—	*	—	8.2	9.5	7.5
Government paramedic	3.5	2.3	*	0.9	—	—	0.2
Other	0.5	0.1	*	—	0.1	0.1	0.1
Private Medical sector	35.5	23.6	*	17.8	8.6	2.6	9.6
Private hospital or clinic	1.6	13.0	*	0.9	7.7	2.0	6.9
Pharmacy/drugstore	26.6	—	*	13.8	—	—	1.3
Private doctor	5.0	10.3	*	1.5	0.8	0.5	1.3
Other	2.4	0.4	*	1.6	0.1	0.1	0.2
Other source	23.5	1.4	*	54.8	0.6	1.7	3.4
Shop	19.9	—	*	26.8	—	—	1.6
Husband	—	—	*	23.6	—	—	0.9
Friend/relative	3.1	—	*	0.9	—	—	0.1
Other	0.6	1.4	*	3.5	0.6	1.7	0.9
Total per cent	100.0	100.0	100.0	100.0	100.0	100.0	100.0
Number	588	725	28	775	16434	2201	20750
			TOTAL				
Public sector	31.0	62.6	(54.8)	15.2	86.1	93.4	79.0
Government/municipal hospital	9.3	38.4	(31.8)	6.1	56.6	52.0	50.2
Primary Health Centre	11.2	17.4	(17.8)	5.5	20.8	29.4	20.1
Sub-centre	6.8	3.9	(0.7)	2.7	0.6	1.1	1.1
Family planning clinic	0.7	0.7	(—)	0.2	0.7	1.2	0.7
Public mobile clinic	0.1	0.2	(4.5)	0.2	0.3	0.5	0.3
Camp	—	—	(—)	—	6.9	9.1	6.0
Government paramedic	2.4	1.3	(—)	0.4	—	—	0.2
Other	0.4	0.6	(—)	0.1	0.2	0.1	0.2
Private medical sector	41.5	35.8	(45.2)	20.3	13.3	4.3	15.0
Private hospital or clinic	3.0	23.8	(14.5)	0.8	12.1	3.3	10.8
Pharmacy/drugstore	30.4	—	(—)	17.3	—	—	2.2
Private doctor	6.6	11.9	(25.6)	1.5	1.1	1.0	1.9
Other	1.6	0.2	(5.1)	0.7	0.1	0.1	0.2
Other source	27.4	1.6	(—)	64.5	0.6	2.3	6.0
Shop	24.3	—	(—)	38.9	—	—	3.4
Husband	—	—	(—)	21.2	—	—	1.4
Friend/relative	2.6	—	(—)	0.9	—	—	0.1
Other	0.6	1.6	(—)	3.5	0.6	2.3	1.0
Total per cent	100.0	100.0	100.0	100.0	100.0	100.0	100.0
Number	1013	1589	33	2055	23136	2916	30741

( ) Based on 25-49 unweighted cases

* Per cent not shown; based on fewer than 25 unweighted cases — Less than 0.05 per cent.

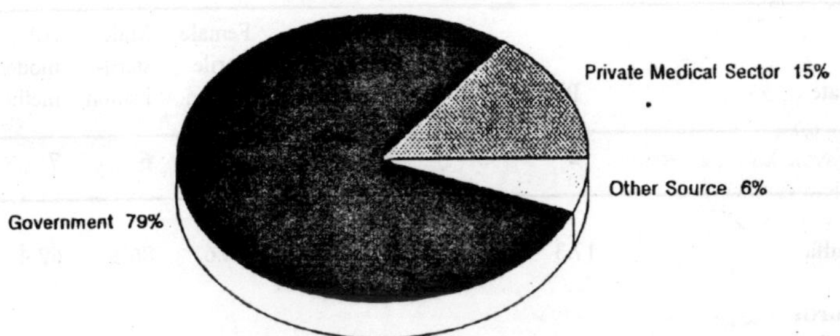

Figure 6.5: Source of Family Planning Among Current Users of Modern Contraceptive Methods

Interstate variations in the extent to which the public sector supplies contraceptive services are shown in Table 6.21. The public sector is the major source for sterilization in both urban and rural areas (particularly the latter) in all the states. In general, sterilization acceptors in the northern, central and eastern states rely more on the public sector for the services than those in the western and southern states. In Himachal Pradesh, Jammu, Punjab, Rajasthan, Orissa, Tripura and Haryana, more than 95 per cent of sterilized women reported having obtained their services from the public sector, whereas in Andhra Pradesh, Kerala, Maharashtra and Gujarat, 77-80 per cent of sterilized women received the services from the public sector. For the modern temporary methods, the utilization of public sector services is relatively low, but there are interstate variations. Ninety-two per cent of IUD insertions in Orissa were done in the public sector, whereas this sector provided services to only 48 per cent of the IUD users in Maharashtra and Tamil Nadu.

Table 6.21: Public sector as source of modern contraceptives
Per centage of current users of modern contraceptive methods who reported the public sector as the source of supply, according to specific method, residence and state, India, 1992-93

State	Pill	Copper T./ IUD	Condom	Female sterile ization	Male steril- ization	All modern methods
1	2	3	4	5	6	7
			URBAN			
India	17.3	52.2	7.8	74.6	86.1	62.4
North						
Delhi	21.7	56.5	7.6	75.4	87.5	45.2
Haryana	*	57.7	14.7	91.6	(97.9)	65.8
Himachal Pradesh	*	83.5	14.2	96.9	98.8	75.2
Jammu Region of J & K	*	69.8	6.8	91.1	(95.6)	62.8
Punjab	*	69.4	9.6	89.1	*	62.7
Rajasthan	*	(80.0)	12.0	96.5	(100.0)	85.6
Central						
Madhya Pradesh	*	73.2	9.2	89.7	90.8	74.9
Uttar Pradesh	(26.2)	49.2	4.4	86.7	93.0	55.2
East						
Bihar	(8.0)	*	4.0	67.7	(66.0)	55.0
Orissa	(22.2)	(85.7)	*	88.0	(81.8)	79.7
West Bengal	(5.0)	*	(6.0)	77.2	*	57.9
Northeast						
Arunachal Pradesh	*	*	*	*	*	(72.2)
Assam	(2.6)	*	12.7	74.5	*	55.8
Manipur	*	(80.0)	*	(93.8)	*	80.4
Meghalaya	*	*	*	(64.9)	*	58.5
Mizoram	*	*	*	94.1	*	87.4
Nagaland	*	*	*	(84.6)	*	(68.9)
Tripura	*	*	*	(93.6)	*	69.6
West						
Goa	*	(43.2)	11.5	76.7	*	62.7
Gujarat	*	44.9	(4.3)	72.6	(85.7)	63.6
Maharashtra	(13.9)	38.9	8.6	62.7	(90.9)	55.2
South						
Andhra Pradesh	*	*	*	62.9	78.9	61.8
Karnataka	*	52.9	(10.3)	75.2	*	68.9
Kerala	*	(65.4)	(13.6)	75.6	86.2	72.1
Tamil Nadu	*	41.0	(2.6)	72.4	*	63.3

{Cont.}

1	2	3	4	5	6	7
			RURAL			
India	41.0	74.9	27 4	90 8	95 7	87 0
North						
Delhi	*	*	8.6	(87.0)	*	46.2
Haryana	*	(76.2)	(22.5)	96.3	98.9	90.1
Himachal Pradesh	*	(84.6)	42.9	98.6	95.8	92.5
Jammu Region of J & K	*	(87.9)	9.2	98.2	100.0	86.2
Punjab	(39.6)	78.2	19.9	98.8	(100.0)	83.1
Rajasthan	*	(81.6)	*	97.1	96.5	95.1
Central						
Madhya Pradesh	(54.1)	*	61.7	96.4	98.4	94.9
Uttar Pradesh	55.5	(72.3)	20.8	95.4	96.6	83.6
East						
Bihar	(17.1)	*	(15.6)	91.2	(92.0)	83.7
Orissa	*	(94.4)	*	98.4	96.9	96.8
West Bengal	23.8	(90.0)	(17.6)	95.0	96.8	87.5
Northeast						
Arunachal Pradesh	*	(96.8)	*	92.6	*	89.6
Assam	(26.1)	*	*	89.8	(90.7)	76.2
Manipur	*	(76.0)	*	93.8	*	83.7
Meghalaya	*	*	*	78.9	*	73.5
Mizoram	*	(92.3)	*	95.0	*	94.0
Nagaland	*	*	*	(82.1)	*	71.6
Tripura	(15.6)	*	*	98.3	*	77.4
West						
Goa	*	(65.7)	(41.7)	85.3	*	80.7
Gujarat	*	(67.5)	*	84.1	89.7	82.3
Maharashtra	*	*	(57.7)	86.7	99.0	87.8
South						
Andhra Pradesh	*	*	*	84.7	92.0	85.6
Karnataka	*	72.6	*	92.4	(97.9)	90.9
Kerala	*	78.0	23.6	77.3	91.9	76.0
Tamil Nadu	*	58.8	*	88.7	92.5	85.8
			TOTAL			
India	31.0	62.6	15.2	86.1	93.4	79.0
North						
Delhi	21.9	56.0	7.7	76.2	86.9	45.2
Haryana	(43.3)	67.9	17.2	95.3	98.6	83.1

(Cont.)......

Himachal Pradesh	*	84.3	35.3	98.4	96.0	90.6
Jammu Region of J & K	(40.0)	79.9	8.3	97.1	99.1	81.1
Punjab	30.6	75.1	15.2	96.5	98.6	77.1
Rajasthan	(48.0)	81.0	28.4	97.0	97.5	92.3
Central						
Madhya Pradesh	(40.2)	76.6	25.9	94.7	96.9	89.2
Uttar Pradesh	46.7	58.6	11.8	93.4	95.4	74.5
East						
Bihar	14.3	(30.6)	9.7	85.8	82.8	76.1
Orissa	(42.8)	91.6	(22.9)	96.5	94.1	93.4
West Bengal	16.2	(82.3)	10.3	90.7	93.9	79.6
Northeast						
Arunachal Pradesh	(66.7)	(97.4)	*	90.7	*	85.7
Assam	22.2	(89.4)	16.6	86.6	90.8	72.0
Manipur	*	78.3	*	93.8	(100.0)	82.3
Meghalaya	*	*	*	73.4	*	68.2
Mizoram	*	(80.4)	*	94.5	*	90.6
Nagaland	*	*	*	83.1	*	70.7
Tripura	15.6	*	*	97.0	*	75.3
West						
Goa	*	53.2	21.1	81.5	(82.8)	72.0
Gujarat	(43.2)	53.2	6.2	80.4	88.4	75.5
Maharashtra	36.5	47.9	21.9	77.7	97.4	74.8
South						
Andhra Pradesh	*	*	(31.0)	78.0	88.3	78.1
Karnataka	*	62.3	(14.6)	86.9	95.1	83.4
Kerala	*	75.0	19.8	76.8	90.0	74.9
Tamil Nadu	*	48.1	5.3	83.6	91.5	78.0

Note: Public sector includes government/municipal hospital, Primary Health Centre, sub-centre, family planning clinic, public mobile clinic, camp and government paramedic.

() Based on 25-49 unweighted cases.

* Per centage not shown; based on fewer than 25 unweighted cases — Less than 0.05 per cent.

6.4 Reasons for Discontinuation

All currently married women who had ever used contraception but who were not using any method at the time of the survey and were not currently pregnant were asked why they had discontinued their use of contraception. Their responses to this question are presented in Table 6.22. Apart from "other" reasons such as the onset of menopause or the absence of the husband (mentioned by 31 per cent), the most commonly mentioned reasons for discontinuing a method are the desire to have a child (28 per cent of discontinuers) and health problems (15 per cent). Another 7 per cent of the discontinuers reported that they discontinued the use because the method created menstrual problems. Method failure was the reason for discontinuation for 5 per cent of the women. With a little motivation and improvement in services, these women may be successfully brought under the programme again.

6.5 Intention to Use Family Planning in the Future

In the NFHS, all currently married women who were not using contraception at the time of the interview (including those who were currently pregnant) were asked about their future intentions regarding the use of family planning and their method preference if they intended to use contraception. This type of information can assist family planning programme administrators in identifying potential groups of users and in providing the types of contraception that are likely to be in demand. Responses to the questions on future use according to past use, place of residence, and number of living children are given in Table 6.23.

Table 6.22: Reasons for discontinuation

Per cent distribution of nonpregnant, currently married ever users who are not currently using a contraceptive method by main reason for stopping use and residence, India, 1992-93

Reason for stopping use	Urban	Rural	Total
Method failed/got pregnant	3.4	6.4	5.3
Lack of sexual satisfaction	1.4	2.1	1.8
Created menstrual problem	7.6	6.0	6.6
Created health problem	20.2	11.6	14.6
Inconvenient to use	3.6	2.2	2.7
Hard to get method	0.7	1.2	1.0
Put on weight	0.6	0.3	0.4
Did not like the method	3.8	4.1	4.0
Wanted to have a child	24.7	30.3	28.4
Wanted to replace dead child	0.2	0.7	0.5
Lack of privacy for use	2.2	1.0	1.4
Other	29.1	32.0	31.0
Don't know/missing	2.6	2.1	2.3
Total per cent	100.0	100.0	100.0
Number	1462	2718	4180

Overall, 58 per cent of currently married nonusers reported that they do not intend to use contraception in the future. Twenty-nine per cent said that they would use in the future, and another 13 per cent were unsure of their intentions. The high proportion of women who do not intend to use family planning suggests that it will be difficult for the family planning programme to succeed without a strong Information, Education and Communication (IEC) component to motivate couples to use contraception.

Among those intending to use family planning, 48 per cent said they would use contraception within the next 12 months, almost an equal proportion said they would use it at a later stage, and 5 per cent were unsure when they would start using contraception. Among women who have never used contraceptive methods before, the majority (60 per cent) reported that they do not intend to use them in the future, and 14 per cent were not sure of their intentions. In contrast, 55 per cent of the smaller number of women who have used contraception in the past, but are not currently using, intend to use contraception again in the future; another 7 per cent are not sure of their intentions.

The proportion of women who intend to use family planning in the future increases gradually with each additional living child up to two, then declines slightly among women with three or more children. For instance, whereas only 15 per cent of women with no living children expressed an intention to use contraceptives in the future, this per centage reaches 36 for those with two living children and then declines to 27 per cent of women with four or more living children. This drop-off in the per centage intending to use family planing among women with four or more children may reflect their relatively advanced ages and consequent infecundability. Intentions to use a contraceptive method in the future do not vary substantially between urban and rural areas.

There are considerable interstate variations in the proportion of women (currently married nonusers) who expressed an intention to use family planning in the future (Table 6.24). In the four large states of Uttar Pradesh, Bihar, Madhya Pradesh and Rajasthan only 19-25 per cent of the current nonusers intend to use a method in the future. It is worth noting that these are the states where the current use of contraception is also low. On the other hand, in Haryana, Himachal Pradesh, Punjab, Gujarat and Kerala, where the contraceptive prevalence rate is 50 per cent or more, a greater proportion of the current nonusers expressed an intention to use contraception in the future.

6.6 Reasons for Nonuse of Contraception

Currently married women who are not using any contraceptive method and who say that they do not intend to use contraception at any time in the future are asked the main reason they do not intend to use a

Table 6.23: Future use

Per cent distribution of currently married women who are currently not using any contraceptive method by intention to use in the future, according to number of living children, residence and whether ever used contraception, India, 1992-93

Past use/ intention to use in future	Number of living children 0	1	2	3	4+	Total
			URBAN			
Never used contraception						
Intends to use in next 12 months	2.2	11.9	13.9	16.1	14.6	11.8
Intends to use later	13.4	16.9	12.8	10.5	3.5	11.7
Intends to use, unsure when	0.4	1.0	1.7	0.6	1.0	1.0
Unsure as to intention	15.0	9.3	6.9	7.7	8.0	9.3
Does not intend to use	64.0	47.3	38.3	42.1	53.8	48.7
Missing	0.2	0.6	0.3	0.1	0.5	0.4
Previously used contraception						
Intends to use in next 12 months	0.1	3.2	9.1	8.1	6.0	5.3
Intends to use later	1.6	4.2	4.7	2.7	1.2	3.0
Intends to use, unsure when	0.2	0.2	0.8	0.4	0.3	0.4
Unsure as to intention	0.9	1.0	1.5	1.6	1.3	1.2
Does not intend to use	2.0	4.2	9.9	10.1	9.8	7.1
Missing	—	0.1	0.2	0.1	0.1	0.1
Total per cent	100.0	100.0	100.0	100.0	100.0	100.0
All currently married nonusers						
Intends to use in next 12 months	2.3	15.2	23.0	24.2	20.6	17.1
Intends to use later	15.0	21.1	17.5	13.2	4.7	14.7
Intends to use, unsure when	0.7	1.2	2.6	1.0	1.3	1.4
Unsure as to intention	15.9	10.3	8.3	9.4	9.3	10.5
Does not intend to use	65.9	51.5	48.2	52.1	63.6	55.8
Missing	0.2	0.7	0.5	0.1	0.6	0.5
Total per cent	100.0	100.0	100.0	100.0	100.0	100.0
Number	1858	2757	2456	1501	2239	10812
			RURAL			
Never used contraception						
Intends to use in next 12 months	1.6	6.7	10.4	14.6	15.3	10.0
Intends to use later	11.2	17.7	14.8	9.6	5.0	11.5
Intends to use, unsure when	0.4	0.9	1.4	1.4	0.9	1.0
Unsure as to intention	17.9	13.6	10.6	12.0	11.8	13.0
Does not intend to use	66.2	54.1	51.1	51.3	55.1	55.3
Missing	0.2	0.1	0.2	0.2	0.3	0.2
Previously used contraception						
Intends to use in next 12 months	0.2	1.8	3.8	4.5	4.5	3.0
Intends to use later	0.8	2.2	2.7	1.9	0.9	1.7

{Cont}....

Intends to use, unsure when		0.2	0.6	0.5	0.4	0.3
Unsure as to intention	0.3	0.5	0.9	0.6	0.8	0.7
Does not intend to use	1.2	2.0	3.6	3.4	4.9	3.2
Missing	—	—	—	0.1	0.1	0.1
Total per cent	100.0	100.0	100.0	100.0	100.0	100.0
All currently married nonusers						
Intends to use in next 12 months	1.8	8.5	14.2	19.1	19.8	13.1
Intends to use later	12.0	19.9	17.4	11.4	5.9	13.1
Intends to use, unsure when	0.4	1.2	1.9	1.8	1.3	1.3
Unsure as to intention	18.2	14.2	11.4	12.6	12.7	13.7
Does not intend to use	67.3	56.1	54.7	54.7	59.9	58.5
Missing	0.2	0.1	0.2	0.3	0.5	0.3
Total per cent	100.0	100.0	100.0	100.0	100.0	100.0
Number	6584	8868	7676	6054	10321	39502
		TOTAL				
Never used contraception						
Intends to use in next 12 months	1.7	8.0	11.3	14.9	15.2	10.4
Intends to use later	11.7	17.5	14.3	9.8	4.7	11.5
Intends to use, unsure when	0.4	0.9	1.5	1.2	0.9	1.0
Unsure as to intention	17.3	12.6	9.7	11.1	11.1	12.2
Does not intend to use	65.7	52.5	48.0	49.5	54.8	53.4
Missing	0.2	0.2	0.2	0.2	0.4	0.3
Previously used contraception						
Intends to use in next 12 months	0.2	2.1	5.1	5.2	4.7	3.5
Intends to use later	1.0	2.7	3.2	2.0	1.0	2.0
Intends to use, unsure when	0.1	0.2	0.6	0.5	0.4	0.4
Unsure as to intention	0.5	0.7	1.0	0.8	0.9	0.8
Does not intend to use	1.4	2.6	5.2	4.8	5.7	4.0
Missing	—	—	0.1	0.1	0.1	0.1
Total per cent	100.0	100.0	100.0	100.0	100.0	100.0
All currently married nonusers						
Intends to use in next 12 months	1.9	10.1	16.3	20.1	19.9	13.9
Intends to use later	12.6	20.2	17.5	11.8	5.7	13.5
Intends to use, unsure when	0.5	1.2	2.1	1.7	1.3	1.3
Unsure as to intention	17.7	13.3	10.7	11.9	12.1	13.0
Does not intend to use	67.0	55.0	53.1	54.2	60.6	57.9
Missing	0.2	0.3	0.3	0.3	0.5	0.3
Total per cent	100.0	100.0	100.0	100.0	100.0	100.0
Number	8441	11625	10132	7555	12560	5031

— Less than 0.05 per cent Includes current pregnancy, if any.

Table 6.24: Future use by state

Per centage of currently married women not currently using contraception who intend to use any time in future, by number of living children, according to state, India, 1992-93

State	Number of living children					
	0	1	2	3	4+	Total
India	15.0	31.5	35.9	33.6	26.9	28.8
North						
Delhi	20.4	41.1	39.7	41.1	42.1	37.4
Haryana	38.1	65.9	68.0	64.1	52.3	58.7
Himachal Pradesh	30.9	56.9	63.0	51.0	40.7	50.0
Jammu Region of J & K	32.3	60.4	61.4	66.5	50.3	54.0
Punjab	23.5	52.7	57.0	49.1	42.9	46.8
Rajasthan	8.6	17.2	26.0	24.9	22.2	19.8
Central						
Madhya Pradesh	11.8	24.6	30.2	32.2	27.5	25.1
Uttar Pradesh	7.1	15.0	20.5	21.9	23.0	18.7
East						
Bihar	11.9	23.4	26.6	28.5	24.9	23.3
Orissa	13.5	28.2	34.0	37.6	29.6	28.8
West Bengal	27.7	55.6	56.3	58.9	37.8	47.1
Northeast						
Arunachal Pradesh	7.9	23.6	29.8	25.0	23.1	23.4
Assam	15.0	39.7	53.8	53.5	47.0	44.4
Manipur	(2.6)	24.0	36.1	41.9	26.6	28.4
Meghalaya	21.4	19.6	20.6	19.8	12.9	17.5
Mizoram	23.8	35.5	36.1	43.7	12.6	30.1
Nagaland	(2.3)	13.6	12.4	9.2	14.6	12.5
Tripura	35.6	58.7	59.6	55.9	43.4	50.9
West						
Goa	27.6	42.0	39.2	31.0	15.5	32.9
Gujarat	31.8	56.3	55.5	40.0	30.5	44.3
Maharashtra	11.1	31.0	38.1	41.6	34.8	31.5
South						
Andhra Pradesh	22.3	32.1	40.9	32.2	24.2	30.5
Karnataka	17.3	37.1	45.3	41.3	21.5	33.0
Kerala	25.5	52.8	51.1	43.1	15.0	41.3
Tamil Nadu	11.9	36.1	39.3	34.1	13.6	28.9

( ) Based on 25-49 unweighted cases.

1 Includes current pregnancy, if any.

Table 6.25: Reasons for nonuse

Per cent distribution of currently married women who are not using any contraceptive method and who do not intend to use in the future by main reason for not intending to use, according to age and residence, India, 1992-93

	Urban			Rural			Total		
Reason	Age <30	Age 30+	Total	Age <30	Age 30+	Total	Age <30	Age 30+	Total
Wants children	64.2	13.8	36.9	63.0	12.5	41.4	63.2	12.8	40.5
Wants a son	12.1	4.2	7.8	15.0	5.7	11.0	14.5	5.3	10.4
Wants a daughter	2.0	0.5	1.2	1.8	0.8	1.4	1.8	0.7	1.4
Worry about side effects	1.8	2.5	2.2	1.2	2.4	1.7	1.3	2.4	1.8
Can't work after sterilization	0.5	1.2	0.9	1.1	3.1	1.9	1.0	2.6	1.7
Lack of knowledge	1.8	2.3	2.1	3.8	6.2	4.8	3.5	5.3	4.3
Afraid of sterilization	1.6	2.6	2.2	1.6	4.5	2.9	1.6	4.0	2.7
Hard to get methods	0.2	0.4	0.3	0.1	0.4	0.2	0.2	0.4	0.3
Cost too much	0.3	0.4	0.4	0 4	0.6	0.5	0.4	0.5	0.4
Against religion	3.2	4.3	3.8	2.7	4.4	3.5	2.8	4.4	3.5
Opposed to family planning	0.3	1.3	0.9	0.9	2.0	1.4	0.8	1.9	1.3
Husband opposed	3.2	3.7	3.4	2.5	4.3	3.2	2.6	4.1	3.3
Other people opposed	0.6	0.5	0.6	0.4	0.4	0 .4	0.5	0. 4	0 .4
Difficult to get pregnant	1.7	14.3	8.5	0.8	8.1	3.9	1.0	9.6	4.9
Menopausal/had hysterectomy	0.4	25.3	13.9	0.1	25.7	11.0	0.2	25.6	11.6
Health does not permit	1.5	7.0	4.5	1.1	7.1	3.7	1.2	7.1	3.9

Inconvenient	0.3	2.9	1.7	0.1	0.9	0.5	0.2	1.4	0.7
Doesn't like existing methods	2.2	5.0	3.7	1.8	4.9	3.1	1.8	4.9	3.2
Other	1.8	7.7	5.0	1.4	6.0	3.3	1.4	6.4	3.7
Total per cent	100.0	100.0	100.0	100.0	100.0	100.0	100.0	100.0	100.0
Number	2763	3271	6034	13250	9858	23108	16013	13129	29142

method. Information on reasons for nonuse is crucial for designing successful information programmes and for understanding the obstacles to further increases in contraceptive prevalence. Reasons for not intending to use any method are indicated in Table 6.25. The largest proportion of women (52 per cent) say they do not intend to use contraception because they want more children, either in general or because they want a child of a specific sex, particularly a son. Not surprisingly, this reason is more common among women under age 30 (80 per cent) than among those 30 or older (19 per cent). It is worth noting that this reason for intended nonuse is almost as prevalent among urban women as among rural women. A small proportion (8 per cent) of women reported that contraception is either against their religion or that they or their husbands are against the use of family planning. A higher proportion of older women (10 per cent) gave these as reasons for not intending to use family planning than younger women (6 per cent). A significant proportion of older women (26 per cent) also reported their actual or perceived sterility as the main reason for not intending to use contraception in the future. Four per cent of all the women do not intend to use family planning methods due to a lack of knowledge. Therefore, there is still some scope for the family planning programme to increase contraceptive use through providing contraceptive information, particularly in rural areas.

6.7 Preferred Future Method of Family Planning

Women currently not using contraception who said they intend to use a method in the future were asked to specify the method of family planning that they want to use. Although female sterilization remains the most preferred method in the future (59 per cent), a sizeable proportion of women (31 per cent) intend to use a modern temporary method (Table 6.26). Among the temporary methods, the pill is the most preferred method (19 per cent), followed by the IUD (6 per cent) and condoms (4 per cent). Only 1 per cent of the intended future users prefer male sterilization.

The choice of preferred methods is slightly different for those who intend to use within 12 months than those who intend to use later, with the modern temporary methods being more popular in the former group and female sterilization being most popular in the latter. The pattern of preferred future methods is generally similar in both urban and rural areas, although the pill is more popular among intended users in rural areas, and condoms and IUDs are more popular in urban areas.

Table 6.26: Preferred method

Per cent distribution of currently married women who are not using a contraceptive method but who intend to use in the future by preferred method, according to whether they intend to use in the next 12 months or later, by residence, India, 1492-93

Preferred method	Next 12 months	Later	Unsure when	All women
	Timing of intended use			
URBAN				
Pill	18.9	7.4	7.8	13.3
Copper T/IUD	12.8	5.2	7.4	9.2
Injection	2.8	0.7	0.2	1.8
Condom	9.5	3.6	6.9	6.7
Female sterilization	45.3	72.7	54.2	57.8
Male sterilization	1.2	0.5	0.6	0.9
Periodic abstinence	3.0	1.5	3.0	2.4
Withdrawal	0.6	0.7	0.8	0.6
Other	1.9	1.9	2.9	1.9
Unsure	3.9	5.8	16.1	5.3
Total per cent	100.0	100.0	100.0	100.0
Number	1848	1594	153	3606
RURAL				
Pill	30.7	11.5	12.5	20.7
Copper T/IUD	7.4	2.2	4.8	4.8
Injection	3.0	1.4	1.5	2.1
Condom	5.3	1.6	2.7	3.4
Female sterilization	43.7	74.8	51.5	58.9
Male sterilization	0.8	1.1	1.0	0.9
Periodic abstinence	3.3	1.4	4.2	2.4
Withdrawal	0.8	0.3	0.5	0.5
Other	1.8	0.8	3.7	1.4
Unsure	3.2	5.1	17.5	4.8
Total per cent	100.0	100.0	100.0	100.0
Number	5166	5189	522	10911
TOTAL				
Pill	27.6	10.5	11.5	18.9
Copper T/IUD	8.8	2.9	5.4	5.9
Injection	3.0	1.2	1.2	2.1
Condom	6.4	2.1	3.6	4.2
Female sterilization	44.1	74.3	52.1	58.6
Male sterilization	0.9	0.9	0.9	0.9
Periodic abstinence	3.2	1.4	4.0	2.4

{Cont.}....				
Withdrawal	0.8	0.4	0.6	0.6
Other	1.8	1.1	3.5	1.5
Unsure	3.4	5.3	17.2	4.9
Total per cent	100.0	100.0	100.0	100.0
Number	7013	6782	675	14516

The contraceptive method mix that intended future users say they would prefer is substantially different from the methods selected by current users. Modern temporary methods are being used by only 14 per cent of current users (Table 6.5), but 31 per cent of intended future users say they would like to use modern temporary methods. These results suggest that the potential demand for modern temporary methods is relatively strong among intended future users and that the family welfare programme should pay increasing attention to these methods as part of a balanced programme to satisfy the contraceptive needs of women.

6.8 Exposure to Family Planning Messages on Radio and Television

For many years, the family welfare programme has been utilizing the electronic mass media to promote family planning. In order to explore the spread of family planning messages through various mass media, respondents were asked whether they had heard such messages on radio or television in the month prior to the survey. Table 6.27 shows the per centage of women who report seeing or hearing a family planning message according to various background characteristics. The effort to disseminate family planning information through the electronic mass media has succeeded in reaching less than half (42 per cent) of ever-married women. This is not surprising, given that only 21 per cent of households in India own televisions and only 39 per cent own radios (Table 3.13). About one in four women (22 per cent) reported hearing a message on both the radio and television in the month preceding the survey. One in seven (15 per cent) reported hearing a family planning message only on the radio, and 6 per cent of women only on television. This suggests-that there is substantial scope for electronic media to play a more significant role in reaching potential users of family planning in the future.

Urban-rural differences in exposure to family planning messages are substantial. While two-thirds (68 per cent) of urban women reported exposure to family planning messages on the radio or television, only one-third (33 per cent) of rural women did so. In urban areas, television and radio are about equally important in conveying family planning messages, but in rural areas, radio is far more important than television.

Table 6.27: Exposure to family planning messages on radio and television
Per cent distribution of ever-married women by whether they heard a radio or television message about family planning in the month prior to the interview, according to selected background characteristics, India, 1992-93

	Heard family planning message on radio/ or television						
Background characteristic Number	Neither	Radio only	Television only	Both	Missing	Total per cent	Number
Age							
13-19	63.2	17.9	4.2	14.6	—	100.0	9448
20-29	56.6	15.3	5.8	22.2	—	100.0	35424
30-39	56.4	13.4	6.6	23.6	—	100.0	27121
40-49	59.2	13.1	5.9	21.8	0.1	100.0	17784
Residbnce							
Urban	31.5	8.3	12.7	47.5	—	100.0	23455
Rural	67.0	16.8	3.5	12.7	—	100.0	66322
Education							
Illiterate	72.5	14.6	3.4	9.5	—	100.0	56656
Lit., < middle complete	44.0	18.3	8.5	29.1	—	100.0	16475
Middle school complete	30.3	15.5	11.5	42.7	—	100.0	6508
High school and above	15.3	7.9	12.0	64.7	—	100.0	10138
Religion							
Hindu	58.3	14.7	5.6	21.4	—	100.0	73648
Muslim	60.0	15.0	5.4	19.6	0.1	100.0	10806
Christian	47.8	17.5	6.3	28.4	—	100.0	2142
Sikh	43.3	5.6	21.4	29.7	—	100.0	1673
Jain	16.5	3.8	11.1	68.5	—	100.0	428
Buddhist	50.1	11.8	8.9	29.1	—	100.0	734
Other	75.3	9.2	3.2	12.2	—	100.0	345
Caste/tribe							
Scheduled caste	65.9	14.8	4.9	14.3	—	100.0	10970
Scheduled tribe	77.9	11.9	2.1	8.0	—	100.0	7934
Other	54.2	14.8	6.5	24.4	—	100.0	70872
Use of contraception							
Ever used	47.7	14.8	8.0	29.6	—	100.0	41172
Never used	66.3	14.4	4.1	15.1	—	100.0	48604
Total	57.8	14.6	5.9	21.7	—	100.0	89777

— Less than 0.05 per cent.

Women's exposure to family planning messages on the radio and television is positively related with educational attainment. Only 27 per cent of illiterate respondents reported having heard a family planning message on the radio or television, whereas 85 per cent of women with at least a high school education have heard a message. The proportion having heard a message on television or on both the radio and television increases sharply with increasing education.

There are almost no differences in the extent of exposure to family planning messages between Hindus and Muslims (40-42 per cent). The exposure to family planning messages on the radio or television is much higher among Christians (52 per cent), Sikhs (57 per cent) and especially Jains (84 per cent). The percentage who recall having heard a family planning message on the radio or television is lowest among scheduled tribe women (22 per cent) and highest among non-SC/ST women (46 per cent). All of these differentials are likely to reflect some combination of greater access to broadcast signals in urban than in rural areas, the greater ability of higher-income groups to own receivers, and the differential attentiveness to media messages associated with differing levels of education and leisure. Media messages on family planning are particularly unlikely to have reached women who have never used contraception, which is the group most in need of obtaining family planning information.

6.9 Acceptability of Family Planning Messages on Radio and Television

Regardless of whether women had heard a family planning message on the radio or television, they were asked whether they considered it acceptable for family planning information to be provided over the airwaves. Two-thirds of the sample women say it is acceptable to have family planning messages on the radio and television. Only 8 per cent say it is not acceptable and the rest (23 per cent) are not sure (Table 6.28). Younger women (under age 20) and older women (over age 39), rural residents, illiterate women, and women belonging to scheduled tribes are less likely than other women to think that it is acceptable to broadcast family planning messages on the radio or television. The acceptance of family planning messages on the electronic media is particularly high among women with at least a middle school education. A higher per centage of Christian, Sikh, Jain and Buddhist women find family planning messages on the radio and television to be acceptable than do the women belonging to other religions. The responses suggest a considerable amount of ambivalence regarding the acceptability of media messages on family planning among illiterate women and those belonging to scheduled tribes and scheduled castes.

Table 6.28: Acceptability of media messages on family planning

Per cent distribution of ever-married women by their attitude toward having messages about family planning on the radio or television, according to selected background characteristics, India, 1992-93

	Acceptability of media messages					
Background characteristic	Acceptable	Not acceptable	Unsure	Missing	Total per cent	Number of women
Age						
13-14	55.0	10.7	34.3	—	100.0	352
15-19	63.4	7.9	28.7	0.1	100.0	9095
20-24	69.6	7.7	22.7	—	100.0	17983
25-29	70.5	7.2	22.2	—	100.0	17441
30-34	70.2	8.1	21.7	—	100.0	14660
35-39	69.9	8.4	21.7	—	100.0	12461
40-44	66.8	9.7	23.4	0.1	100.0	9748
45-49	62.8	10.0	27.1	0.1	100.0	8036
Residence						
Urban	81.3	8.5	10.2	—	100.0	23455
Rural	63.7	8.1	28.1	—	100.0	66322
Education						
Illiterate	57.3	9.4	33.3	0.1	100.0	56656
Lit. ,< middle complete	83.9	6.2	9.9	—	100.0	16475
Middle school complete	90.2	4.6	5.1	—	100.0	6508
High school and above	90.6	7.0	2.3	—	100.0	10138
Religion						
Hindu	68.3	7.6	24.1	—	100.0	73648
Muslim	64.3	12.5	23.2	0.1	100.0	10806
Christian	76.8	8.0	15.2	—	100.0	2142
Sikh	79.6	5.3	15.1	—	100.0	1673
Jain	84.5	13.7	1.8	—	100.0	428
Buddhist	79.3	8.9	11.8	—	100.0	734
Other	49.0	14.6	36.4	—	100.0	345
Caste/tribe						
Scheduled caste	63.8	6.7	29.4	0.1	100.0	10970
Scheduled tribe	51.4	11.0	37.5	—	100.0	7934
Other	70.9	8.1	20.9	—	100.0	70872
Total	68.3	8.2	23.4	—	100.0	89777

— Less than 0.05 per cent.

6.10 Discussion of Family Planning Among Couples

Among nonsterilized couples, all currently married women who know a contraceptive method were asked how often they talked with their husbands about family planning in the year before the survey. The extent of such communication is fairly high. Overall, 51 per cent of women said they had discussed this topic with their husbands in the previous year (Table 6.29). Thirty-seven per cent discussed family planning once or twice and 13 per cent discussed it more often. A relatively high per centage (58 per cent) of women age 25-34 reported that they had discussed family planning with their husbands. Women in the early and late reproductive years are least likely to have communicated with their husbands on family planning, probably because younger women are still early in the family building process and hence are not yet interested in limiting family size, and older women no longer believe themselves to be at high risk of pregnancy (see Table 6.25).

Substantial differences in the extent of discussion of family planning among couples are also observed according to the place of residence, respondent's level of education, her husband's education, and the ever use of family planning. Women in urban areas are more likely to have discussed family planning with their husbands than those in rural areas (60 per cent compared to 47 per cent). As expected, the extent of husband-wife communication about family planning is positively related to the educational attainment of women, as well as the education of their husbands. For example, 71 per cent of women who completed high school had discussed family planning with their husbands compared to only 42 per cent of illiterate women. Similarly, interspousal communication was more common among women whose husbands had continued schooling beyond high school (68 per cent) than among those whose husbands were illiterate (41 per cent).

Around one-half of Hindus, Muslims and women belonging to "other" religions have discussed family planning with their husbands, compared to 56-75 per cent of Christian, Buddhist, Sikh and Jain women. The non-SC/ST women are more likely than scheduled caste and scheduled tribe women to have discussed family planning in the year preceding the survey.

Tabte 6.29: Discussion of family planning with husband
Per cent distribution of nonsterilized currently married women knowing a contraceptive method by the number of times they discussed family planning with their husbands in the past year, according to selected background characteristics, India, 1992-93.

Background characteristic	Number of times family planning discussed					
	Never	Once or twice	More often	Missing	Total per cent	Number of women
Age						
13-14	68.5	24.1	7.4	—	100.0	237
15-20	56.6	33.3	10. 0	0.1	100.0	7927
20-24	45.2	41.1	13.6	0.2	100.0	14747
25-29	40.8	42. 9	16.1	0.2	100.0	11280
30-34	43 2	40 3	16.2	0.3	100.0	7483
35-39	50.9	34.5	13.9	0 7	100.0	5436
40-44	62 1	26.2	11.2	0.5	100.0	4189
45-49	71.2	21.2	7.2	0.4	100.0	3700
Residence						
Urban	39.9	42.6	17.1	0.4	100.0	14369
Rural	52.7	35.1	12.0	0.2	100.0	40667
Respondent 's education						
Illiterate	57.5	33.0	9 2	0.3	100 0	34187
Lit., < middle complete	42 2	41 7	15.9	0.3	100.0	9218
Middle school complete	35.0	44.3	20.5	0.2	100.0	4167
High school and above	29.0	45.9	24.9	0.2	100.0	7464
Religion						
Hindu	50.1	37.0	12.6	0.3	100.0	43837
Muslim	49.7	35.3	14.8	0.2	100.0	8153
Christian	43.8	34.7	21.0	0.5	100.0	1171
Sikh	32.8	46.6	20.5	--	100.0	1070
Jain	24.6	53.5	20.9	0.9	100.0	266
Buddhist	41.3	47.9	10.8	--	100.0	365
Other	49.5	39.0	11.5	--	100.0	173
Caste/tribe						
Scheduled caste	54.4	34.9	10.5	0.3	100.0	6914
Scheduled tribe	58.0	32.0	9.7	0.2	100.0	4207
Other	47.8	37.8	14.1	0.3	100.0	43915
Use of contraception						
Ever used	24.2	48.4	27.2	0.2	100.0	13687
Never used	57.7	33.2	8.7	0.3	100.0	41350
Husband 's education						
Illiterate	59.1	31.7	8.9	0.3	100.0	18697

{Cont}.........						
Lit.,< primary complete	53.5	33.7	12.4	0.3	100.0	4954
Primary school complete	51.2	36.7	11.9	0.2	100.0	7982
Middle school complete	44.9	40.1	14.8	0.2	100.0	7016
High school complete	41.2	42.7	15.8	0.3	100.0	10606
Above high school	31.9	43.7	24.2	0.2	100.0	5673
Missing	48.7	30.4	14.1	6.8	100.0	109
Total	49.4	37.0	13.3	0.3	100.0	55036

Note: Table excludes women who are sterilized or whose husbands are sterilized.
— Less than 0.05 per cent.

A large majority (76 per cent) of the women who have ever used a family planning method discussed the topic with their husbands in the last year, 48 per cent having discussed it once or twice and 27 per cent having discussed it more often. Among those who have never used family planning, however, only 42 per cent have discussed family planning with their husbands in the past year.

6.11 Attitudes of Couples Toward Family Planning

Information on attitudes toward family planning was obtained by asking women whether they and their husbands approved or disapproved of couples using a method to delay or avoid pregnancy. Table 6.30 shows the degree of consensus between women's attitudes and those of their husbands. Of course, women may not accurately report their husband's actual attitudes toward contraception. However, a wife's perception of her husband's attitude is important since it may affect her own decisions.

Table 6.30 shows that 77 per cent of currently married, nonsterilized women who know of a contraceptive method approve of family planning use and only 22 per cent disapprove. Whereas 21 per cent of women say they do not know their husband's attitude, 19 per cent think that their husbands disapprove of family planning. There is a substantial amount of consensus between individual husbands and wives regarding the approval of family planning. In fact, 58 per cent of female respondents reported that both they and their husbands approve of family planning and 12 per cent said they both disapprove. This pattern of consensus among couples in favour of family planning makes the task of family planning administrators much easier.

Table 6.30: Attitudes of couples toward family Planning

For nonsterilized currently married women who know of a contraceptive method, the percentage who approve of family planning by their perception of their husband's attitude, according to selected background characteristics, India, 1992-93

	Respondent approves			Respondent disapproves					
Background characteristic	Husband approves	Husbands disap-proves	Husband attitude unknown'	Husband approves	Husbands disap-proves	Husbands attitude unknowns	Respon-dent unsure	Total percent	Number of women
1	2	3	4	5	6	7	8	9	10
Respondent's age									
13-14	42.0	3.7	24.2	2.2	8.8	16.9	2.2	100.0	273
15-19	56.5	5.6	16.9	1.2	8.9	10.0	0.8	100.0	7927
20-24	63.2	6.2	11.7	1.1	9.3	7.5	0.9	100.0	14747
25-29	63.9	6.7	9.3	1.3	10.2	7.7	0.9	100.0	11280
30-34	59.2	7.6	8.6	1.2	13.4	8.9	1.2	100.0	7483
35-39	55.1	8.4	9.8	1.6	14.0	10.0	1.1	100.0	5436
40-44	46.9	9.1	12.1	1.6	16.9	12.5	1.0	100.0	4189
45-49	44.4	8.2	14.0	1.7	15.7	14.8	1.2	100.0	3700
Residence									
Urban	70.7	7.4	7.7	1.3	8.6	3.6	0.7	100.0	14369
Rural	54.1	6.8	13.0	1.3	12.5	11.3	1.1	100.0	40667
Respondent's education									
Illiterate	47.9	7.3	14.4	1.4	14.6	13.4	1.1	100.0	34187
Lit. < middle complete	67.7	8.3	8.9	1.5	8.9	4.0	0.8	100.0	9218
Middle school complete	76.6	6.5	7.3	1.2	5.3	2.1	1.0	100.0	4167

1	2	3	4	5	6	7	8	9	10
High school and above	85.2	4.2	4.7	0.8	3.7	0.9	0.6	100.0	7464
Religion									
Hindu	59.2	6.6	12.0	1.3	10.2	9.6	1.0	100.0	43837
Muslim	49.3	9.2	10.1	1.6	19.5	9.4	0.9	100.0	8153
Christian	65.3	8.1	10.8	1.5	9.1	4.2	1.0	100.0	1171
Sikh	83.4	2.5	9.1	0.9	2.6	1.4	0.1	100.0	1070
Jain	83.3	3.8	3.9	1.7	5.0	1.3	1.1	100.0	266
Buddhist	60.0	12.0	7.4	1.2	12.1	6.2	1.1	100.0	365
Other	54.2	3.3	11.4	1.9	18.5	10.4	0.3	100.0	173
Caste/tribe									
Scheduled caste	55.0	6.9	14.1	1.2	10.1	11.7	1.0	100.0	6914
Scheduled tribe	50.0	4.8	14.3	2.2	13.0	14.7	1.0	100.0	4207
Other	59.8	7.2	10.9	1.2	11.5	8.4	1.0	100.0	43915
Use of contraception									
Ever used	85.4	5.8	2.8	1.3	3.4	0.8	0.6	100.0	13687
Never used	49.5	7.4	14.5	1.3	14.1	12.1	1.1	100.0	41350
Family planning discussed with husband in last year									
Never	37.6	7.0	20.1	1.4	16.1	17.0	0.9	100.0	27177
Once or twice	77.3	7.7	3.7	1.3	7.8	1.6	0.7	100.0	20377
More often	84.6	4.8	2.4	1.2	4.3	2.1	0.5	100.0	7331
Don't knowmissing	1.8	3.1	3.0	1.6	0.8	2.0	87.7	100.0	151

1	2	3	4	5	6	7	8	9	10
Husband's education									
Illiterate	45.9	7.9	14.7	1.3	14.9	14.4	1.0	100.0	18697
Lit., < primary complete	54.1	8.6	11.6	1.9	14.1	8.7	1.0	100.0	4954
Primary school complete	56.6	8.2	12.0	1.5	11.6	9.0	1.1	100.0	7982
Middle school complete	62.7	6.9	11.3	1.3	9.8	7.1	0.9	100.0	7016
High school complete	68.5	5.3	9.3	1.3	8.6	5.9	1.0	100.0	10606
Above high school	82.0	3.9	5.5	0.9	4.9	2.0	0.7	100.0	5673
Missing	47.5	9.4	14.0	—	7.1	14.7	7.3	100.0	109
Total	58.4	7.0	11.6	1.3	11.5	9.3	1.0	100.0	55036

Note: Table excludes women who are sterilized or whose husbands are sterilized.
— Less than 0.05 percent
1 Respondent does not know her husband's attitude
2 Includes women with missing information on approval of contraception

Table 6.31: Exposure to and acceptance of family planning messages and discussion and approval of famlly planning

Per centage of ever-married women who have heard a family planning message on the radio or television, who approve of media messages on family planning, and the percentage of nonsterilized currently married women knowing a contraceptive method who have discussed family planning with their husbands, and who approve and perceive that their husbands approve of family planning, according to state, India, 1992-43

State	Heard family planning message on the radio or television	Accept media messages on family planning	Discussed family planning with husband	Both husband and wife approve of family planning
1	2	3	4	5
India	42.2	68.3	50.3	58.4
North				
Delhi	74.3	76.2	66.9	76.4
Haryana	52.5	82.2	67.3	79.4
Himachal Pradesh	45.2	84.1	58.0	77.8
Jammu Region of J & K	60.4	79.9	62.1	80.2
Punjab	59.9	81.8	69.5	86.0
Rajasthan	33.3	55.1	44.2	59.1
Central				
Madhya Pradesh	34.3	50.0	36.3	50.3
Uttar Pradesh	32.7	50.3	47.8	42.3
East				
Bihar	26.6	37.5	34.6	46.0
Orissa	26.1	71.5	30.8	61.1
West Bengal	34.2	83.5	58.7	70.0
Northeast				
Arunachal Pradesh	29.9	48.5	53.4	52.1
Assam	23.7	85.3	78.7	76.3
Manipur	63.3	66.7	71.7	59.2
Meghalaya	35.4	34.7	48.2	44.4
Mizoram	50.8	70.7	55.9	60.6
Nagaland	38.6	41.5	79.5	57.9
Tripura	38.1	89.3	64.7	80.7
West				
Goa	74.2	83.4	58.5	67.1
Gujarat	47.4	81.4	58.5	70.1
Maharashtra	51.5	77.4	59.7	57.8

{Cont.}....

South				
Andhra Pradesh	58.4	86.7	41.6	77.1
Karnataka	66.8	77.8	56.9	63.2
Kerala	55.9	87.4	60.9	62.6
Tamil Nadu	51.9	92.5	47.9	63.7

The per centage of women approving family planning decreases slowly with the age of the woman. Urban women are more likely to approve of family planning than rural women (86 per cent versus 74 per cent). The approval of family planning by both husband and wife is 71 per cent in urban areas and 54 per cent in rural areas. Rural women are less likely to know their husband's attitude than urban women, a fact which is consistent with the lower level of interspousal communication about family planning in rural areas.

Education of women as well as their husbands is an important determinant of the approval of family planning by both husband and wife. Overall, 70 per cent of illiterate women approve of family planning compared to 94 per cent of women who have completed high school. Approval by both husband and wife is the lowest (48 per cent) among illiterate women. A similar relationship is observed with the level of husband's education. As the education of the husband increases, the proportion of women who reported that both they and their husbands approve of family planning increases, from 46 per cent in the case of illiterates to 82 per cent for those having more than a high school education.

Approval is lower among those belonging to scheduled tribes than among other groups. Eighty-five per cent of the women who have ever used family planning reported that both they and their husbands approve of family planning, compared with 50 per cent of never users. Among never users who approve of family planning, only 10 per cent said their husbands do not approve of family planning.

Table 6.30 also reveals that as expected, the approval of family planning by both the husband and wife is positively related to the number of times family planning was discussed between the husband and the wife in the past year. The per centage of women who reported that both they and their husbands approve family planning is 38 for those who did not discuss family planning, 77 for those who discussed the topic once or twice and 85 for those who had more frequent discussions about family planning with their husbands. The per centage of women who are not aware of their husband's attitude is greatest (37 per cent) among those who did not discuss family planning with their husbands in the last year.

Interstate variations in exposure to mass media, acceptance of media messages, discussion of family planning between husband and wife and approval of family planning are summarized in Table 6.31. States differ widely on each of these indices. There is a particularly pressing need to evolve state-specific Information, Education and Communication (IEC) activities in the larger, demographically backward states of Uttar Pradesh, Bihar, Madhya Pradesh and Rajasthan. Exposure to family planning messages is limited in these states (only 27-34 per cent of women heard recent family planning messages on the radio or television), a relatively small proportion of women feel that media messages are acceptable (38-55 per cent), husband-wife communication is low (36-48 per cent having discussed family planning with their husband in the last year) and a relatively small proportion of the couples approve of family planning (42-59 per cent). The situation is much better in Punjab, Haryana, Delhi, Himachal Pradesh, and Jammu where a larger proportion of women than the national average have heard family planning messages and are favourable toward such media messages. Husband-wife communication is also relatively high in these states as is the approval of family planning. All of the states in the southern and western regions also score above average on the two media indicators and most of them are also well above average on the indicators of interspousal communication and the approval of family planning.

Notes

1 For a method with negligible use in India, it is perhaps surprising that 19 per cent of women say they have heard of the method. One possible explanation for the unexpectedly high reported knowledge of contraceptive injections in North India is that the Hindi word for injections (suit is also often used in reference to IUD insertions.

2 In the NFHS, no specific reference period was defined for current use. The woman was asked whether she or her husband was currently using a method. 135

7

FERTILITY REFERENCES

Fertility behaviour is a complex phenomenon resulting from an interplay of various social and cultural patterns related to marriage, child-birth, child rearing and familial or kinship affiliation. In the case of India, the cultural importance of the kinship network, coupled with high mortality among children, is considered to be one of the main obstacles to rapid fertility decline. The traditional desire for a large family is embedded in the perceived values and roles that children perform in their families. Children are valued for their role in perpetuating tradition and the ancestral line, providing economic and social support for parents in their old age, and strengthening the marital bond. Although Indian couples traditionally desire many children, with a particular preference for sons, fertility preferences are not immutable. In fact, the two to three child norm is becoming firmly established in many parts of India, as indicated by the NFHS findings on the fertility preferences of women.

Interpretation of data on fertility preferences as a measure of women' s future childbearing intentions is a subject of considerable controversy. Survey questions have been criticized on the grounds that answers may be misleading for a number of reasons. Attitudes toward child-bearing may not be fully formed, they may be held with little conviction, and they may change over time. Moreover, the responses may not take into account the effect of social or community pressures or the attitudes of the husband and other family members, who may have a strong influence on a woman's reproductive decisions. Finally, a woman's preference for limiting her family size can only be implemented if she has the means to fulfil her desires. Nevertheless, in the aggregate, data on fertility preferences can be useful as an indicator of general fertility attitudes and the possible future course of fertility. Fertility preferences data also facilitate the assessment of the need for family planning and the extent of unwanted fertility.

The National Family Health Survey included several questions on women's desire for children in the future. Specifically, these questions dealt with: (a) whether a woman wanted another child, and if so, how soon she wanted her next child; and b) how many children she would want in her lifetime if she could start all over again. The extent of sex preference was ascertained from questions on the preferred sex of the next child and the ideal number of children by sex. These questions are analyzed in this chapter.

7.1 Desire for More Children

In the NFHS, information on future childbearing intentions was sought from currently married women, who were asked, "Would you like to have another child or would you prefer not to have any more children?" Women who did not have any children were asked whether or not they wanted to have any children. If a woman was pregnant, she was asked whether or not she wanted another child after the one she was expecting. Women who wanted another child were then asked about the preferred timing and sex of their next child.

The fertility preferences of currently married women are presented in Table 7.1 and illustrated in Figure 7.1. Overall, only 34 per cent of women say they want another child at some time in the future and more than half of these women say they would like to wait at least two years before having their next birth. Less than two-fifths of women who desire an additional child say they would like another child soon (that is, within two years). Four per cent of women believe decisions pertaining to the number of children are "up to God". More than one-quarter of women (26 per cent) say they do not want any more children and 31 per cent of women (or their husbands) are sterilized. These two groups together constitute 57 per cent of all currently married women in India.

In the NFHS, it is assumed that women do not want any more children if they or their husbands are sterilized. However, some dissatisfaction is expected with sterilization and has been observed among the sterilized populations in other countries, although the extent of sterilization regret is usually less than 10 per cent (Loaiza, 1995). The NFHS included questions on sterilization regret and the reasons for the regret. Overall, 6 per cent of sterilized women (or women whose husbands are sterilized) regret that the sterilization was performed (Table 7.2). However, less than half of these women regret the sterilization because they or their husbands want more children or because they want to replace a dead child. A major cause of sterilization regret is side effects of the operation. Therefore, the assumption that women (or their husbands) who are sterilized do not want any more children will only slightly underestimate preferences to have another child and overestimate the desire to stop childbearing.

From the point of view of understanding the total desire to limit or space births, it is of interest to add together women who do not want any more children (including those who have already been sterilized) and women who want to delay their next birth for two years or longer (as well as women who are unsure of the preferred timing of their next child). Overall, as shown in Table 7.1, 78 per cent of women fall in this category (81 per cent in urban areas and 76 per cent in rural areas).

Among women who want another child, there is a strong preference for having a son as the next child. Forty-nine per cent say they want a son, only 11 per cent express a desire for a daughter, and the rest say that the sex of the child does not matter (24 per cent) or that it is "up to God" (16 per cent). The desire for a son is particularly strong in rural areas and among high parity women. Women who do not have any children are extremely unlikely to want a daughter for their first child, with 2 per cent expressing a desire for a daughter compared to 36 per cent who want a son.

As expected, the desire for more children declines rapidly as the number of children increases (Table 7.1 and Figure 7.2). Eighty-four per cent of women with no children say they want a child and less than 3 per cent say they do not want any children or are sterilized. The proportion who want another child drops to 32 per cent for women who have two living children and 15 per cent for those with three living children. The desire to have a child within two years drops even more rapidly, from 58 per cent for women without any living children to 9 per cent or less for women with two or more living children. Interestingly, the desire to space is very strong for women who have fewer than three children. Twenty-one per cent of women with no children say that they would like to wait at least two years before having their first child. The proportion more than doubles to 54 per cent among women with one child. Similarly, 23 per cent of women with two children would like to wait at least two years before having their next child. Since nearly 50 per cent of all women have fewer than three living children, the strong expressed desire for spacing among these women cannot be ignored. The family planning programme in India needs to increase access to temporary methods if it is to satisfy the needs of a large segment of the population who wish

Table 7.1 Fertility preferences
Per cent distribution of currently married women by desire for children and preferred sex of additional child, according to number of living children and residence, India, 1992-93

Desire for children	Number of living children[1]							
	0	1	2	3	4	5	6+	Total
1	2	3	4	5	6	7	8	9
				URBAN				
Desire for additional child								
Have another soon[2]	59.6	18.4	5.2	2.8	2.0	1.0	0.3	11.1
Have another later[3]	20.3	49.0	13.6	5.7	3.1	1.6	2.0	16.0
Have another, undecided when	4.2	1.7	0.4	0.3	0.2	0.1	0.1	0.9
Undecided	1.3	2.6	1.7	1.1	0.8	0.8	0.4	1.4
Up to God	4.0	2.4	1.9	1.7	2.2	2.7	2.3	2.3
Want no more	1.7	18.4	44.9	31.6	30.9	33.1	45.6	30.8
Sterilized	1.0	3.9	29.7	54.2	57.3	55.6	39.6	33.6
Declared infecund	7.3	3.4	2.4	2.4	3.2	4.9	9.5	3.7
Missing	0.6	0.1	0.1	0.1	0.3	0.2	0.2	0.2
Total per cent	100.0	100.0	100.0	100.0	100.0	100.0	100.0	100.0
Number	2014	4000	5586	4601	2954	1506	1416	22077
Preferred sex of additional child								
Boy	25.0	34.6	54.4	68.1	78.2	59.6	(63.3)	39.1

Girl	4.5	18.8	17.1	12.6	7.1	16.0	(9.1)	13.8
Doesn't matter	49.4	32.3	17.1	11.1	6.7	15.7	(14.5)	32.1
Up to God	21.2	14.3	11.4	8.1	8.0	8.7	(13.0)	15.1
Total per cent	100.0	100.0	100.0	100.0	100.0	100.0	100.0	100.0
Number wanting more	1695	2767	1075	407	157	42	35	6177
			RURAL					
Desire for additional child								
Have another soon[2]	57.4	22.8	10.2	4.9	2.3	1.3	0.9	13.7
Have another later[3]	21.7	55.4	26.7	11.8	6.7	4.1	2.6	20.9
Have another, undecided when	4.7	3.0	1.3	0.7	0.5	0.3	0.3	1.5
Undecided	2.5	1.3	2.0	1.7	1.2	1.5	1.8	1.7
Up to God	5.7	3.8	4.1	3.9	3.8	3.9	5.0	4.2
Want no more	1.8	6.9	23.6	26.4	33.4	40.2	51.1	24.2
Sterilized	0.9	4.3	29.7	47.5	47.6	43.0	29.9	29.8
Declared infecund	5.2	2.3	2.4	3.1	4.4	5.4	8.0	3.9
Missing	0.1	0.1	0.1	0.1	0.2	0.3	0.4	0.2
Total per cent	100.0	100.0	100.0	100.0	100.0	100.0	100.0	100.0
Number	6902	10292	12705	13094	8933	5401	52n	62601
Preferred sex of additional child								
Boy	39.7	45.7	60.9	69.4	71.1	70.1	54.0	51.1
Girl	1.6	13.7	14.7	11.8	10.1	5.6	4.9	10.3
Doesn't matter	36.6	23.7	12.6	8.3	7.6	9.6	18.7	22.2
Up to God	22.2	16.9	11.8	10.5	11.2	14.7	22.4	16.3
Total per cent	100.0	100.0	100.0	100.0	100.0	100.0	100.0	100.0
Number wanting more	5786	8360	4840	2266	855	310	201	22617

1	2	3	4	5	6	7	8	9
			TOTAL					
Desire for additional child								
Have another soon[2]	57.9	21.6	8.7	4.3	2.3	1.2	0.8	13.0
Have another later[3]	21.4	53.6	22.7	10.2	5.8	3.6	2.4	19.6
Have another, undecided when	4.6	2.6	1.0	0.6	0.5	0.3	0.3	1.4
Undecided	2 2	1.7	1.9	1.5	1.1	1.3	1.5	1.6
Up to God	5.3	3.4	3.5	3.4	3.4	3.6	4.4	3.7
Want no more	1.8	10.1	30.1	27.7	32.8	38.6	49.9	25.9
Sterilized	0.9	4.2	29.7	49.2	50.0	45.7	31.9	30.8
Declared infecund	5.7	2.6	2.4	2.9	4.1	5.3	8.3	3.8
Missing	0 2	0 1	0 1	0 1	0 2	0.3	0.3	O.2
Total per cent	100.0	100.0	100.0	100.0	100.0	100.0	100.0	100.0
Number	8916	14292	18292	17695	11887	6907	6690	84678
Preferred sex of additional child								
Boy	36.3	42.9	59.7	69.2	72.2	68.9	55.4	48.6
Girl	2.2	15.0	15.1	11.9	9.6	6.9	5.5	11.0
Doesn't matter	39.5	25.8	13.4	8.7	7.5	10.3	18.1	24.3
Up to God	21.9	16.2	11.8	10.2	10.7	14.0	21.0	16.1
Total per cent	100.0	100.0	100.0	100.0	100.0	100.0	100.0	100.0
Number wanting more	7481	11126	5915	2673	1011	352	236	28795

( ) Based on 25-49 unweighted cases.
I Includes current pregnancy, if any.
2 Wants next birth within 2 years.
3 Wants to delay next birth for 2 or more years.

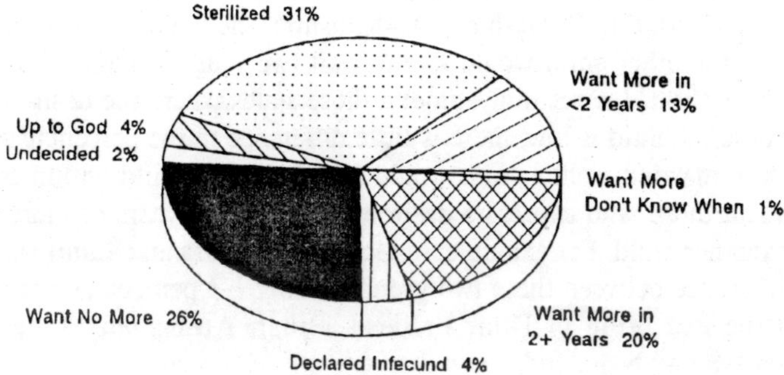

NFHS, India, 1992-93

Figure 7.1 Fertility Preferences Among Currently Married Women Age 13-49

to space their births. Increasing access to spacing methods for women who want more children is likely to lower overall fertility and population growth, as well as provide health benefits to both mothers and their children.

Table 7.2: Sterlization regret

Percentage of sterilized couples who regret sterlization (according to the wife's report) and per cent distribution of reasons for regret sterilization, India, India 1992-93

Sterilization regret/reasons	Urban	Rural	Total
Percertage of sterilized			
couples who regret sterilization	4.0	6.1	5.5
Number of sterilized couples	7417	18635	26051
Reasons fair regret			
Respondent wants another child	35.2	2 .1	28 8
Wants to replace child who died	13.8	13.3	13.4
Husband wants another child	5.7	4.5	4.8
Side effects	40 7	49.2	.47.4
Other	4.5	5.8	5.6
Total per cent	100.0	100.0	100.0
Number of couples who regret sterilization	300	1140	1439

Table 7.3 shows variations in fertility preferences by state. The percentage of currently married women who want to have another child varies considerably from a high of 53 in Arunachal Pradesh and Meghalaya to a low of 25 in Himachal Pradesh and Punjab. In every state except Andhra Pradesh and Maharashtra, the majority of women who want another child would like to wait two years or more to have their next child. Interestingly, among those states where the desire for an additional child is low, there is little difference in the percentage of currently married women who would like to have a child within two years and those who express a desire to wait for two years or more to have another child. For example, in Goa, Maharashtra and Tamil Nadu the difference between these two groups is only 1-3 percentage points. With the exception of Uttar Pradesh, Bihar, Arunachal Pradesh, Meghalaya and Nagaland, more than one out of two currently married women in all states say they do not want any more children or they or their husbands are sterilized. At least two out of three currently married women in Delhi, Himachal Pradesh, Punjab, Tripura, Kerala and Tamil Nadu do not want any more children (including sterilized women and women whose husbands are sterilized). Nineteen per cent of women in Nagaland believe that decisions pertaining to childbearing are "up to God",but this response is rare in most other states.

Table 7.4 provides information about subgroup variations in the potential demand for family planning. As before, women who are sterilized (or whose husbands are sterilized) are added to those who say they want no more children to derive this measure. Overall, there is little subgroup variation among women who have no children, except that older women are more likely to express a desire not to have any children. Differences by subgroups emerge as the number of living children increases and are especially marked for women who have 2-3 children. As expected, the desire to have no more children increases with age, from 2 per cent among women age 13-14 to 84 per cent among women age 35-44 and then falls slightly to 77 per cent among women age 45-49. Urban women are more likely to want to stop childbearing than rural women, and this difference is especially marked among women with fewer than three children. Educational attainment is strongly related to fertility desires for women who have at least 2 children, but this difference narrows as the number of living children increases. The desire to have no more children is lowest among Muslim women (49 per cent) and highest among Sikhs and Gains (70 per cent). Scheduled tribe women are least likely to want no more children, but even in this group nearly one out of two women do not want any more children. It is also evident

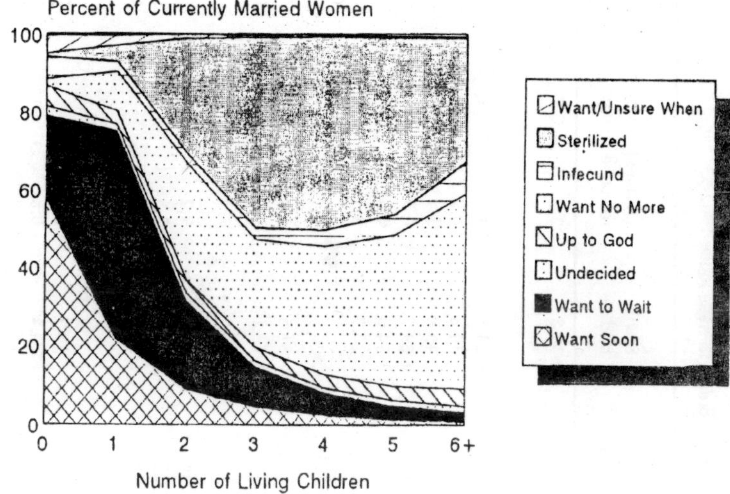

Figure 7.2 Fertility Preferences by Number of Living Children

from Table 7.4 that the sex composition of living children is strongly related to the fertility preferences of women. For example, the desire to have no more children among women with three children is twice as high for those who have all sons as for those who have all daughters. The table shows a strong desire for at least one son, but the inverted U-shaped pattern for women with three or more living children also shows a weak desire to have at least one daughter. The desire to have a daughter may be related to the importance of the Hindu religious obligation of *kanyadan*, which provides an opportunity to make merit by giving one's daughter away at the time of her marriage.

7.2 Need for Family Planning Services

Assessing the demand for family planning is crucial to the success of a country's population and family planning programmed It enables policymakers and programme planners to estimate the market for family planning services and assess programme effectiveness. In this report the demand for family planning is estimated as the sum of the unmet need for family planning and the current prevalence of contraceptive use. Unmet need has been measured in various ways in past studies (Westoff and Ochoa, 1991). Here, currently married women who say

Table 7.3: Fertility preferences by state

Per cent distribution of currently married women by desire for children, according to state, India, 1992-93

State	Want within 2 years	Want after 2 years	Want, undecided when	Undecided	up to God	Want no more	Sterilized	Declared infecund	Missing	Total percent
India	13.0	19.6	1.4	1.6	3.7	25.9	30.8	3.8	0.2	100.0
North										
Delhi	9.8	16.6	0.5	1.4	1.6	45.4	23.3	1.3	0.1	100.0
Haryana	14.8	17.3	0.5	1.9	0.5	29.3	34.8	0.9	—	100.0
Himachal Pradesh	9.3	15.9	0.2	1.4	0.3	25.7	45.8	1.4	—	100.0
Jammu Region of J & K	14.8	17.5	0.1	1.3	0.1	35.6	29.7	0.9	—	100.0
Punjab	11.4	13.3	0.2	1.3	0.4	37.8	34.0	1.6	—	100.0
Rajasthan	12.7	20.3	1.2	3.1	7.1	24.2	27.7	3.5	0.2	100.0
Central										
Madhya Pradesh	12.3	25.3	2.8	2.2	4.2	19.6	31.5	1.8	0.2	100.0
Uttar Pradesh	12.4	25.6	1.0	1.6	9.7	31.5	13.1	4.9	0.3	100.0
East										
Bihar	16.7	24.0	1.1	1.8	6.3	24.1	18.6	7.2	0.2	100.0
Orissa	13.7	18.1	1.9	3.1	2.2	25.9	31.6	3.5	—	100.0
West Bengal	10.0	20.5	0.8	0.7	0.8	34.5	30.6	2.1	—	100.0
Northeast										
Arunachal Pradesh	20.5	30.3	2.4	3.5	5.4	24.0	10.7	3.4	—	100.0
Assam	11.2	22.7	0.9	1.0	1.1	47.8	14.4	0.8	—	100.0
Manipur	8.5	29.1	0.6	1.5	2.4	41.4	13.8	2.8	—	100.0

Meghalaya	14.7	35.0	3.5	4.6	8.7	17.0	10.0	6.6	—	100.0
Mizoram	12.9	24.3	0.7	2.2	2.4	10.2	44.6	2.8	—	100.0
Nagaland	5.6	18.7	1.8	6.4	19.0	35.1	6.4	7.0	—	100.0
Tripura	12.6	15.2	0.7	1.1	0.3	50.2	19.1	0.8	—	100.0
West										
Goa	12.9	13.8	0.8	2.7	0.6	33.3	30.5	5.3	0.1	100.0
Gujarat	13.7	17.2	0.7	1.4	1.8	20.6	41.0	3.5	0.1	100.0
Maharashtra	11.7	13.5	2.3	1.2	0.7	20.4	46.1	4.0	—	100.0
South										
Andhra Pradesh	17.7	12.8	2.6	1.6	1.4	13.6	44.8	5.3	0.4	100.0
Karnataka	12.4	16.7	0.9	1.5	1.7	20.6	42.5	3.4	0.3	100.0
Kerala	10.8	16.1	1.1	1.3	1.1	19.3	48.3	1.8	0.2	100.0
Tamil Nadu	12.0	14.6	1.0	0.7	0.6	27.1	39.5	4.2	0.2	100.0

— Less than 0.05 percent

that they either do not want any more children or that they want to wait two or more years before having another child, but are not using contraception, are defined as having an *unmet need* for family planning. Current users of family planning methods are said to have a *met need* for family planning. The total demand for family planning is the sum of the met need and the unmet need for family planning. Table 7.5 shows the unmet need, met need and total demand for family planning, according to whether there is a need for spacing or limiting births*. The table also contains detailed definitions of these concepts.

According to these definitions, 20 per cent of women in India have an unmet need for family planning. The unmet need for spacing births (11 per cent) is slightly greater than the unmet need for limiting births (9 per cent). Together with the 41 per cent of currently married women who are using contraception, a total of 60 per cent of currently married women have a demand for family planning. If all of the women who say they want to space or limit their births were to use family planning, the contraceptive prevalence rate would increase from 41 per cent to 60 per cent of married women. This means that 68 per cent of the demand for family planning is being met by current programmed as seen in the last column of Table 7.5. If the level of unmet need indicated in the table is assumed to reflect the needs of all currently married women age 13-49 in India, then about 30 million women in India have an unmet need for family planning.

The unmet need for limiting childbearing increases steadily until age 30-34 and decreases thereafter. The unmet need for spacing, on the other hand, is particularly strong for women under age 25. This is the segment of the population whose family planning needs are least likely to be met by current programmes. Only 12 per cent and 19 per cent of the family planning needs of currently married women age 13-14 and 15-19, respectively, are being met. Although this per cent increases steadily from 43 per cent for women age 20-24 to 85 per cent for women age 40-44, it is only being nearly fully satisfied for women age 45-49.

Rural areas have a slightly greater unmet need for family planning than urban areas, with a greater unmet need for spacing than limiting in rural areas. Although the use of and demand for family planning is higher in urban than in rural areas, the per cent of demand satisfied is also somewhat higher in urban areas. There is little difference in the unmet need for family planning by educational attainment of women,

* Women with an unmet need or a met need are allocated to the "spacing" or "limiting" group depending on their fertility preference responses, not according to the contraceptive method being used or preferred.

but both the use of and the demand for family planning is lower among illiterate women than among women with some education. Accordingly, the total needs of illiterate women are less likely to be satisfied by current family planning programmed. Among the religious groups, unmet need is highest among Muslim women, who are least likely to have their total demand satisfied. Differences in the unmet need for family planning services by caste/tribe are not marked. The final panel in Table 7.5 indicates that current family planning services are particularly inadequate for satisfying the childspacing needs of women with fewer than two living children. Consequently, the percentage of total need satisfied is much lower among women with no living children (19 per cent) or one living child (42 per cent) than among those who have two or more living children.

The most populous state, Uttar Pradesh, has the highest total unmet need for family planning (30 per cent), followed closely by Nagaland, Bihar and Meghalaya (Table 7.6 and Figure 7.3). In fact, more than one-quarter of all Indian women with an unmet need for family planning reside in Uttar Pradesh. The total unmet need is lowest in Andhra Pradesh (10 per cent). With the exception of Delhi, Punjab, Nagaland, Tripura and Goa, the unmet need for spacing is greater than the unmet need for limiting in every state. There is no difference in the unmet need for spacing and limiting in Punjab. Less than 20 per cent of currently married women in Nagaland and Uttar Pradesh are using family planning and women in these two states are also least likely to have their demand for family planning satisfied. On the other hand, more than 80 per cent of the overall demand for family planning in Punjab, Mizoram, Tripura, Andhra Pradesh and Kerala is being met by current programmed

7.3 Ideal Number of Children

The above analysis has focused on the respondent's reproductive desires for the future, implicitly taking into account the number of sons and daughters that she already has. Another measure of fertility preferences is a woman's ideal family size. In determining the ideal number of children, the respondent is asked to perform a more difficult abstract task of stating the number of children she would like to have if she could start childbearing all over again. In the NFHS, women with no children were asked, "If you could choose exactly the number of children to have in your whole life, how many would that be?" Women who already had children were asked, "If you could go back to the time you did not have any children and could choose exactly the number of children to have in your whole life, how many would that be?" Some women had difficulty in answering these hypothetical questions and often the questions had to be repeated to ensure that they were understood by the respondent. Despite the widespread criticism that asking women to quantify the number of children they would like to have may be an alien concept in many developing countries, 90 per cent of respondents were able to give a numeric response when asked for their ideal number of children.

Table 7.4: Desire to have no more children by background characteristics
Percentage of currently married women who want no more children by number of living children and selected background characteristics, India, 1992-93

Background characteristic	Number of living children							
	0	1	2	3	4	5	6+	Total
Age								
13-14	1.1	4.4	*	NC	NC	NC	NC	1.8
15-19	1.1	3.0	31.9	60.5	*	*	NC	6.9
20-24	1.4	5.9	39.0	59.0	67.3	79.9	89.2	27 3
25-29	2.0	17.0	60.1	70.0	75.5	78.4	79.2	57 4
30-34	5.7	39.4	79.0	82.7	83.0	82.9	81.7	76.5
35-39	11.2	54.7	84.1	90.4	90.4	87.3	84.7	83.5
40-44	15.7	58.3	85.7	89.0	88.9	89.1	83.8	83.9
45-49	13.8	58.8	78.1	80.4	81.6	81.7	77.4	76.6
Residence								
Urban	2.7	22.3	74.6	85.8	88.2	88.6	85.1	64.3
Rural	2.7	11.2	53.2	73.9	81.0	83.2	80.9	53.9
Education								
Illiterate	2.6	11.4	45.8	70.0	79.6	82.2	80.7	54.0
Literate, < middle complete	2.9	13.1	67.2	86.3	90.9	92.3	86.3	63.0
Middle school complete	2.5	14.0	75.3	90.3	89.0	89.3	87.9	58.5
High school and above	2.6	24.0	83.0	91.4	91.1	92.9	90.2	59.7
Religion								
Hindu	2.8	14.7	60.9	78.3	84.2	85.6	83.2	57.2
Muslim	2.3	9.5	38.6	60.1	70.5	76.6	77.8	49.2
Christian	2.3	15.7	74.2	79.8	78.9	79.6	76.4	60.2
Sikh	1.2	10.2	74.4	89.0	94.7	96.4	95.0	69.6
Jain	(0.8)	39.5	82.7	90.8	(94.6)	*	*	70.4
Buddhist	(2.6)	17.1	67.1	86.1	94.4	(95.9)	(99.2)	64.5
Other	0.4	23.2	60.1	72.6	74.0	66.8	65.1	50.0
Caste/tribe								
Scheduled caste	2.2	9.6	46.1	72.5	81.0	85.4	86.0	53.1
Scheduled tribe	2.9	10.8	47.1	65.3	77.0	79.3	77.4	49.4
Other	2.7	15,4	62.8	78.9	83.8	84.8	81.6	58.0

{Cont}.....

Number of living sons[2]								
None	2.7	13.7	36.9	41.3	56.5	55.3	56.0	15.6
1	NA	18.6	66.0	73.4	76.1	81.9	79.4	57.6
2	NA	NA	71.5	88.0	88.4	87.9	84.6	83.8
3	NA	NA	NA	82.6	89.5	86.7	84.1	86.0
4	NA	NA	NA	NA	82.5	87.4	81.8	83.6
5	NA	NA	NA	NA	NA	83.2	82.7	82.8
6+	NA	NA	NA	NA	NA	NA	82.4	82.4
Number of living daughters[2]								
None	2.7	18.6	71.5	82.6	82.5	83.2	75.3	32.5
1	NA	13.7	66.0	88.0	89.5	87.4	85.7	64.6
2	NA	NA	36.9	73.4	88.4	86.7	81.7	73.0
3	NA	NA	NA	41.3	76.1	87.9	83.6	75.3
4	NA	NA	NA	NA	56.5	81.9	83.3	78.9
5	NA	NA	NA	NA	NA	55.3	81.6	77.8
6+	NA	NA	NA	NA	NA	NA	79.0	79.0
Total	2.7	14.3	59.7	77.0	82.8	84.4	81.8	56.7

Note: Women who have been sterilized, or whose-husbands have been sterilized, are considered to want no more children.
NA: Not applicable.
NC: Not calculated because there are no cases on which to base a percentage.
( ) Based on 25-49 unweighted cases.
* Percentage not shown; based on fewer than 25 unweighted cases.
1 Includes current pregnancy, if any,
2 Excludes pregnant women.

Table 7.7 shows that for a large majority (66 per cent) of women, the ideal number of children falls within the narrow range of 2-3 children. A relatively small percentage of women (3 per cent) think that one child is ideal and one in five women consider four children or more as ideal. For those who gave numeric responses, the average number of children considered ideal is 2.9. The Third All India Survey conducted in 1988-89 found the ideal family size to be 3.0 (Operations Research Group, 1990). The mean ideal number of children in the NFHS ranges from 2.4 to 2.6 for women with fewer than three children to 4.0 for women who already have six or more children, and is slightly higher in rural areas than in urban areas. Thus, although the "two-child family" norm can not be said to exist in India at this time, the majority of women giving a numeric response to the ideal family size questions consider a small or moderate size family as ideal rather than a very large one.

Some critics argue that women tend to adjust their fertility ideals upwards in keeping with increases in their actual family size (Lightbourne and MacDonald, 1982). However, it is evident that in India a large proportion of women say that their ideal number of children is less than the

Table 7.5: Need for family planning services

Percent of currently married women with unmet need, met need, and total demand for family planning (FP) services by selected background characteristics, India, 1992-93

Background characteristic	Unmet need for FP[1]			Net need-currently using[2]			Total demand for FP			Percent of need satis fied
	To space	To limit	Total	To space	To Limit	Total	To space	To limit	Total	
Age										
13-14	29.6	3.6	33.2	3.9	0.8	4.7	33.5	4.4	37.9	12.4
15-19	28.2	2.3	30.4	5.1	2.1	7.1	33.2	4.3	37.6	18.9
20-24	22.8	5.1	27.9	7.0	14.0	21.0	29.8	19.1	48.9	43.0
25-29	11.2	10.5	21.6	4.9	37.5	42.4	16.1	47.9	64.0	66.2
30-34	4.4	13.2	17.6	1.8	54.1	55.9	6.2	67.3	73.5	76.0
35-39	1.5	12.0	13.5	0.7	60.3	61.0	2.2	72.3	74.5	81.9
40-44	0.7	9.0	9.7	0.1	56.2	56.3	0.7	65.2	65.9	85.3
45-49	0.2	4.1	4.4	0.1	45.7	45.8	0.3	49.8	50.2	91.3
Residence										
Urban	8.6	8.4	17.1	5.2	45.8	51.0	13.8	54.2	68.1	74.9
Rural	11.9	8.5	20.3	2.7	34.2	36.9	14.6	42.6	57.2	64.5
Education										
Illiterate	11.0	9.3	20.3	1.5	32.4	33.9	12.5	41.6	54.1	62.6
Lit., < middle complete	10.8	7.2	18.1	4.0	46.4	50.4	14.8	53.6	68.4	73.6
Middle school complete	12.7	6.5	19.3	6.8	44.0	50.8	19.5	50.6	70.1	72.5
High school and above	10.5	7.3	17.8	10.2	44.5	54.7	20.7	51.8	72.5	75.5

Religion										
Hindu	10.9	8.0	18.9	3.1	38.6	41.6	14.0	46.5	60.5	68.8
Muslim	12.9	12.9	25.8	4.6	23.2	27.8	17.5	36.1	53.6	51.8
Christian	8.6	6.7	15.3	5.5	42.9	48.4	14.1	49.6	63.7	76.0
Sikh	7.9	6.2	14.1	5.6	51.9	57.5	13.5	58.1	71.6	80.3
Jain	5.8	5.4	11.2	8.5	54.2	62.7	14.3	59.6	73.8	84.9
Buddhist	7.3	7.3	14.6	2.9	47.9	50.9	10.2	55.2	65.5	77.7
Other	15.7	6.5	22.1	3.8	30.0	33.8	19.5	36.5	56.0	60.5
Caste/tribe										
Scheduled caste	12.3	9.5	21.8	2.2	32.4	34.5	14.5	41.9	56.3	61.3
Scheduled tribe	11.2	7.2	18.4	1.6	31.4	33.0	12.8	38.6	51.4	64.1
Other	10.8	8.4	19.3	3.8	38.6	42.4	14.6	47.0	61.6	68.8
Number of living children										
None	16.0	1.6	17.6	3.4	0.8	4.2	19.4	2.4	21.8	19.3
1	24.4	2.5	27.0	11.0	8.3	19.3	35.4	10.8	46.2	41.7
2	12.6	7.7	20.3	3.6	42.5	46.1	16.2	50.2	66.4	69.5
3	6.7	8.4	15.1	1.2	57.7	58.9	7.9	66.2	74.1	79.6
4	4.0	11.5	15.5	0.6	58.2	58.8	4.6	69.7	74.3	79.1
5	2.6	15.8	18.4	0.5	52.8	53.2	3.0	68.6	71.6	74.3
6+	2.2	22.3	24.5	0.3	39.9	40.2	2.5	62.1	64.7	62.1
Total	11.0	8.5	19.5	3.4	37.2	40.6	14.4	45.7	60.1	67.6

1 *Unmet need for spacing* includes pregnant women whose pregnancy was mistimed, amenorrhoeic women whose last birth was mistimed, and women who are neither pregnant nor amenorrhoeic and who are not using any method of family planning and say they want to wait 2 or more years for their next birth. Also included in unmet need for spacing are women who are unsure whether they want another child or who want another child but are unsure when to have the birth. Unmet need for limiting refers to pregnant women whose pregnancy was unwanted, amenorrhoeic women whose last child was unwanted and women who are neither pregnant nor amenorrhoeic and who are not using any method of family planning and who want no more children.

2 *Using for spacing* refers to women who are using some method of family planning and say they want to have another child or are undecided whether to have another. Using for limiting refers to women who are using and who want no more Children. Note that the specific methods used are not taken into account here.

Table 7.6 :Need for family planning services by state

Per cent of currently married women with unmet need, met need, and total demand for Family Planning (FP) services by state, India, 1992-93

State	Unmet need for FP[1]			Net need-currently using[2]			Total demand for FP			Per cent of need satis fied
	To space	To limit	Total	To space	To Limit	Total	To space	To limit	Total	
India	11.0	8.5	19.5	3.4	37.2	40.6	14.4	45.7	60.1	67.6
North										
Delhi	7.6	7.9	15.4	10.7	49.6	60.3	18.2	57.5	75.7	79.6
Haryana	8.8	7.6	16.4	4.4	45.2	49.7	13.2	52.8	66.0	75.2
Himachal Pradesh	9.2	5.6	14.9	3.7	54.7	58.4	12.9	60.3	73.2	79.7
Jammu Region of J & K	8.9	8.6	17.5	5.4	44.0	49.4	14.3	52.6	66.9	73.9
Punjab	6.5	6.5	13.0	5.4	53.4	58.7	11.8	59.9	71.7	81.9
Rajasthan	10.8	9.0	19.8	1.6	30.2	31.8	12.4	39.2	51.6	61.7
Central										
Madhya Pradesh	13.1	7.4	20.5	2.0	34.6	36.5	15.1	42.0	57.1	64.0
Uttar Pradesh	16.7	13.4	30.1	2.0	17.8	19.8	18.6	31.2	49.9	39.7
East										
Bihar	14.4	10.6	25.1	1.9	21.1	23.1	16.4	31.8	48.1	47.9
Orissa	12.7	9.7	22.4	1.5	34.7	36.3	14.3	44.4	58.6	61.8
West Bengal	9.4	8.0	17.4	10.2	47.2	57.4	19.6	55.2	74.8	76.7
Northeast										
Arunachal Pradesh	12.9	7.4	20.4	5.3	18.3	23.6	18.2	25.7	44.0	53.7
Assam	11.0	10.7	21.7	8.6	34.2	42.8	19.5	44.9	64.5	66.3
Manipur	11.7	10.0	21.7	7.4	27.5	34.9	19.1	37.5	56.6	61.7

Meghalaya	20.6	4.6	25.1	5.0	15.7	20.7	25.5	20.3	45.8	45.1
Mizoram	9.2	2.8	11.9	7.1	46.7	53.8	16.2	49.4	65.7	81.8
Nagaland	12.9	13.8	26.7	1.9	11.1	13.0	14.7	25.0	39.7	32.7
Tripura	5.3	8.2	13.5	9.8	46.4	56.1	15.1	54.5	69.6	80.7
West										
Goa	7.8	7.9	15.7	5.7	42.1	47.8	13.5	49.9	63.5	75.3
Gujarat	7.6	5.5	13.1	2.6	46.7	49.3	10.2	52.2	62.4	79.0
Maharashtra	7.3	6.8	14.1	3.1	50.7	53.7	10.4	57.5	67.9	79.2
South										
Andhra Pradesh	6.3	4.1	10.4	0.9	46.1	47.0	7.2	50.3	57.4	81.9
Karnataka	11.8	6.4	18.2	2.3	46.8	49.1	14.1	53.2	67.3	73.0
Kerala	7.2	4.5	11.7	6.6	56.6	63.3	13.9	61.1	75.0	84.4
Tamil Nadu	7.8	6.7	14.6	3.3	46.5	49.8	11.1	53.2	64.4	77.4

1 *Unmet need for spacing* includes pregnant women whose pregnancy was mistimed, amenorrhoeic women whose last birth was mistimed, and women who are neither pregnant nor amenorrhoeic and who are not using any method of family planning and say they want to wait 2 or more years for their next birth. Also included in unmet need for spacing are women who are unsure whether they want another child or who want another child but are unsure when to have the birth. Unmet need for limiting refers to pregnant women whose pregnancy was unwanted, amenorrhoeic women whose last child was unwanted and women who are neither pregnant nor amenorrhoeic and who are not using any method of family planning and who want no more children.

2 *Using for spacing* refers to women who are using some method of family planning and say they want to have another child or are undecided whether to have another. Using for limiting refers to women who are using and who want no more Children. Note that the specific methods used are not taken into account here.

number they already have. For example, among women who have six living children or more, 65 per cent state that their ideal family would consist of fewer than six children. Similarly, 66 per cent of women with five living children think that fewer than five children is ideal. Thus, family size norms are relatively low and nearly half of women with more than two children actually have more children than they consider ideal. This may be taken as another indicator of surplus or unwanted fertility.

Table 7.8 shows the mean ideal number of children for ever-married women by age and selected background characteristics. The mean ranges between 2.7 and 2.8 for women below age 30 and then increases steadily to 3.2 for women age 45-49. Rural women in India on average desire half a child more than urban women. The mean ideal family size declines as educational attainment increases, from 3.1 for illiterate women to 2.1 for women with at least a high school education. The ideal family size for Muslims is one child higher than for pains and about half a child higher than for Hindus and Christians. Similarly, women belonging to scheduled tribes have an ideal family size that is half a child larger than the non-SC/ST women. There is little difference in the ideal family size by women's work status. Women whose husbands are illiterate desire one child more than women whose husbands have studied beyond high school.

The ideal family size varies considerably by state, as shown in Table 7.9. Women in four of the seven northeastern states (Arunachal Pradesh, Meghalaya, Mizoram and Nagaland) state that at least four children are ideal. In contrast, two children are considered ideal in Tamil Nadu. In general, states in the southern, western and northern regions of the country have a lower ideal family size than states in the central, eastern and northeastern regions of the country.

In the NFHS, women who gave a numerical response to the question about the ideal number of children were further asked how many of these children they would like to be boys and how many they would like to be girls. Parental attitudes and aspirations regarding the sex of their children have attracted considerable research interest because of the belief that sex preference may sustain higher fertility levels than would be the case if parents are indifferent to the sex of their children (Cleland *et al.*, 1983). Researchers argue that childbearing may continue beyond a preferred family size if women (or couples) desire a particular combination of sons and daughters. Empirical support for a strong influence of son preference on fertility, however, is rather weak (Arnold, 1987; Bairagi and Langsten, 1986). Numerous research studies in India have found a strong preference for sons, particularly in North India (Das Gupta, 1987;

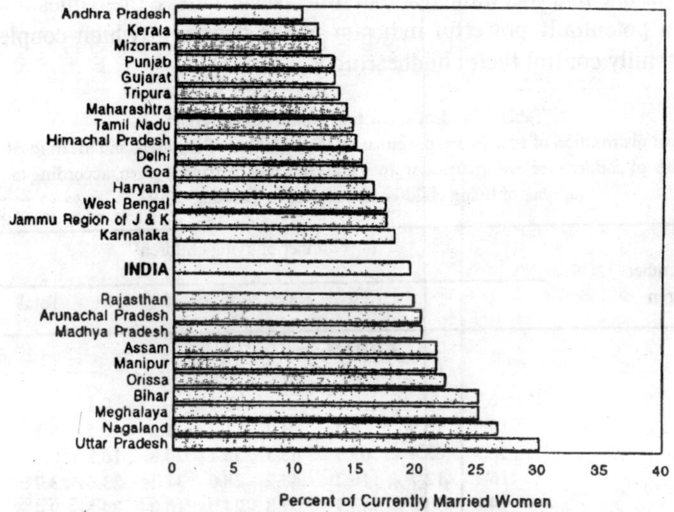

Figure 7.3 Unmet Need for Family Planning by State

Miller, 1981; Population Research Centre, CRRID, 1993; Rastogi and Raj Kumari, 1992; Basu, 1989; Khan *et al.*, 1989).

Stated preferences about the sex composition of children in the ideal family (Table 7.10) confirm the existence of a strong son preference in India that was observed earlier in the discussion of the preferred sex of the next child. Overall, the ideal family size consists of 1.6 sons, 1.1 daughters and 0.2 children of either sex. son preference is stronger in rural areas than in urban areas. Sons are preferred to daughters in both urban and rural areas irrespective of the number and sex composition of a woman's living children. There is a general tendency for women who have more daughters at each parity to indicate a weaker preference for sons.

7.4 Fertility Planning

Another way to gauge the extent of unwanted fertility is to focus on recent births. For each child born in the four years before the survey and for each current pregnancy, women were asked whether the pregnancy was wanted at that time (planned), wanted at a later time (mistimed), or not wanted at all (unwanted). Information from these questions may result in underestimation of unplanned pregnancy due to rationalization. A woman may retrospectively declare an unplanned pregnancy as one that was wanted at that time. Nevertheless, these questions form a potentially powerful indicator of the degree to which couples successfully control their childbearing.

Table 7.7: Ideal and actual number of children
Per cent distribution of ever-married women by ideal number of children, and mean ideal number of children for ever-married women and currently married women, according to number of living children and residence, India, 1992-93

Ideal number of children	Number of living children[1]							
	0	1	2	3	4	5	6+	Total
URBAN								
None	0.2	—	—	—	0.1	—	0.1	—
1	10.9	15.9	6.3	3.2	1.7	1.2	0.5	6.5
2	58.3	62.4	69.5	40.3	35.1	24.8	16.2	50.1
3	16.1	12.7	16.2	40.9	28.0	31.3	23.6	23.7
4	4.0	3.2	3.9	7.8	24.0	16.0	24.5	9.4
5	1.3	0.6	0.4	1.4	2.0	10.1	5.3	1.9
6+	0.4	0.3	0.3	0.5	1.1	2.8	10.9	1.3
Non-numeric responses	8.9	4.9	3.4	5.9	8.1	13.8	18.8	7.0
Total per cent	100.0	100.0	100.0	100.0	100.0	100.0	100.0	100.0
Number of women	2250	4266	5880	4828	3110	1619	1503	23455
Mean ideal number[2]								
Ever-married women	2.2	2.1	2.2	2.6	2.9	3.2	3.7	2.5
Currently married women	2.2	2.1	2.2	2.6	2.9	3.2	3.7	2.5
RURAL								
None	0.1	—	—	—	—	—	—	—
1	3.3	4.6	1.5	1.4	0.8	0.5	0.5	2.0
2	40.6	46.2	47.6	25.6	21.3	14.8	10.1	32.4
3	28.1	28.3	29.7	44.2	25.3	26.7	20.7	30.6
4	11.4	9.6	11.1	15.3	33.0	22.1	24.5	16.9
5	2.1	2.1	2.1	3.0	5.1	13.0	7.9	4.1
6+	0.7	0.8	0.9	1.3	2.9	5.5	14.6	2.7
Non-numeric responses	13.7	8.4	7.0	9.0	11.6	17.4	21.7	11.2
Total per cent	100.0	100.0	100.0	100.0	100.0	100.0	100.0	100.0
Number of women	7622	11123	13407	13676	9352	5625	55186	6322
Mean ideal number[2]								
Ever-married women	2.7	2.6	2.7	3.0	3.4	3.6	4.1	3.0
Currently married women	2.7	2.6	2.7	3.0	3.4	3.6	4.1	3.0

{Cont.}

				TOTAL				
None	0.1	—	—	—	—	—	—	—
1	5.0	7.7	3.0	1.9	1.0	0.6	0.5	3.1
2	44.6	50.7	54.3	29.5	24.7	17.0	11.5	37.0
3	25.3	23.9	25.6	43.3	25.9	27.7	21.3	28.8
4	9.7	7.8	8.9	13.4	30.8	20.8	24.5	14.9
5	1.9	1.7	1.6	2.6	4.3	12.4	7.3	3.6
6+	0.6	0.7	0.7	1.1	2.4	4.9	13.8	2.4
Non-numeric responses	12.6	7.4	5.9	8.2	10.7	16.6	21.1	10.1
Total per cent	100.0	100.0	100.0	100.0	100.0	100.0	100.0	100.0
Number of women	9872	15389	19286	18503	12461	7244	7021	89777
Mean ideal numbers[2]								
Ever-married women	2.6	2.4	2.5	2.9	3.2	3.5	4.0	2.9
Currently married women	2.6	2.4	2.5	2.9	3.2	3.5	4.0	2.9

— Less than 0.05 per cent

1 includes current pregnancy, if any.

2 Means are calculated excluding the women giving non-numeric responses.

Table 7.11 shows the percentage distribution of births during the four years preceding the survey and current pregnancies by fertility planning status, according to selected background characteristics. Almost one out of four births in India (including current pregnancies) in the four years preceding the survey was not wanted at the time the woman became pregnant. Nine per cent were unwanted and 14 per cent were mistimed. Differentials in fertility planning by residence and caste/tribe are not very substantial. Although fertility planning does not show a clear trend by education, more educated women are less likely to have unwanted births. However, mistimed births are more common among literate than illiterate women. Muslim women are most likely to have unwanted births and Christian women and women belonging to other religious groups not otherwise classified are most likely to have mistimed births. Major differences are apparent by birth order and the age of the mother at the time of the birth. First births are relatively well planned, second and third births are most likely to be mistimed, and fourth and higher order births are particularly likely to be unwanted. Similarly, the percentage of pregnancies that were unplanned increases steadily with increasing age to a level of 45 per cent for women age 40-44. Mistimed births are more common among younger women (below age 30), whereas older women are more likely to have unwanted births.

Table 7.8 Ideal number of Children by background characteristics
Mean ideal number of children for ever-married women by age and selected background characteristics, India, 1992-93

Background characteristic	Current age								
	13-14	15-19	20-24	25-29	30-34	35-39	40-44	45-49	Total
Residence									
Urban	(2.5)	2.5	2.4	2.4	2.5	2.6	2.7	2.8	2.5
Rural	2.9	2.7	2.8	2.9	3.1	3.1	3.3	3.4	3.0
Education									
Illiterate	2.9	2.9	2.9	3.1	3.2	3.3	3.4	3.5	3.1
Lit., < middle complete	2.5	2.5	2.5	2.6	2.7	2.7	2.8	2.9	2.6
Middle school complete	*	2.4	2.3	2.3	2.4	2.5	2.5	2.6	2.4
High school and above	*	2.2	2.1	2.1	2.1	2.2	2.2	2.3	2.1
Religion									
Hindu	2.8	2.7	2.6	2.7	2.8	2.9	3.0	3.2	2.8
Muslim	(2.9)	3.0	3.0	3.3	3.5	3.6	3.8	3.8	3.3
Christian	*	2.7	2.8	2.8	2.8	3.0	3.1	3.4	2.9
Sikh	*	2.4	2.4	2.4	2.5	2.6	2.8	2.8	2.5
Jain	NC	*	2.1	2.0	2.1	2.5	(2.6)	2.7	2.3
Buddhist	*	2.6	2.3	2.4	2.8	2.7	2.7	(3.3)	2.6
Other	*	3.0	2.9	3.3	3.0	3.7	4.1	4.3	3.3
Caste/tribe									
Scheduled caste	(2.8)	2.7	2.8	2.9	3.1	3.1	3.3	3.3	3.0
Scheduled tribe	(3.0)	2.9	3.0	3.3	3.4	3.5	3.6	3.8	3.3
Other	2.8	2.7	2.6	2.7	2.8	2.9	3.0	3.2	2.8

Work status									
Not working	2.8	2.7	2.7	2.8	2.9	3.0	3.2	3.3	2.9
Working in family farm/business	(2.7)	2.7	2.8	2.9	3.0	3.0	3.2	3.4	3.0
Employed by someone else	(2.9)	2.7	2.7	2.7	2.8	2.8	2.8	3.0	2.8
Self employed	*	2.6	2.7	2.8	2.8	2.9	2.9	3.3	2.8
Husband's education									
Illiterate	3.0	2.9	3.0	3.1	3.3	3.3	3.5	3.5	3.2
Lit., < primary complete	(3.0)	2.7	2.8	2.8	2.9	3.0	3.1	3.2	2.9
Primary school complete	(2.4)	2.6	2.6	2.8	2.9	3.0	3.1	3.1	2.9
Middle school complete	*	2.6	2.6	2.6	2.8	2.9	3.0	3.2	2.8
High school complete	(2.7)	2.6	2.5	2.6	2.6	2.7	2.7	2.8	2.6
Above high school	*	2.3	2.2	2.2	2.2	2.3	2.4	2.6	2.3
Don't know, missing	*	*	*	(2.8)	*	*	*	*	2.9
Total	2.8	2.7	2.7	2.8	2.9	3.0	3.1	3.2	2.9

Note: Means are calculated excluding women who gave non-numeric responses.
NC: Not calculated because there are no cases on which to base a mean.
( ) Based on 25-49 unweighted cases.
* Mean not shown; based on fewer than 25 unweighted cases.

Table 7.9: Ideal number of children by age and state

Mean ideal number of children for ever-married women by age and state, India, 1992-93

	Current age								
State	13-14	15-19	20-24	25-29	30-34	35-39	40-44	45-49	Total
India	2.8	2.7	2.7	2.8	2.9	3.0	3.1	3.2	2.9
North									
Delhi	NC	2.5	2.4	2.4	2.5	2.6	2.6	2.8	2.5
Haryana	*	2.4	2.5	2.5	2.6	2.6	2.7	2.8	2.6
Himachal Pradesh	NC	2.2	2.2	2.3	2.3	2.5	2.6	2.7	2.4
Jammu Region of J & K	*	2.7	2.5	2.7	2.7	2.9	3.1	3.1	2.8
Punjab	*	2.4	2.3	2.4	2.5	2.7	2.9	2.8	2.6
Rajasthan	*	2.6	2.7	3.0	3.1	3.2	3.4	3.4	3.0
Central									
Madhya Pradesh	*	2.7	2.8	3.1	3.2	3.4	3.5	3.8	3.1
Uttar Pradesh	*	3.0	3.1	3.3	3.5	3.6	3.7	3.8	3.4
East									
Bihar	(3.2)	3.2	3.1	3.3	3.5	3.5	3.8	3.8	3.4
Orissa	*	2.9	2.8	2.9	3.0	3.1	3.5	3.6	3.0
West Bengal	(2.8)	2.5	2.5	2.5	2.6	2.7	2.8	2.8	2.6
Northeast									
Arunachal Pradesh	*	3.8	4.3	4.5	4.8	4.9	5.6	(5.9)	4.7
Assam	*	3.0	2.9	3.1	3.2	3.3	3.5	3.7	3.2
Manipur	NC	*	3.2	3.5	3.7	4.0	4.2	4.4	3.7
Meghalaya	*	3.6	4.2	4.4	4.7	5.1	5.2	5.4	4.6
Mizoram	NC	(3.5)	3.8	3.8	4.1	4.5	4.9	5.1	4.3
Nagaland	NC	(3.0)	3.4	3.7	4.2	4.5	4.7	4.2	4.0
Tripura	*	2.5	2.4	2.5	2.5	2.7	2.9	2.6	2.6
West									
Goa	*	(2.6)	2.4	2.3	2.4	2.8	3.0	3.1	2.7
Gujarat	*	2.6	2.5	2.5	2.6	2.5	2.7	2.8	2.6
Maharashtra	(3.0)	2.5	2.4	2.5	2.5	2.6	2.6	2.8	2.5
South									
Andhra Pradesh	(2.6)	2.5	2.5	2.7	2.8	2.9	3.2	3.3	2.7
Karnataka	*	2.5	2.4	2.4	2.5	2.6	2.8	2.9	2.5
Kerala	*	2.7	2.5	2.4	2.5	2.7	2.9	3.2	2.6
Tamil Nadu	*	2.1	2.1	2.0	2.0	2.1	2.1	2.2	2.1

Note: Means are calculated excluding women who gave non-numeric responses.

NC: Not calculated because there are no cases on which to base a mean.

() Based on 25-49 unweighted cases.

* Mean not shown; based on fewer than 25 unweighted cases.

Table 7.10: Ideal sex composition of children by actual sex composition of living children

Mean ideal number of sons and daughters for ever-married women by sex composition of living children, according to residence, India, 1992-93

	Urban			Rural			Total		
Sex composition of living children	Sons	Daughters	Doesn't matter	Sons	Daughters	Doesn't matter	Sons	Daughters	Doesn't matter
None	0.9	0.7	0.5	1.4	1.0	0.3	1.3	0.9	0.3
1 child	0.9	0.7	0.4	1.4	0.9	0.2	1.3	0.9	0.3
1 son	1.0	0.7	0.4	1.4	0.9	0.2	1.3	0.8	0.3
No sons	0.9	0.8	0.4	1.4	1.0	0.2	1.3	0.9	0.3
2 children	1.0	0.8	0.4	1.5	1.0	0.2	1.3	0.9	0.3
2 sons	1.1	0.7	0.5	1.5	0.8	0.3	1.4	0.8	0.3
1 son	1.0	0.9	0.3	1.5	1.0	0.2	1.3	1.0	0.2
No sons	1.0	0.9	0.4	1.4	1.2	0.2	1.3	1.1	0.3
3 children	1.4	1.0	0.3	1.7	1.1	0.2	1.6	1.1	0.2
3 sons	1.5	0.8	0.3	1.9	0.9	0.2	1.8	0.9	0.2
2 sons	1.5	0.9	0.3	1.7	1.0	0.2	1.7	1.0	0.2
1 son	1.3	1.0	0.3	1.6	1.2	0.2	1.5	1.2	0.2
No sons	1.2	1.1	0.4	1.6	1.3	0.2	1.5	1.2	0.2
4+ children	1.7	1.2	0.3	2.1	1.4	0.2	2.0	1.3	0.2
2 or more sons	1.8	1.2	0.3	2.1	1.4	0.2	2.1	1.3	0.2
1 son	1.5	1.2	0.2	1.8	1.3	0.2	1.7	1.3	0.2
No sons	1.4	1.2	0.4	1.8	1.4	0.2	1.7	1.3	0.2
Total	1.2	0.9	0.4	1.7	1.1	0.2	1.6	1.1	0.2

Note: Table excludes women who gave non-numeric responses to the questions on the ideal number of sons and daughters.

Table 7.11: Fertility planning

Per cent distribution of births during the four years preceding the survey and current pregnancies by fertility planning status, according to selected background characteristics, India, 1992-93

Planning status of pregnancy

Background characteristic	Wanted then	Wanted later	Wanted no more	Missing	Total per cent	Number of births
Residence						
Urban	75.2	15.2	9.3	0.3	100.0	12878
Rural	77.4	13.4	8.6	0.5	100.0	44299
Education						
Illiterate	78.2	11.7	9.6	0.5	100.0	37845
Lit., < middle complete	72.4	18.2	9.1	0.3	100.0	9509
Middle school Complete	73.8	19.6	6.5	0.2	100.0	4089
High school and above	78.2	16.8	4.7	0.2	100.0	5 734
Religion						
Hindu	77.4	13.6	8.5	0.5	100.0	45412
Muslim	73.6	14.7	11.4	0.2	100.0	8765
Christian	76.2	17.2	6.3	0.3	100.0	1174
Sikh	82.7	11.3	6.0	—	100.0	970
Jain	84.1	11.2	4.7	—	100.0	177
Buddhist	80.1	13.4	6.4	0.1	100.0	398
Other	75.6	19.0	5.3	0.1	100.0	281
Caste/tribe						
Scheduled caste	77.0	13.0	9.2	0.8	100.0	7750
Scheduled tribe	82.6	10.7	6.1	0.6	100.0	5483
Other	76.2	14.4	9.0	0.4	100.0	43944
Birth order[1]						
1	89.0	10.2	0.4	0.4	100.0	15934
2	79.1	19.0	1.5	0.4	100.0	13754
3	75.8	15.9	7.9	0.4	100.0	9983
4	71.7	14.0	13.6	0.6	100.0	6621
5	66.7	12.1	20.7	0.5	100.0	4293
6+	56.6	9.7	33.0	0.6	100.0	6592
Mother's age at birth[2]						
13-14	83.4	16.0	0.4	0.2	100.0	471
15-19	83.3	14.9	1.2	0.6	100.0	12699
20-24	79.6	15.7	4.3	0.4	100.0	21675
25-29	75.0	13.3	11.4	0.3	100.0	13206
30-34	68.0	9.3	22.3	0.4	100.0	6136
35-39	57.6	7.3	34.2	0.9	100.0	2245
40-44	53.5	6.1	39.3	1.0	100.0	645
45-49	54.6	6.3	36.4	2.8	100.0	98
Total	76.9	13.8	8.8	0.5	100.0	57177

{Cont}.....

— Less than 0.05 per cent.
1 Includes current pregnancy, if any.
2 For current pregnancy, estimated maternal age at birth.

The impact of unwanted fertility can be estimated by comparing *wanted fertility rates* with the total fertility rates presented in Chapter 5. The wanted fertility rate is calculated in the same way as the total fertility rate, except that unwanted births are excluded from the numerator. A birth is considered unwanted if the number of living children at the time of conception was greater than or equal to the current ideal number of children, as reported by the respondent. Women who gave a non-numeric response to the question on the ideal number of children were assumed to want all their births. The wanted fertility rate represents the level of fertility that theoretically would result if all unwanted births were prevented. A comparison of the total fertility rate with the total wanted fertility rate indicates the potential demographic impact of the elimination of all unwanted births. Table 7.12 provides information on wanted fertility rates.

The wanted TFR for India of 2.6 is lower by three-quarters of a child (or 22 per cent) than the TFR of 3.4. Large differences between these two measures are evident for all population subgroups, and especially Muslims, scheduled castes, illiterate women, and rural women.

Table 7.13 provides similar information for each state. In Haryana, Assam and Uttar Pradesh, the wanted TFR is at least one child less than the TFR. On the other hand, the smallest differences between the wanted TFR and TFR are seen in Kerala and Mizoram (0.2 child). In general, the northern states show the largest percentage difference between the two rates (23-31 per cent). In contrast, the difference between the two rates is 10 per cent or less in Kerala and in four of the seven northeastern states (Arunachal Pradesh, Meghalaya, Mizoram and Nagaland).

For India as a whole, the total fertility rate would drop by 22 per cent if unwanted pregnancies could be eliminated. A reduction of this magnitude would bring the TFR down more than halfway between its current level and the replacement level of approximately 2.1 children per woman. Similarly, the contraceptive prevalence rate would increase from 41 per cent to 60 per cent if the unmet need for family planning could be totally satisfied. These underlying facts (based on women's stated preferences) provide a clear opportunity for improving the results of the family welfare programme. If women's expressed needs can be satisfied, then the quality of their lives and their children's lives will improve and considerable progress will be made toward achieving the country's population goals.

Table 7.12: Wanted fertility rates

Total wanted fertility rates and total fertility rates for the three years preceding the survey, by selected background characteristics, India, 1992-93

Background characteristic	Total wanted fertility rate	Total fertility rate
Residence		
Urban	2.09	2.70
Rural	2.86	3.67
Education		
Illiterate	3.15	4.03
Literate, < middle complete	2.31	3.01
Middle school complete	1.95	2.49
High school and above	1.78	2.15
Religion		
Hindu	2.58	3.30
Muslim	3.35	4 41
Christian	2.41	2.87
Sikh	1.79	2.43
Other	2.20	2.77
Caste/tribe		
Scheduled caste	2.93	3.92
Scheduled tribe	2.94	3.55
Other	2.57	3.30
Total	2.64	3.39

Note: Rates are calculated based on births in the period 1-36 months before the interview to women age 15-49. The total fertility rates are the same as those presented in Table 5.3.

Table 7.13: Wanted fertility rates
Totat wanted fertility rates and total fertility rates for the three years preceding the survey, by state, India, 1992-93.

State	Total wanted fertility rate	Total fertility rate
India	2.64	3.39
North		
Delhi	2.20	3.02
Haryana	2.81	3.99
Himachal Pradesh	2.04	2.97
Jammu Region of J & K	2.21	3.13
Punjab	2.15	2.92
Rajasthan	2.78	3.63
Central		
Madhya Pradesh	3.21	3.90
Uttar Pradesh	3.82	4.82
East		
Bihar	3.18	4.00
Orissa	2.32	2.92
West Bengal	2.20	2.92
Northeast		
Arunachal Pradesh	3.84	4.25
Assam	2.52	3.53
Manipur	2.29	2.76
Meghalaya	3.39	3. 73
Mizoram	2.09	2.30
Nagaland	2.95	3.26
Tripura	1.98	2.67
West		
Goa	1.60	1.90
Gujarat	2.33	2.99
Maharashtra	2.13	2.86
South		
Andhra Pradesh	2.09	2.59
Karnataka	2.18	2.85
Kerala	1.82	2.00
Tamil Nadu	1.76	2.48

Note: Rates are calculated based on births in the period 1-36 months before the interview to women age 15-49. The total fertility rates are the same as those presented in Table 5.2.

8

MORBIDITY AND MORTALITY

The data on the prevalence ,of certain diseases as well as mortality rates, especially for infants and young children is presented in this chapter. This type of information is relevant both to the demographic assessment of the population and to health policies and programmes. Mortality estimates are also useful (in conjunction with fertility estimates) for projecting the future size of the population. Detailed information on the mortality of children can be used to identify sectors of the population that are at high risk and in need of health services.

The NFHS collected information on mortality and morbidity in both the Household and Woman's Questionnaires. The Household Questionnaire includes questions on individuals in the household suffering from blindness, tuberculosis, leprosy, physical impairment of the limbs, and malaria. The Household Questionnaire also includes a question on deaths occurring in the household during the past two years. The Woman's Questionnaire collects information on the survival status of all births, the age at death if the child died, and the prevalence of common childhood diseases for children under 4 years of age. The prevalence and treatment of childhood diseases are discussed in *Chapter 9*.

8.1 MORBIDITY AND PHYSICAL IMPAIRMENTS

Because demographic sample surveys generally do not include questions on the prevalence of diseases, there is little experience on which to base an assessment of the validity and reliability of such questions. The patterns shown by the morbidity data analyzed in this section are generally plausible, suggesting that the questions have provided useful information. At the same time, there is little to indicate whether the overall prevalence levels are correct. It is certainly possible that the results of the survey substantially understate the prevalence of certain conditions because some survey respondents fail to report them.

It is worth noting some of the possible reasons for failure to report particular health conditions. Conditions carrying a stigma, such as leprosy, may be underreported due to intentional concealment by respondents or embarrassment on the part of interviewers about asking these questions. Respondents are aware of certain conditions, such as blindness and physical impairment, but may be unaware of others unless they have been diagnosed by medical personnel. Moreover, given the linguistic diversity in India, locally as well as nationally, respondents may know that a household member suffers from a given condition but fail to report it because they do not recognize the words used by the interviewer in asking the question.

Table 8.1 shows, for all India, the prevalence in the household population of the five health conditions listed in the Household Questionnaire. Of the five, malaria has the highest incidence, afflicting 3,324 per 100,000 population during the three months prior to the survey. Blindness (partial or complete), reported for 3,001 per 100,000 population, is second most prevalent. The remaining diseases all show an overall incidence of less than 700 per 100,000.

Malaria

In the NFHS, more than 3 per cent of the population was reported to have malaria in the three months before the survey. It should be noted that the NFHS was not undertaken at the same time of the year in all states and, hence, the calendar dates of the reference period (three months prior to the survey) for the assessment of the prevalence of malaria vary from state to state. Since there is seasonal variation in the incidence of malaria, the prevalence rates of malaria for any state cannot be assumed to reflect the situation throughout the year in that state. However, the data collection was conducted in three phases throughout the year, and hence the prevalence rate for total India may be taken as more representative of the situation throughout the year.

The prevalence of malaria is more than twice as high in rural areas (3,896 per 100,000) than in urban areas (1,729 per 100,000), and is slightly higher for males than for females (3,363 per 100,000 compared with 3,283 per 100,000). The sex differential is very small in both urban and rural areas. Differences in prevalence among age groups are modest but suggest that prevalence is higher for those age 60 and over than for those below age 60 for India as a whole. This is also true for rural areas, which constitute the bulk of India's population, but in urban areas the prevalence of malaria is highest among children age 0-4.

Table 8.1: Morbidity and physical impairments

Number of persons per 100,000 household population suffering from blindness, tuberculosis, leprosy, physical impairment of the limbs, and malaria, according to age, sex and residence, India, 1992-93

Demographic characteristic	Number of persons per 100,000 suffering from:						Number of usual residents
	Blindness						
	Partial	Complete	Tuberculosis	Leprosy	Physical impairment of limbs	Malaria during the last three months	
URBAN							
Age							
0 - 4	97	164	140	42	366	2072	13964
5 - 14	366	698	181	74	512	1789	31174
15-59	2055	177	368	104	521	1634	77904
60-69	12747	877	998	150	900	1800	5669
70+	17772	2035	1033	72	2141	1817	3341
Sex							
Male	1972	366	397	104	671	1655	68595
Female	2666	386	286	79	439	1810	63456
Total	2306	375	344	92	559	1729	132051
RURAL							
0 - 4	220	195	81	29	461	3650	47207
5 - 14	324	525	117	68	688	4026	96109
15-59	2210	204	617	152	598	3749	195415
60-69	15096	1244	1812	371	1183	5005	18666
70+	21222	3252	1731	297	1721	4546	11044

Sex							
Male	2482	411	625	162	814	3984	188843
Female	2900	450	393	95	513	3804	179599
Total	2686	430	512	130	667	3896	368441
TOTAL							
Age							
0 - 4	192	188	95	32	440	3290	61172
5 -14	334	567	132	69	645	3478	127283
15-59	2166	196	546	138	576	3146	273319
60-69	14549	1159	1623	320	1117	4258	24335
70+	20421	2970	1569	245	1818	3912	14384
Sex							
Male	2346	399	564	147	776	3363	257438
Female	2839	433	365	91	494	3283	243055
Total	2585	416	467	120	639	3324	500492

Note: Table excludes persons with missing information on sex.

Partial and Complete Blindness

The overall prevalence of partial blindness is 2,585 per 100,000 population, with slightly lower prevalence in urban than in rural areas (2,306 compared with 2,686 per 100,000). Prevalence rates range from 192 per 100,000 for persons age 0-4 to 20,421 per 100,000 for persons age 70 and over. The much higher prevalence among older persons is striking and probably reflects a combination of historical improvements in the prevention of blindness and the tendency for blindness to increase with age at all periods in history. In both urban and rural areas, females are more prone to partial blindness than are males. In the country as a whole, the prevalence of partial blindness is 2,839 per 100,000 for females and 2,346 per 100,000 for males.

The overall prevalence of complete blindness is 416 per 100,000 population. The NFHS estimate of total blindness is considerably higher than the 1981 Census estimate of 73 per 100,000 (Office of the Registrar General and Census Commissioner, 1983). This is probably indicative of relatively high underenumeration in the census rather than a substantial increase in blindness between 1981 and 1992-93.

The prevalence of complete blindness is slightly higher in rural areas (430 per 100,000) than in urban areas (375 per 100,000). Females are more prone than males to total blindness in both urban and rural areas, although the differences between the sexes are small. As expected, complete blindness is also far more prevalent among the old than among the young or middle-aged.

Physical Impairment of the Limbs

The overall prevalence of persons with physically impaired limbs is 639 per 100,000, with a slightly higher prevalence in rural areas than in urban areas. Physical impairment of the limbs is more common among males (776 per 100,000) than among females (494 per 100,000). The sex differential is similar in urban and rural areas. As with blindness, impairment of the limbs is much more prevalent among those age 60 and over than among younger people: 440 to 645 per 100,000 at ages 0-4 and 5-14 compared with 1,818 per 100,000 at age 70 and over.

Tuberculosis

Tuberculosis, which is becoming an increasing problem worldwide has an overall prevalence of 467 per 100,000, with rural areas once again having a higher prevalence than urban areas (512 per 100,000 compared with 314 per 100,000). The prevalence of tuberculosis is higher among males (564 per 100,000) than among females (365 per 100,000).

Age differences are marked, ranging from 95 per 100,000 at age 0-4 to about 1,600 per 100,000 at ages 60 and over.

Leprosy

The reported prevalence of leprosy is only 120 per 100,000. The observed sex difference is small, with higher prevalence for males than for females in both urban and rural areas. The prevalence of leprosy tends to rise with age, but is slightly lower at age 70 and over than at age 60-69. This pattern prevails in both urban and rural areas. It is not clear why prevalence falls off after age 70, but it could be due to lower probabilities of survival for persons who contracted leprosy further in the past.

Comparisons by State

Table 8.2 shows comparisons of prevalence rates for morbidity and physical impairments by state. The prevalence of partial blindness varies considerably by state, from a low of 557 per 100,000 in Meghalaya to a high of 5,142 per 100,000 in Andhra Pradesh. The states with prevalence rates below 1,000 per 100,000 are Meghalaya, Jammu, Tamil Nadu, Punjab, Haryana, Arunachal Pradesh, West Bengal, Assam and Himachal Pradesh. The states with prevalence rates above 2,500 per 100,000 are Andhra Pradesh, Karnataka, Rajasthan, Madhya Pradesh, Maharashtra, Orissa, Gujarat and Uttar Pradesh.

Variation in the prevalence rate for complete blindness is also large. In this case the prevalence rate ranges from 115 per 100,000 in Mizoram to 842 per 100,000 in Andhra Pradesh. The states with prevalence rates below 200 per 100,000 are Mizoram, Manipur, Nagaland, Haryana, West Bengal, Assam and Punjab. The states with prevalence rates above 400 per 100,000 include Andhra Pradesh, Uttar Pradesh, Rajasthan, Bihar, Madhya Pradesh, Himachal Pradesh and Gujarat. The prevalence of partial blindness and the prevalence of complete blindness are positively correlated at 0.75; in most cases, the higher the prevalence of partial blindness, the higher the incidence of complete blindness.

State differentials are also substantial for the other conditions examined. Physical impairment of the limbs is most common in Nagaland but it is also a substantial problem in Punjab and the southern states of Andhra Pradesh, Karnataka and Tamil Nadu. Levels of tuberculosis are particularly high in Manipur, Arunachal Pradesh and Rajasthan and leprosy is reported to be relatively high in Uttar Pradesh and Manipur.

Table 8.2: Morbidity and physical impairments by state

Number of persons per 100,000 household population suffering from blindness, tuberculosis, leprosy, physical impairment of the limbs, and malaria by state, India, 1992-93

	Number of persons per 100,000 suffering from:					
State	Blindness Partial	Complete	Tuberculosis	Liprosy	Physical impairment of limbs	Malaria during the last three months
India	**2585**	**416**	**467**	**120**	**639**	**3324**
North						
Delhi	1269	208	192	101	240	554
Haryana	679	145	327	14	681	933
Himachal Pradesh	929	455	242	56	562	1141
Jammu Region of J & K	620	249	245	18	663	853
Punjab	664	199	238	28	841	2546
Rajasthan	4182	479	724	128	593	5103
Central						
Madhya Pradesh	3353	478	435	136	73 3	4728
Uttar Pradesh	2557	544	560	222	632	7395
East						
Bihar	2270	479	595	123	712	1428
Orissa	2842	319	555	96	583	5148
West Bengal	753	161	357	47	386	678
Northeast						
Arunachal Pradesh	718	294	938	110	460	4213
Assam	914	192	638	36	406	2707
Manipur	1319	123	951	199	460	1641
Meghalaya	557	202	321	17	590	4723
Mizoram	1409	115	311	33	459	4636
Nagaland	1237	136	491	153	1101	2778
Tripura	1141	289	289	0	482	2619
West						
Goa	2456	258	179	16	532	243
Gujarat	2819	447	308	29	539	3228
Maharashtra	3214	320	293	72	573	3742
South						
Andhra Pradesh	5142	842	407	118	785	1944
Karnataka	4517	383	136	132	795	457
Kerala	1104	300	586	18	662	112
Tamil Nadu	632	204	703	209	759	576

The prevalence of malaria varies widely across the states, at least partly because of seasonal variations in the timing of the survey fieldwork. Malaria was most often reported in the belt extending from Rajasthan through Uttar Pradesh and Madhya Pradesh to Orissa. On the other hand, there were very few reports of malaria in Kerala, Goa and Delhi. No state is worse than the national average for all of the diseases or medical conditions, but three states (West Bengal, Tripura and Goa) consistently have lower prevalence than the national average.

8.2 Crude Death Rates and Age-Sex-Specific Death Rates

Table 8.3 shows crude death rates (CDRs) and age-sex-specific death rates by residence for the usual resident population of India, as estimated from both the NFHS and the Sample Registration System (SRS), which is maintained by the Office of the Registrar General. The death rates from the NFHS are based on deaths occurring to usual residents of the household during the two years preceding the survey (approximately 1991-92) as obtained from the Household Questionnaire, and the death rates from the SRS are the average rates for 1991-92. The death rates from the NFHS are calculated as the annual number of deaths in each age group in the two-year period before the date of interview per 1,000 usual residents. The denominator of this measure is calculated by projecting the number of usual residents at the time of the survey back to the mid-point of the time period on the basis of the intercensal population growth rate in the state. The urban intercensal growth rate is assumed to be the same for all age and sex groups in urban areas. Similarly, the rural intercensal growth rate is applied to all rural age and sex groups and the total intercensal growth rate is applied to the total population in each age and sex group.

Questions on the number of deaths occurring to usual residents in each household during a particular time period have been included in demographic surveys in many countries, and have generally resulted in a substantial understatement of deaths. We, therefore, begin by considering the evidence on the completeness of reporting of deaths. The Sample Registration System (SRS) provides a useful comparison.

Table 8.3 shows an estimated CDR for India of 9.7 per 1,000 in the NFHS, compared with 10.0 per 1,000 from the SRS. Therefore, overall estimates from the two sources agree quite well. The rural estimates are also quite similar (10.4 per 1,000 in the NFHS and 10.8 per 1,000 in the SRS). The NFHS estimate for urban areas (7.6 per 1 ,000) is slightly higher than the SRS estimate (7.1 per 1,000). The urban CDR estimated by the NFHS is 27 per cent lower than the rural CDR. The NFHS estimate of the CDR may be subtracted from the earlier NFHS estimate of the crude birth rate from the household birth record (Table 5.1 in Chapter 5) to calculate the rate of natural increase of the population of India. The rate of natural increase so estimated is 18.3 per 1,000 population per year for the two-year period before the survey. These estimates imply a doubling time of 38 years for India's population in the absence of net international migration. At this rate of growth, India's population will reach one billion in the year 2000 and 1.5 billion in 2022.

By sex, the male CDR (10.0 in both the NFHS and the SRS) is slightly higher than the female CDR in the NFHS (9.4) and the same as the female CDR in the SRS (10.0). Table 8.3 also compares age-sex-specific death rates by residence from the NFHS and the SRS. On the whole, the two sets of estimates agree rather well, with a tendency for age-specific death rates from the NFHS to be slightly lower than corresponding rates from the SRS. In both cases, death rates are relatively high for the youngest children (age 0-4), uniformly low at ages 5-44, and rapidly increasing at ages 45 and above.

In most countries, male death rates are higher than female death rates at nearly all ages. South Asia generally has been an exception in this respect, with higher death rates for females over much of the age span (Preston, 1990; Ghosh, 1987). In the NFHS, females have higher age-specific death rates up to age 35, after which males generally have higher rates.

Comparisons among the NFHS estimates of the CDR by state (Table 8.4) show that the CDR ranges from 1.9 per 1,000 in Nagaland to 11.9 per 1,000 in Uttar Pradesh, with most estimates falling in the range of 8-12 per 1,000. The estimates for Nagaland and Mizoram seem implausibly low, as does the estimate for urban residents of Arunachal Pradesh. It should be pointed out, however, that the sampling errors are relatively large in these areas due to the small size of the samples. Delhi, Jammu, Punjab, Meghalaya, Mizoram and Tripura are the only exceptions to the general tendency of the rural CDR to exceed the urban CDR.

Table 8.4 also shows the average CDRs for the year 1991-92 from the SRS for 23 states for which the SRS has published estimates. The NFHS and SRS estimates differ by less than 1 per 1,000 in 9 of the 17 major states. In the remaining major states, the NFHS estimates are higher than the SRS estimates for Delhi, Bihar and West Bengal and lower than the SRS estimates for Rajasthan, Madhya Pradesh, Orissa, Andhra Pradesh and Karnataka. In the six small states for which comparisons can be made, two states have estimates that differ by less than 1 per 1,000 and the SRS estimates are higher in three of the four remaining states.

Table 8.3: Crude death rates and age-sex specific death rates
Crude Death Rates (CDR) and age-sex specific death rates from the NFHS and the SRS, by residence, India, 1991-92

	NFHS (1991-92)			SRS (1991-92)		
Age	Male	Female	Total	Male	Female	Total
			URBAN			
0 - 4	14.4	15.8	15.1	15.4	16.3	15.8
5 - 9	1.6	1.9	1.7	1.4	1.6	1.5
10-14	1.6	0.3	1.0	0.8	0.9	0.9
15-19	1.3	1.7	1.5	1.3	1.6	1.4
20-24	1 8	1.4	1.6	1.8	2.1	2.0
25-29	2 5	2.4	2.5	2.2	2.2	2.3
30-34	2.3	2.8	2.5	2.5	2.1	2.3
35-39	4 0	2.1	3.1	3.5	2.9	3.3
40-44	4 5	2.3	3.5	4.9	3.2	4.1
45-49	5.7	4.9	5.4	8.3	4.2	6.4
50-54	11 7	5.4	8.9	12.6	7.9	10.5
55-59	16 5	10.1	13.2	20.2	13.7	17.1
60-64	33.6	15.5	24.3	31.4	20.6	26.0
65-69	41.2	22.9	32.3	41.2	34.3	37.6
70+	95.8	94.1	95.0	88.7	78.2	83.1
CDR	8.3	6.9	7.6	7.4	6.8	7.1
			RURAL			
0 - 4	25.4	25.9	25.7	27.7	30.7	29.1
5 - 9	2.3	2.6	2.5	2.8	3.5	3.2
10-14	1.6	2.2	1.9	1.5	1.8	1.6
15-19	2.2	3.4	2.8	2.0	2.8	2.4
20-24	2.9	3.2	3.0	2.6	3.6	3.1
25-29	2.4	3.1	2.8	2.8	3.5	3.1
30-34	2.7	3.4	3.0	3.5	3.4	3.4
35-39	4.0	3.3	3.7	4.3	3.9	4.1
40-44	5.3	3.9	4.7	5.9	4.7	5.3
45-49	8.2	4.6	6.5	9.5	6.1	7.8
50-54	10.1	10.9	10.5	13.5	9.8	11.7
55-59	14.0	9.8	11.7	20.8	14.9	17.9
60-64	24.2	20.3	22.3	33.1	25.3	29.2
65-69	30.8	29.7	30.3	48.0	40.1	44.0
70+	91.0	99.9	94.9	98.1	89.7	93.7
CDR	10.6	10.3	10.4	10.7	10.8	10.8
			TOTAL			
0 - 4	23.0	23.6	23.3	25.3	27.9	26.5

{Cont}.....

5 - 9	2.1	2.5	2.3	2.5	3.1	2.8
10-14	1.6	1.7	1.6	1.4	1.6	1.5
15-19	2.0	2.9	2.5	1.9	2.6	2:2
20-24	2 5	2.7	2.6	2.4	3.2	2.8
25-29	2 4	2.9	2.7	2.7	3.2	2.9
30-34	2.6	3.2	2.9	3.3	3.1	3.2
35-39	4.0	3.0	3.5	4.1	3.6	3.9
40-44	5.1	3.4	4.3	5.4	4.2	5.0
45-49	7.5	4.7	6.2	9.2	5.7	7.5
50-54	10.6	9.4	10.0	13.3	9.4	11.4
55-59	14.7	9.9	12.1	20.7	14.6	17.7
60-64	26.2	19.1	22.8	32.7	24.3	28.6
65-69	33.2	28.0	30.8	46.7	39.0	42.7
70+	92.1	98.5	95.0	96.1	87.3	91.5
CDR	10.0	9.4	9.7	10.0	10.0	10.0

Note: Crude death rates and age-sex specific death rates from the NFHS are based on the annual number of deaths reported for the *de jure* population during the two years prior to the Survey. The SRS rates are the average rates for 1991-92, based on the *de jure* population.
Source for the SRS: Office of the Registrar General (1993a, 1994)

8.3 Infant and Child Mortality

Definitions of Infant and Child Mortality

All respondents in the NFHS were asked to provide a complete birth history, including sex, date of birth, survival status, and age at the time of the survey or age at death for each live birth. For children who had died, age at death was recorded in days for children dying in the first month of life, in months for children dying before their second birthday, and in years for children dying at later ages. This information was used to calculate the following direct estimates of infant and child mortality[1]:

Neonatal mortality: the probability of dying in the first month of life;

Postneonatal mortality: the difference between infant and neonatal mortality;

Infant mortality ($_1q_0$) the probability of dying before the first birth day;

Child mortality ($_4q_1$): the probability of dying between the first and fifth birthday;

Under-five mortality($_5q_0$): the probability of dying before the fifth birth day.

Table 8.4: Crude death rates by state

Crude death rates from the NFHS and the SRS, by state and residence, India, 1991-92

	NFHS (1991-92)			SRS (1991-92)		
State	Urban	Rural	Total	Urban	Rural	Total
India	7.6	10.4	9.7	7.1	10.8	10.0
North						
Delhi	8.0	4.1	7.8	6 2[a]	7.9[a]	6.3[a]
Haryana	8.1	9.3	9.0	6.9	8.9	8.5
Himachal Pradesh	6.5	8.6	8.4	6.5[b]	8.7[b]	8.6b
Jammu Region of J & K	8.9	8.6	8.7	U	U	U
Punjab	7.2	7.0	7.1	6.1	8.7	8.0
Rajasthan	7.2	7.9	7.8	7.7	10.6	10.1
Central						
Madhya Pradesh	9.1	10.7	10.3	9.2[b]	14.9[b]	13.8[b]
Uttar Pradesh	7.7	13.0	11.9	8.3	12.0	11.3
East						
Bihar	9.0	12.0	11.5	6.3	10.2	9.8
Orissa	7.4	11.6	11.0	6.5	13.5	12.8
West Bengal	8.6	10.2	9.7	6.7[b]	8.9[b]	8.3[b]
Northeast						
Arunachal Pradesh	0.8	9.1	8.2	3.3	12.8[a]	9.3[a]
Assam	7.0	11.9	11.3	6.9	11.8	11.5
Manipur	5.3	6.1	5.8	6.1	5.5[a]	5.6
Meghalaya	6.6	6.1	6.2	3.4	9.4[a]	8.4
Mizoram	4.2	2.7	3.4	U	U	U
Nagaland	1.7	2.0	1.9	0.8	4.4[a]	3.7[a]
Tripura	13.0	11.6	11.8	5.3	7.6[a]	7.4[a]
West						
Goa	5.9	7.1	6.5	6.0	7.8[a]	7.2[a]
Gujarat	7.2	10.2	9.1	7.9	8.8	8.5
Maharashtra	7.3	8.1	7.7	6.2	9.3	8.2
South						
Andhra Pradesh	7.4	9.2	8.7	6.7[b]	10.5[b]	9.7[b]
Karnataka	6.2	8.1	7.5	6.9	9.8	9.0
Kerala	6.1	6.3	6.2	5.3	6.2	6.0
Tamil Nadu	7.3	11.0	9.7	7.6[b]	9.5[b]	8.8[b]

Note: Crude death rates from the NFHS are based on the annual number of deaths reported for the *de jure* population during the two years prior to the survey. The SRS rates are the average rates for 1991-92, based on the *de jure* population.

U: Not available.

[a] Three years moving average, 1990-92. [b] Average rates for 1990-91.

Source for the SRS: Office of the Registrar General (1993 [a], 1993[b], 1994).

Assessment of Data Quality

The reliability of mortality estimates calculated from retrospective birth histories depends upon the completeness with which deaths of children are reported and the extent to which birth dates and ages at deaths are accurately reported and recorded. Estimated rates of infant and child mortality are subject to both sampling and nonsampling errors. This section describes the results of various checks for nonsampling errors — in particular, underreporting of deaths in early childhood (which would result in an underestimate of mortality) and misreporting of the date of birth or age at death (which could distort the age pattern of under-five mortality). Both problems are likely to be more pronounced for children born long before the survey than for children born recently. Failure to report deaths will result in mortality figures that are too low. If underreporting is more severe for children born longer ago, the estimates will tend to understate any decline in mortality that has occurred.

Underreporting of infant deaths, in particular, is usually most severe for deaths which occur very early in infancy. If deaths in the early neonatal period are selectively underreported, then there will be an abnormally low ratio of deaths under seven days to all neonatal deaths and an abnormally low ratio of neonatal to infant mortality. Changes in these ratios over time can be examined to test the hypothesis that underreporting of early infant deaths is more common for births that occurred longer before the survey. Results fir suggest that early infant deaths have not been severely underreported in India as a whole in the NFHS, since the ratios of deaths under seven days to all neonatal deaths are quite high (a ratio of less than 25 per cent is often used as a guideline to indicate underreporting of early neonatal deaths). The ratios decline slightly over time, from 70 in the five years preceding the survey to 66 in the period 10-14 years preceding the survey, indicating that some early infant deaths may not have been reported by older women. The ratios of infant deaths that occurred during the neonatal period are also quite high, and again they increase slightly over time.

One problem that is inherent in most retrospective surveys is heaping of ages at death on certain digits, *e.g.*, 6, 12 and 18 months. Misreporting of the age at death will bias estimates of the age pattern of mortality if the net result of misreporting is the transference of deaths between age segments for which the rates are calculated; for example, an overestimate of child mortality relative to infant mortality may result if children dying during the first year of life are reported as having died at age one or older. Thus, heaping at 12 months can bias the mortality estimates because a certain fraction of these deaths, which are reported to have occurred after infancy (i.e., at ages 12-23 months), may have actually occurred during infancy (i.e., at ages 0-11 months). In this case, heaping would bias the infant mortality rate ($_1q_0$) downward and child mortality ($_4q_1$) upward.

In the NFHS, there was some misreporting of age at death due to a preference for reporting age at death at 3, 6, 8, 10, 12, 15, 20 and 25 days. Examination of the distribution of deaths under age two years during the 15 years prior to the survey by month of death indicates that the calculated infant mortality rates for India as a whole are not likely to be understated by more than 1-2 per cent because of age heaping. There was some heaping on 12 months of death, but due to strong emphasis during interviewer trainings[2], there were few deaths reported to have occurred at age one year. This brief check on internal consistency of the NFHS childhood mortality data for all India suggests that although there is some evidence of heaping in age at death at certain ages, the bias in infant and child mortality rates arising from this heaping is negligible.

However, an examination of the distribution of births and deaths since 1982 suggests that there may be some underreporting of deaths in the most recent five-year period. The proportion of deaths to births decreases from 13 per cent in 1982-87 to 9 per cent since 1987. Some of this decrease undoubtedly reflects a real reduction in mortality during that period and some reflects the fact that younger children have had less exposure to the risk of mortality. However, the sharp disjuncture in the proportion of deaths between 1987 and 1988 may be due partly to underreporting of deaths relative to births during the most recent period.

It is seldom possible to establish, with confidence, mortality levels for a period more than 15 years before a survey. Even within the recent 15-year period considered here, apparent trends in mortality rates should be interpreted with caution for several reasons. First, there may be differences in the completeness of death reporting related to the length of time before the survey. Second, the accuracy of reports of age at death and of date of birth may deteriorate systematically with time. Third, sampling variability for mortality rates is relatively high especially for groups with relatively few births. The fourth reason relates to truncation of mortality rates further back in time, because women currently age 50 and over who were bearing children during these periods were not included in the survey. This truncation particularly affects mortality trends. For example, for the period 10-14 years before the survey, the rates do not include any births for women age 40-49 since these women were over age 50 at the time of the survey and not eligible to be interviewed.

Since these excluded births to older women were likely to be at a somewhat greater risk of dying than births to younger women, the mortality levels for the period may be slightly underestimated. However, the estimates for later periods are less affected by the truncation bias since fewer older women are excluded. The extent of this bias depends on the proportion of births omitted, however, and Table 8.9 shows that among children born in the five years before the survey, only S per cent were born to women over age 34 years. Given this small proportion of births excluded, selection bias for infant and child mortality statistics as far back as 15 years before the survey should be negligible.

Levels and Trends in Infant and Child Mortality

Table 8.5 and Figure 8.1 show various measures of infant and child mortality by residence group for the three quinquennial periods preceding the survey. Infant mortality rates in India declined by 22 per cent during the 15 years prior to the NFHS. The infant mortality rate for the total population declined from 101 per 1,000 births 10-14 years prior to the survey (approximately 1978-82) to 79 per 1,000 births 0-4 years prior (approximately 1988-92), an average rate of decline of 2 infant deaths per 1,000 live births per year. There was a steady decline in all of the mortality measures over the three S-year periods preceding the survey. The percentage decline in mortality was not the same for all five measures of mortality. The largest proportionate decline is observed for child mortality (31 per cent) and the smallest for neonatal mortality (18 per cent). Postneonatal mortality fell by 27 per cent and under-five mortality by 24 per cent. Most of the decline in child mortality occurred between the periods 10-14 years and 5-9 years preceding the survey, but for neonatal and postneonatal mortality, the rate of decline accelerated between the two most recent periods.

In all instances, urban mortality rates are lower than rural mortality rates. In the fiveyear period preceding the survey, infant mortality was 52 per cent higher in rural areas than in urban areas and child mortality was nearly twice as high in rural areas. Urban-rural differences in the rate of decline of mortality depend on the mortality measure examined. Postneonatal mortality and infant mortality declined by a larger percentage in rural areas than in urban areas, whereas neonatal mortality and child mortality fell by about the same percentage in the two areas. Overall, under-five mortality fell slightly faster in rural areas (25 per cent) than in urban areas (22 per cent).

Table 8.5: Infant and child mortality

Neonatal, postneonatal, infant, child and under-five mortality for five-year periods preceding the survey, by residence, India, 1992-93

Years prior to survey	Neonatal mortality (NN)	Postneonatal mortality[1] (PNN)	Infant mortality $({}_1q_0)$	Child mortality $({}_4q_1)$	Under-five mortality $({}_5q_0)$
		URBAN			
0-4 years	34.1	22.0	56.1	19.6	74.6
5-9 years	36.8	25.7	62.4	20.6	81.8
10-14 years	42.5	26.1	68.7	29.0	95.7
		RURAL			
0-4 years	52.9	32.2	85.0	37.6	119.4
5-9 years	62.2	40.7	102.9	43.3	141.8
10-14 years	65.1	46.2	111.3	55.0	160.2
		TOTAL			
0-4 years	48.6	29.9	78. 5	3.4	109.3
5-9 years	56.4	37.2	93.6	37.7	127.8
10-14 years	59.5	41.2	100.7	48.2	144.0

[1] Computed as the difference between the infant and neonatal mortality rates.

Despite the improvements in infant and child mortality, 1 in every 13 children still dies in the first year of life, and 1 in 9 dies before reaching age five. Clearly child survival programmes in India need to be intensified to produce further reductions in the level of infant and child mortality.

The estimated NFHS infant mortality rate of 79 in 1988-92 is virtually identical to the 1990 SRS value of 80 infant deaths per 1,000 live births, but slightly lower than the average SRS infant mortality rate of 85 for the period 1988-92 (Office of the Registrar General, 1993b, 1994). In rural areas, the NFHS estimate (85) is lower than the average SRS estimate of 92 for 1988-92, but in urban areas the NFHS rate of 56 is almost identical to the SRS rate of 55. For earlier periods also, the overall NFHS estimates of infant mortality are somewhat lower than the SRS estimates—5 per cent lower in 1983-87 (94 compared with 99) and 12 per cent lower in 1978-82 (101 compared with 115).

Socioeconomic Differentials in Infant and Child Mortality

Table 8.6 and Figure 8.2 show infant and child mortality statis-

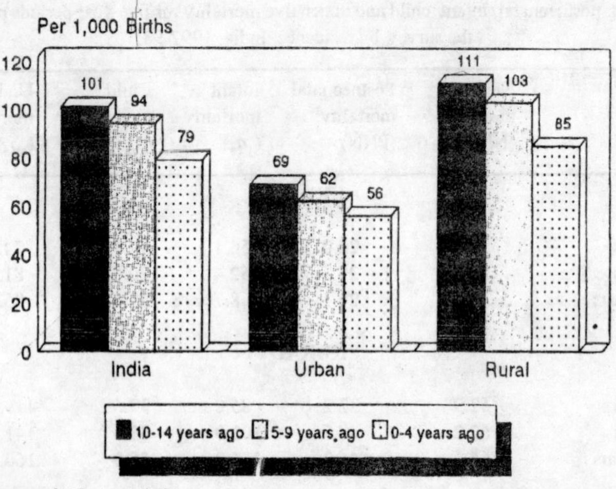

Figure 8.1: Infant Mortality Rates for Five-Year Periods by Residence

tics for the 10-year period preceding the survey, by selected background characteristics. As one would expect, infant mortality declines sharply with increasing education of mothers, from a high of 101 per 1,000 for illiterate mothers to a low of 37 for mothers with at least a high school education. The other mortality indicators vary by education in a similar fashion. Scheduled castes have higher levels of infant mortality than scheduled tribes, who in turn have higher levels than non-SC/ST women. Hindus have higher infant and child mortality than Muslims, and other religious groups (Christians, Sikhs, Jains and Buddhists) have substantially lower rates.

Antenatal or delivery care by a trained health professional is associated with greatly reduced infant and child mortality risks. Infant mortality rates range from 97 per 1,000 for births with neither antenatal or delivery care, to 64 per 1,000 for births with either type of care, and 44 per 1,000 for births with both types of care. One might expect the effect of antenatal and delivery care to be most pronounced for mortality risks immediately following birth (neonatal mortality), but this is not the case. The impact of antenatal and delivery care is considerably greater for child mortality (with a 76 per cent reduction if both types of care are received, relative to neither type of care) than for neonatal mortality (48 per cent reduction). It seems unlikely that the presence of antenatal or delivery care can explain fully its apparent impact. Utilization of antenatal and delivery care services is undoubtedly associated with other circumstances favourable to child survival, which might explain the apparently large effect of antenatal and delivery care on child mortality.

The impact of antenatal and delivery care on survival during the first month of life is nonetheless very large. Children of mothers who received no such care have a neonatal mortality rate that is almost twice that experienced by children whose mothers received both antenatal and delivery care, 58 compared with 30 per 1,000 live births. The differential is all the more impressive because women who have pregnancy-related complications (whose babies have a relatively high risk of dying) are usually more likely to seek antenatal and delivery care in the first place (see Table 9.9 in Chapter 9).

Table 8.6 also shows that the place of delivery is associated with substantial differences in infant and child mortality. Births delivered at home have the highest infant and child mortality rates, followed by births delivered in public facilities. Binhs delivered in private facilities have considerably lower mortality rates. Again, these differences undoubtedly reflect socioeconomic differences as well as the direct effects of place of delivery. For example, those who give birth in private facilities tend to come from higher socioeconomic groups.

The pattern of socioeconomic differentials in infant and child mortality just described typifies both urban and rural areas as well as the whole country. However, absolute levels of infant and child mortality are considerably lower in urban areas than in rural areas.

Demographic Differentials in Infant and Child Mortality

This section examines differentials in infant and child mortality by demographic characteristics of both the child and the mother. Table 8.7 and Figure 8.3 present mortality rates for the 10 years preceding the survey by sex of the child, age of the mother at the time of the child's birth, birth order, length of the previous birth interval and size of the child at birth.

The data on death rates in Table 8.3 indicated that the female death rate for the age group 0-4 exceeds the male rate by 3 per cent. Table 8.7 suggests that, within this age group, excess female mortality occurs only after the neonatal period. During the neonatal period, males have a higher risk of dying than females (57 compared with 48 deaths per 1,000 births). Higher neonatal mortality among boys than girls is found in most populations and reflects greater underlying male frailty. Postneonatal mortality, however, is 13 per cent higher for females than for males, and child mortality (ages 1-4) is 43 per cent higher for

Table 8 6: Infant and child mortal1ty by backgrgund characteristics
Neonatal, postneonatal, infant, child and under-five mortality by selected background characteristics for the 10-year period preceding the survey, India, 1992-93

Background characteristic	Neonatal mortality (NN)	Posts-neonatal mortality (PNN)	Infant ortality (${}_4q_0$)	Child mortality (${}_aq_1$)	Under-five mortality (${}_5q_0$)
		URBAN			
Mother's education					
Illiterate	46.2	34.4	80.6	31.0	109.1
Literate, < middle complete	29.0	20.6	49.7	18.7	67.4
Middle school complete	33.6	19.7	53.4	8.8	61.7
High school and above	22.3	8.8	31.1	5.2	36.2
Religion					
Hindu	38.6	25.4	64.0	20.6	83.2
Muslim	28.4	22.9	51.3	19.9	70.2
Christian	28.3	9.4	37.8	10.3	47.7
Sikh	14.1	22.0	36.0	6.0	41.8
Jain	(25.9)	(4.0)	(29.8)	(6.4)	(36.1)
Buddhist	(36.1)	(12.3)	(48.4)	*	(94.2)
Caste/tribe					
Scheduled caste	45.0	35.7	80.6	33.2	111.2
Scheduled tribe	43.9	11.7	55.5	25.2	79.3
Other	34.1	23.0	57.1	18.4	74.4
Medical maternity care[2]					
No antenatal or delivery care	55.9	35.1	90 9	57 9	143 6
Either antenatal or delivery care	27.5	22.3	49 8	9 7	59 0
Both antenatal and delivery care	25.8	13.1	38 8	8 3	46 8
Place of delivery[3]					
Public health facility	31.3	16.6	47.9	13.6	60.9
Private health facility	21.7	8.4	30.1	1.5	31.5
Home	34.1	27.1	61.2	30.9	90.2
Total	35.5	23.9	59.4	20.1	78.3
		RURAL			
Mother's education					
Illiterate	63.1	40.9	104.0	46.7	145.9

{Cont}......

Literate, < middle complete	43.0	25.0	68.0	24.8	91.1
Middle school complete	40.5	17.6	58.1	9.5	67.0
High school and above	30.4	17.2	47.6	8.0	55.2
Religion					
Hindu	59.1	38.0	97.1	41.3	134.4
Muslim	56.6	33.0	89.6	38.8	124.9
Christian	34.3	20.5	54.8	23.1	76.6
Sikh	31.9	18.7	50.6	22.7	72.2
Buddhist	(37.1)	(26.7)	(63.8)	(42.8)	(103.8)
Other	58.4	34.5	92.9	53.7	141.6
Caste/tribe					
Scheduled caste	66.9	46.0	112.9	50.0	157.2
Scheduled tribe	55.6	38.1	93.7	51.5	140.5
Other	56.3	34.5	90.8	36.9	124.4
Medical maternity care[2]					
No antenatal or delivery care	57.7	39.7	97.4	54.0	146.1
Either antenatal or delivery care	44.4	22.6	67.0	26.2	91.4
Both antenatal and delivery care	33.9	15.9	49.8	18.8	67.7
Place of delivery[3]					
Public health facility	48.4	20.7	69.1	25.2	92.5
Private health facility	35.3	14.6	49.8	7.4	56.8
Home	48.4	31.5	79.9	41.3	117.9
Total	57.7	36.6	94.3	40.4	130.9
		TOTAL			
Mother's education					
Illiterate	60.6	40.0	100.6	44.3	140.5
Literate, < middle complete	38.8	23.7	62.5	22.8	83.9
Middle school complete	37.6	18.5	56.1	9.2	64.8
High school and above	25.3	11.9	37.2	6.2	43.2
Religion					
Hindu	55.0	35.4	90.4	36.9	124.0
Muslim	47.1	29.6	76.6	32.2	106.3
Christian	32.6	17.3	49.9	19.4	68.4
Sikh	27.7	19.5	47.2	18.5	64.8

{Cont}.......

Jain	(20.7)	(2.8)	(23.5)	(13.8)	(37.0)
Buddhist	36.6	19.8	56.4	45.4	99.3
Other	57.3	28.6	85.9	46.4	128.3
Caste/tribe					
Scheduled caste	63.1	44.2	107.3	46.9	149.1
Scheduled tribe	54.6	35.9	90.5	49.1	135.2
Other	50.6	31.6	82.2	32.0	111.5
Medical Maternity care[2]					
No antenatal or delivery care	57.5	39.3	96.8	54.3	145.8
Either antenatal or delivery care	41.2	22.5	63.7	22.9	85.1
Both antenatal and delivery care	29.8	14.5	44.2	13.2	56.8
Place of delivery[3]					
Public health facility	40.3	18.7	59.1	19.3	77.2
Private health facility	27.5	11.0	38.5	3.9	42.3
Home	46.5	30.9	77.5	39.9	114.3
Total	52.7	33.7	86.3	35.5	118.8

Note: Total includes the mortality experience of "other" religious groups in urban areas and Jains in rural areas, Which is not shown separately.

( ) Based on 250-499 unweighted children surviving to the beginning of the age interval.

* Rate not shown; based on fewer than 250 unweighted children surviving to the beginning of the age interval.

1 Computed as the difference between the infant and neonatal mortality rates

2 Rates for the four-year period preceding the survey. Medical care is that given by a doctor, nurse trained midwife, or other health professional in a hospital, clinic, or health centre or care received at home from a health worker.

3 Rates for the four-year period preceding the survey.

females than for males. This reversal of sex differentials in mortality after the age of weaning has been observed in other studies conducted in South Asia and is thought to reflect the relative nutritional and medical neglect of girls after breastfeeding has ceased. In fact, child mortality is somewhat higher for females than males in most less developed countries, but the differentials are much larger in India than elsewhere (United Nations Secretariat, 1988; Arnold, 1992). In fact, the maximum extent to which female child mortality exceeded male child mortality in any of the 28 Demographic and Health Surveys examined in a recent study was 23 per cent (Sullivan *et al.*, 1994).

For both social and biological reasons, infant and child mortality often exhibit a U-shaped pattern with respect to mother's age at childbirth, with children of both very young and very old mothers at higher risk of dying than children whose mothers are in the prime reproductive ages. This pattern is also seen in India. As Table 8.7 shows, infant

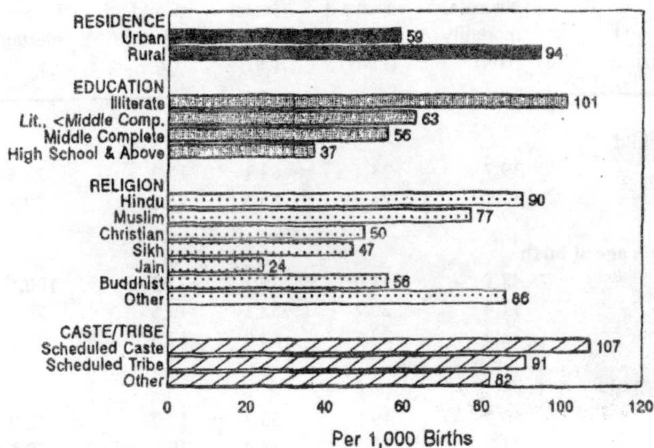

Figure 8.2: Infant Mortality Rates by Selected Background Characteristics

mortality is higher for children of mothers under age 20 (107 per 1,000) or age 40-49 (112 per 1,000) and is lowest for children of mothers age 20-29 (76 per 1,000). A similar age pattern is also observed for the other infant and child mortality rates. It should be noted that infants born to young mothers are more likely to be of low birth weight, which is probably an important factor contributing to their higher neonatal mortality rate. Similarly, children born to mothers above age 30 are at higher risk of experiencing congenital malformations.

Birth order also has a U-shaped relationship to infant deaths. Neonatal mortality rates are relatively high for first births and high order births. However, postneonatal mortality and child mortality (ages 1-4) do not show a U-shaped pattern; for these measures, mortality tends to increase with birth order. The steady increase in child mortality with birth order may reflect the more intense competition for nutritious food faced by higher birth order children once they are weaned. It is also likely that higher birth order children are disproportionately from lower socioeconomic groups, in which mortality is higher.

Table 8.7: Infant and child mortality by demographic characteristics
Neonatal postneonatal, infant child and under-five mortality by selected demographic characteristics for the 10-year period preceding the survey, India, 1992-93

Background characteristic	Neonatal mortality (NN)	Post-neonatal mortality[1] (PNN)	Infant mortality ($_1q_0$)	Child mortality ($_4q_1$)	Under-five mortality ($_5q_0$)
URBAN					
Sex of child					
Male	39.7	23.4	63.1	15.3	77.5
Female	31.1	24.4	55.5	25.2	79.3
Mother's age at birth					
< 20	48.1	31.0	79.1	23.3	100.5
20-29	31.4	20.7	52.1	19.6	70.7
30-39	36.4	27.6	64.0	17.3	80.2
Birth order					
1	40.9	19.5	60.3	12.7	72.2
2	31.0	23.5	54.4	19.2	72.6
3	29.1	21.9	51.0	19.6	69.5
4	36.9	25.2	62.2	27.1	87.6
5	33.6	35.5	69.1	29.4	96.5
6	36.6	35.0	71.6	27.5	97.2
7+	49.5	32.6	82.1	33.5	112.9
Previous birth interval					
< 24	45.5	40.4	86.0	30.7	114.0
24-47	27.4	20.8	48.2	21.3	68.5
48+	23.0	11.3	34.2	12.5	46.3
Birth size[2]					
Large	26.9	15.8	42.7	13.9	56.0
Average	19.5	15.9	35.5	18.1	52.9
Small	61.5	30.6	92.1	18.7	109.1
Total	35.5	23.9	59.4	20.1	78.3
RURAL					
Sex of Child					
Male	62.1	34.1	96.2	33.9	126.8
Female	53.1	39.2	92.2	47.3	135.1
Mother's age at birth					
< 20	76.0	37.8	113.8	41.2	150.3
20-29	49.3	34.5	83.8	40.0	120.4
30-39	58.4	40.1	98.5	39.2	133.8
40-49	53.5	63.9	117.4	62.5	172.5

{Cont}.........

Birth order					
1	71.3	33.2	104.5	31.0	132.3
2	52.3	31.9	84.2	36.7	117.8
3	46.5	32.1	78.7	42.7	118.0
4	49.5	38.9	88.5	42.8	127.5
5	53.0	43.0	96.0	49.7	140.9
6	58.6	44.2	102.8	42.4	140.9
7+	73.4	53.9	127.3	58.7	178.6
Previous birth interval					
< 24	84.8	57.4	142.2	62.7	196.0
24-47	41.3	31.4	72.7	39.1	109.0
48+	27.2	17.3	44.5	16.9	60.7
Birth size[2]					
Large	40.0	19.1	59.1	37.8	94.7
Average	32.2	25.5	57.8	35.7	91.4
Small	94.5	48.5	143.0	44.3	181.0
Total	57.7	36.6	94.3	40.4	130.9
TOTAL					
Sex of child					
Male	57.0	31.7	88.6	29.4	115.4
Female	48.1	35.8	83.9	42.0	122.4
Mother's age at birth					
< 20	70.8	36.5	107.3	37.6	140.9
20-29	44.8	31.0	75.8	34.6	107.8
30-39	53.7	37.4	91.1	34.3	122.3
40-49	51.0	60.8	111.8	57.5	162.9
Birth order					
1	63.4	29.6	93.0	26.0	116.6
2	46.9	29.7	76.6	32.0	106.2
3	42.6	29.8	72.4	37.1	106.7
4	46.9	36.1	83.0	39.4	119.1
5	49.4	41.6	90.9	45.7	132.5
6	55.0	42.7	97.7	39.8	133.6
7+	69.8	50.5	120.3	54.3	168.1
Previous birth interval					
< 24	76.0	53.6	129.6	55.0	177.5
24-47	38.4	29.2	67.6	35.2	100.5
48+	26.2	15.9	42.1	15.8	57.2
Birth size[2]					
Large	36.8	18.2	55.0	31.7	84.9
Average	29.3	23.3	52.7	31.7	82.7
Small	87.4	44.6	132.1	38.8	165.7

{Cont}.........

Total	52.7	33.7	86.3	35.5	118.8

Note: Total includes the mortality experience of children whose size at birth is unknown and urban children whose mothers were age 40-49 at the time of birth which is not shown separately.

1 Computed as the difference between the infant and neonatal mortality rates.

2 Rates for the four-year period preceding the survey.

Childspacing patterns have a powerful effect on the survival chances of children in India. Infant and child mortality risks increase sharply as the length of the preceding birth interval decreases. Infant mortality is more than three times as high for children with a preceding birth interval of less than 24 months as for children with a preceding interval of 48 months or more (130 compared with 42 per 1,000). Lengthening the birth interval from less than 24 months to 24-47 months has a much stronger association with child survival than does lengthening the interval from 24-47 months to 48 months or more. Note, however, that although the length of the preceding birth interval is likely to affect mortality risks directly, a substantial portion of the total association between birth intervals and mortality risks may reflect other risk factors that are correlated with birth intervals. For example, shorter intervals are likely to occur in larger families, and larger families tend to come from lower socioeconomic groups and also are more likely to reside in rural areas where medical facilities and other survival-enhancing resources are less readily available. Nevertheless, multivariate analyses of birth intervals and child survival that control for socioeconomic background commonly find short intervals (less than 24 months) to be damaging to a child's survival chances.

Another important determinant of the survival chances of children is the baby's weight at the time of birth. Many studies have found that low birth weight babies (under 2,500 grams) have a substantially increased risk of mortality. Because most babies in India are not weighed at the time of birth, mothers were asked whether babies born during the four years preceding the interview were "large, average, or small" at birth. The last panel of Table 8.7 shows infant and child mortality statistics for births classified in this way. Children who are perceived by their mothers to be smaller than average at birth experience much higher mortality risks than children perceived to be average or larger. Once again, the pattern of demographic differentials in infant and child mortality just described typifies urban and rural areas as well as the whole country.

Infant mortality rates vary dramatically from one state to another,

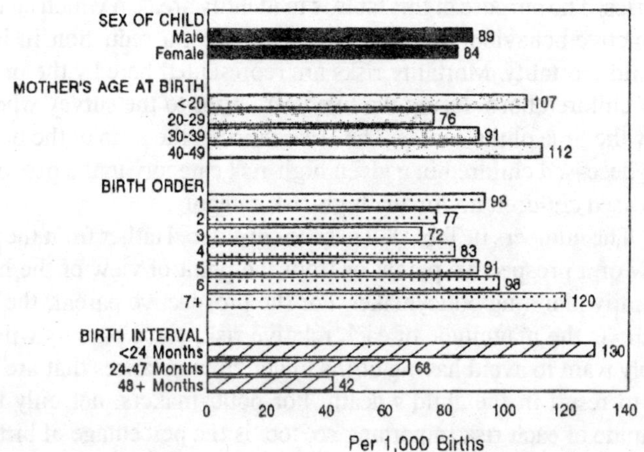

Figure 8.3: Infant Mortality Rates by Selected Demographic Characteristics

ranging from 15 in Mizoram to 112 in Orissa (Table 8.8 and Figure 8.4). Orissa also recorded the highest infant mortality rate in the SRS in every year between 1988 and 1992. Other large states with infant mortality rates above the national average are Uttar Pradesh (100), Bihar and Assam (89 each), and Madhya Pradesh (85). These same states have the highest under-five mortality rates in India. The infant mortality rates seem implausibly low in Nagaland and Mizoram (17 and 15, respectively), but the NFHS rate for Nagaland is consistent with the SKS estimate of 18 for 1989-91 (the SRS did not report an infant mortality rate for Mizoram for those years). All of the mortality rates are also relatively low in Kerala and Goa, the two states with the lowest levels of fertility.

8.4 High-Risk Fertility Behaviour

In theory, the mother's age at the time of birth, the interval between births, and the order of a birth (all factors with a high risk of mortality for the children) can be controlled by the parents if they want to increase the probability of survival of their children. Understanding the prevalence of high-risk births in India is, therefore, of interest for health and family planning policymakers and programme managers. Table 8.9 shows the percentages of births in the five years preceding the interview that fall into different child survival risk categories, as well as the distribution of all currently married women across these categories. It also shows the relative risks of children dying across the different risk categories. The purpose of this table is to identify areas in which changed reproductive behaviour would be likely to effect a reduction in infant and child mortality. Mortality risks are represented here by the proportion of children born during the five years prior to the survey who had died by the time of the survey. The "risk ratio" is the ratio of the proportion of deceased children in a given high-risk category to the proportion of deceased children not in any high-risk category.

The numbers in Table 8.9 may be considered either from the point of view of a prospective parent or from the point of view of the health and family planning policymaker. For the prospective parent, the critical issue is the magnitude of each relative risk, since parents will presumably want to avoid having births under circumstances that are more likely to result in the child's death. For policymakers, not only is the magnitude of each risk important; so, too, is the percentage of births or women in each of the high-risk categories. The latter is important because it determines whether particular types of high-risk births are likely to occur frequently or only rarely; presumably, policymakers will want to target their efforts toward the types of high-risk births that occur most frequently.

In terms of the magnitudes of the risks associated with each risk factor, Table 8.9 suggests that the most vulnerable births are high order births that occur to older women within 24 months of a previous birth (risk ratio of 3.16). However, less than 1 per cent of all births occur to women in this group. Although the risk ratio is smaller for women under 18 years of age, 9 per cent of all births occur to women with this single risk factor. In the aggregate, therefore, infant mortality rates would undoubtedly decline if early childbearing could be curtailed. In addition, individual couples would be well advised to avoid having children until the wife reaches age 18, as the risks of a child dying if the mother is younger are relatively high. Short birth intervals should also be discouraged (based on a consideration of both the risk ratios and the percentage of births in each category).

Although mortality risks to children can be reduced by changing women's childbearing behaviour, the risk ratios shown in Table 8.9 almost certainly overstate the magnitude of the potential effect. This is because a mother's demographic characteristics are not the only causal factors influencing the risks of mortality experienced by her children. Women who have many children at short birth intervals almost certainly tend, for example, to live in rural areas, which will raise mortality risks

Table 8.8: Infant and child mortality by state

Neonatal, postneonatal, infant, child and under-five mortality by state for the 5-year period preceding the survey, India, 1992-93

Background characteristic	Neonatal mortality (NN)	Post-neonatal mortality[1] (PNN)	Infant mortality ($_1q_0$)	Child mortality ($_4q_1$)	Under-five mortality ($_5q_0$)
India	48.6	29.9	78.5	33.4	109.3
North					
Delhi	34.9	30.5	65.4	19.0	83.1
Haryana	38.4	34.9	73.3	27.4	98.7
Himachal Pradesh	34.2	21.7	55.8	14.1	69.1
Jammu Region of J & K	31.9	13.5	45.4	14.3	59.1
Punjab	31.2	22.5	53.7	15.0	68.0
Rajasthan	37.2	35.4	72.6	32.3	102.6
Central					
Madhya Pradesh	53.2	32.0	85.2	49.3	130.3
Uttar Pradesh	59.9	40.0	99.9	46.0	141.3
East					
Bihar	54.8	34.4	89.2	42.0	127.5
Orissa	64.7	47.4	112.1	21.3	131.0
West Bengal	51.8	23.5	75.3	26.0	99.3
Northeast					
Arunachal Pradesh	17.5	22.5	40.0	33.3	72.0
Assam	50.9	37.8	88.7	58.7	142.2
Manipur	25.1	17.3	42.4	20.2	61.7
Meghalaya	37.8	26.3	64.2	24.3	86.9
Mizoram	8.3	6.3	14.6	14.9	29.3
Nagaland	10.0	7.2	17.2	3.6	20.7
Tripura	43.6	32.3	75.8	31.2	104.6
West					
Goa	20.6	11.3	31.9	7.2	38.9
Gujarat	42.3	26.4	68.7	37.9	104.0
Maharashtra	36.4	14.0	50.5	20.9	70.3
South					
Andhra Pradesh	45.3	25.0	70.4	22.4	91.2
Karnataka	45.3	20.2	65.4	23.5	87.3
Kerala	15.5	8.2	23.8	8.4	32.0
Tamil Nadu	46.2	21.5	67.7	20.1	86.5

1 Computed as the difference between the infant and neonatal mortality rates

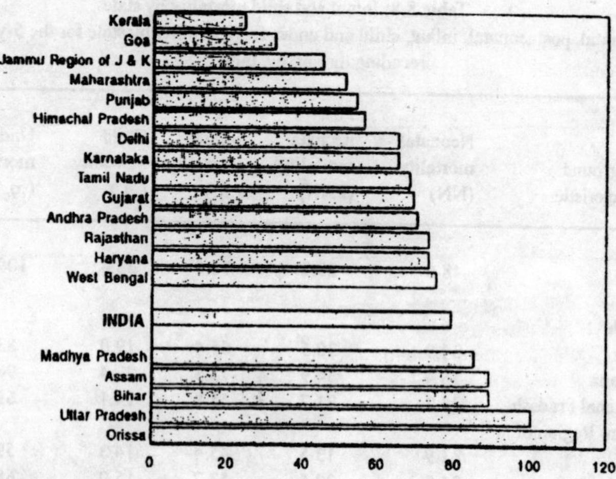

Note: Rates are for the 5-year period preceding the survey; excludes 6 small northeastern states

NFHS, India, 1992-93

Figure 8.4: Infant Mortality Rates by State

to their children independently of their childbearing behaviour. However, a multivariate analysis designed to assess the effects of the demographic factors, while controlling for the potentially confounding effects of residence, education, and other correlated socioeconomic factors, is beyond the scope of this report.

Table 8.10 shows how high-risk fertility behaviour varies by state. For India as a whole, 52 per cent of children born during the last five years are in at least one elevated risk category. The percentage tends to be higher in high-fertility states, such as Uttar Pradesh (59 per cent) and Bihar (58 per cent). The low-fertility state of Kerala has the lowest percentage in any risk category (27 per cent). The percentage of children born to mothers less than 18 years of age (10 per cent for India as a whole)[3] reflects patterns in the age at marriage. The proportion exceeds 15 per cent in Maharashtra, Andhra Pradesh and Karnataka, which are states with relatively low median ages at first marriage. The percentage born to mothers older than 34 is 5 per cent for India and is highest in Meghalaya (12 per cent). The percentage born with a previous birth interval less than 24 months is 20 per cent for India and the percentage with a birth order higher than three is 31 per cent. Overall, there is substantial scope in all states for improving child survival by avoiding high-risk births.

Table 8.9: High-risk fertility behaviour

Percentage of children born in the last five years at elevated risk of mortality and percentage of currently married women at risk of conceiving a child with an elevated risk of mortality according to category of increased risk and residence India 1992-93

High-risk category	Births in last 5 years: Per cent of births	Births in last 5 years: Risk ratio	Percentage of currently married women
URBAN			
Not in any high-risk category	55.8	1.00	56.1[b]
Single high-risk category			
Age<18: Age under 18 years at birth	5.9	2.08	1.0
Age>34: Age over 34 years at birth	0.6	0.69	7.5
BI <24 : Birth interval under 24 months	12.2	1.48	8.7
BO>3 : Birth order higher than 3	15.0	1.17	7.7
Subtotal	33.8	1.43	25.0
Multiple high-risk category			
Age<18 & BI <24[C]	0.8	2.86	0.3
Age>34 & BI <24	—	*	0.1
Age>34 & BO>3	2.9	1.37	13.4
Age>34 & BI<24 & BO>3	0.4	1.57	0.8
BI <24 & BO>3	6.3	2.54	4.4
Subtotal	10.4	2.20	19.0
In any high-risk category	44.2	1.61	43.9
Total per cent	100.0	NA	100.0
Number	13872	NA	22075
RURAL			
Not in any high-risk category	45.3	1.00	49 5[b]
Single high-risk category			
Age<18: Age under 18 years at birth	9.9	1.65	2.9
Age>34: Age over 34 years at birth	0.3	0.80	3.3
BI <24 : Birth interval under 24 months	9.6	1.74	8.6
Bo 3 : Birth order higher than[3]	20.5	1.07	10.6
Subtotal	40.3	1.37	25.3
Multiple high-risk category			
Age<18 & BI<24[C]	1.4	2.57	0.7
Age>34 & BI<24	—	*	-
Age>34 & Bo>3	4.5	1.40	15.6
Age>34 & BI<24 & Bo>3	0.7	3.17	1.4

{Cont}.......

BI<24 & BO>3	7.7	2.17	7.5
Subtotal	14.4	2.02	25.2
In any high-risk category	54.7	1.54	50.5
Total per cent	100.0	NA	100.0
Number	47239	NA	62603
	TOTAL		
Not in any high-risk category	47.7	1.00	51.2[b]
Single high-risk category			
Age<18: Age under 18 years at birth	9.0	1.78	2.4
Age>34: Age over 34 years at birth	0.4	0.73	4.4
BI<24 : Birth interval under 24 months	10.2	1.68	8.6
BO>3 : Birth order higher than 3	19.2	1.12	9.9
Subtotal	38.9	1.42	25.2
Multiple high-risk category			
Age<18 & BI<24[c]	1.3	2.72	0.6
Age>34 & BI<24	—	*	0.1
Age>34 & BO>3	4.1	1.45	15.0
Age>34 & BI<24 & BO>3	0.6	3.16	1.2
BI<24 & BO>3	7.4	2.28	6.7
Subtotal	13.5	2.11	23.5
In any high-risk category	52.3	1.59	48.8
Total per cent	100.0	NA	100.0
Number	61111	NA	84678

Note: Risk ratio is the ratio of the proportion dead of births in a specific highrisk category to the proportion dead of births in the "not in any high-risk" category.

NA: Not applicable.

* Risk ratio not shown; denominator of the upper proportion in the risk ratio is fewer than 50 unweighted births.

— Less than 0.05 per cent

[a] Women are placed into the categories according to the status they would have at the birth of a child if they were to conceive at the current time: current age less than 17 years and 3 months or older than 34 years and 2 months, last birth occurred less than 15 months ago, or last birth was order 3 or higher.

[b] Includes sterilized women and women whose husbands are sterilized.

[c] Also includes category age under 18 and birth order greater than. 3

8.5 Maternal Mortality

It has been estimated by the World Health Organization that world-wide at least one-half million women die every year from causes related to pregnancy and childbirth and 99 per cent of these deaths occur in developing countries (World Health Organization, 1991). Although reliable national estimates of maternal mortality are not available for most countries, South Asia is thought to have among the highest maternal mortality rates in the world. Most demographic surveys do not have samples which are large enough to produce reliable estimates of maternal mortality. The NFHS sample, however, is sufficiently large to estimate maternal mortality at the national level for the two-year period preceding the survey. The NFHS estimates are based on a series of questions in the Household Questionnaire about deaths occurring to usual residents of the household and visitors since January (or since *Pongal* or *Makar Sankranti)* of the second calendar year preceding the start of the survey in each state. In the case of deaths to women age 13-49, a series of follow-up questions was asked about whether the woman was pregnant when she died, whether the death occurred during childbirth, whether she died within two months after the end of a pregnancy or childbirth, and whether the death was due to a complication of the pregnancy or childbirth.

On the basis of this information, it is possible to calculate the *Maternal Mortality Rate* (MMR), which is defined here as the number of maternal deaths per 100,000 live births. This measure is based on the annual number of female deaths to usual residents of the sample households that occurred during childbirth or within two months after the end of a pregnancy or childbirth. The average maternal mortality rate at the national level for the 2-year period preceding the NFHS is 437 deaths per 100,000 live births. The rural MMR (448) is 13 per cent higher than the urban MMR (397). There is no way to assess the completeness and accuracy of these estimates, but it should be pointed out that direct survey estimates of this type often underenumerate maternal deaths. It should also be noted that despite the large size of the NFHS sample, sampling errors for the maternal mortality estimates are quite large. The 95 per cent confidence interval for the maternal mortality rate ranges from 334 to 540 per 100,000 live births and the confidence intervals are even wider for the urban and rural estimates. Because of the large sampling errors, reliable maternal mortality rates can not be calculated for individual states or population subgroups.

The maternal mortality rate of 437 deaths per 100,000 live births implies that more than 100,000 women in India die every year from causes related to pregnancy and childbirth. This finding reinforces the urgency of insuring that all pregnant women receive adequate antenatal care during pregnancy and that deliveries take place under hygienic conditions with the assistance of a trained medical practitioner.

Table 8.10: High-risk fertility behaviour by state
Percentage of children born in the last five years at elevated risk of mortality, according to category of increased risk and state, India, 1992-93

State	Not in any high-risk category	Single high-risk category: Age<18	Age>34	BI<24	BO>3	Sub-total	Multiple high-risk category: Age<18 & BI<24ᵃ	Age>34 & BI<24	BI<34 & B0>3	Age>34 & BI<24 & BO>3	BI<24 & B0>3	Sub-total	In any high-risk category	Total Per cent
India	47.7	9.0	0.4	10.2	19.2	38.9	1.3	—	4.1	0.6	7.4	13.5	52.3	100.0
North														
Delhi	57.1	3.2	0.4	13.3	14.9	31.8	0.6	—	2.5	0.5	7.4	11.0	42.9	100.0
Haryana	46.7	8.0	0.3	15.2	17.3	40.9	0.6	—	3.2	0.3	8.3	12.5	53.3	100.0
Himachal Pradesh	58.3	2.7	0.4	16.9	12.3	32.3	0.4	0.1	2.7	0.4	5.8	9.4	41.7	100.0
Jammu Region of J & K	55.8	3.3	0.4	14.0	16.6	34.4	0.3	—	3.6	0.3	5.5	9.7	44.2	100.0
Punjab	57.5	3.4	0.7	16.8	12.9	33.7	0.2	0.1	2.2	0.2	6.2	8.8	42.5	100.0
Rajasthan	47.8	8.1	0.5	9.1	21.4	39.0	1.0	—	4.5	0.8	6.9	13.2	52.2	100.0
Central														
Madhya Pradesh	46.1	10.6	0.2	8.8	20.7	40.4	0.9	—	4.0	0.6	8.0	13.5	53.9	100.0
Uttar Pradesh	41.3	6.0	0.3	9.7	23.6	39.6	0.7	—	7.4	1.2	9.9	19.2	58.7	100.0
East														
Bihar	41.7	8.6	0.4	9.0	25.2	43.1	1.1	—	5.6	0.6	7.9	15.2	58.3	100.0
Orissa	52.3	7.7	0.4	9.7	18.1	36.0	1.5	—	3.0	0.5	6.8	11.7	47.7	100.0
West Bengal	47.6	13.0	0.2	8.4	18.6	40.2	1.6	—	3.3	0.4	6.9	12.2	52.4	100.0

Northeast														
Arunachal Pradesh	42.9	7.4	1.1	10.9	21.1	40.5	1.0	—	5.5	2.4	7.7	16.6	57.1	100.0
Assam	36.0	11.7	0.3	8.2	24.1	44.3	2.4	—	4.5	1.0	11.9	19.8	64.0	100.0
Manipur	52.7	1.9	1.0	10.0	20.7	33.6	—	0.3	4.6	0.7	8.2	13.8	47.3	100.0
Meghalaya	43.1	5.3	0.2	12.9	16.9	35.3	0.9	0.1	8.3	3.0	9.3	21.6	56.9	100.0
Mizoram	53.0	3.1	0.5	18.1	14.4	36.2	—	0.2	4.2	0.7	5.7	10.8	47.0	100.0
Nagaland	48.8	4.1	0.8	13.0	17.4	35.3	0.3	0.3	5.0	2.2	8.2	15.9	51.2	100.0
Tripura	48.5	10.7	0.9	8.Z	18.6	38.4	1.3	0.1	5.5	0.6	5.6	13.1	51.5	100.0
West														
Goa	66.6	2.3	3.4	11.2	10.3	27.2	0.4	0.1	2.7	0.8	2.2	6.3	33.4	100.0
Gujarat	56.6	4.6	0.1	12.9	15.8	33.4	0.6	—	2.7	0.4	6.2	10.0	43.4	100.0
Maharashtra	49.7	12.4	0.4	11.7	14.5	39.0	2.8	—	1.3	0.5	6.7	11.3	50.3	100.0
South														
Andhra Pradesh	49.1	17.0	0.3	8.5	15.9	41.7	2.5	—	1.9	0.1	4.7	9.2	50.9	100.0
Karnataka	47.1	13.1	0.6	10.3	17.2	41.1	2.1	0.1	1.9	0.4	7.2	11.7	52.9	100.0
Kerala	72.7	3.0	1.2	11.2	7.3	22.8	0.3	0.1	2.0	0.1	2.1	4.6	27.3	100.0
Tamil Nadu	62.3	7.6	0.6	12.9	10.3	31.4	0.9	0.2	2.1	0.2	2.9	6.3	37.7	100.0

BI: Birth interval, BO: Birth order.
— Less than 0.05 per cent.
– Less than 0.05 per cent
ᵃ Also includes category age under 18 and birth order greater than 3.

NOTES

1 A detailed description of the method for calculating the probabilities presented here is given in Rutstein (1984). The mortality estimates are not rates, but are probabilities, calculated according to the conventional life table approach. For any calendar period, deaths and exposure in that period are first tabulated for the age intervals 0, 1-2, 3-5, 6-11, 12-23, 24-35, 36-47, and 48-59 months. Then age interval-specific probabilities of survival are calculated. Finally, probabilities of mortality for larger age segments are produced by multiplying the relevant age interval survival probabilities together and subtracting the product from 1.00: ${}_nq_x = 1 - \Pi(1\text{-}qi)$

2 Interviewers in the NFHS were instructed to probe for the exact number of months lived by the chilfl if the age at death was reported as "1 year".

3 The percentage born to mothers less than IX years of age is calculated by adding together the percentages in the two columns that include women in this age group. A similar procedure is used to calculate the percentage of women in the other risk groups.

9

MATERNAL AND CHILD HEALTH

Safe motherhood practices and child survival programmes are critically important in a country that is experiencing high infant and child mortality and maternal mortality. Realizing the importance of maternal and child health care services, the Ministry of Health, Government of India, took concrete steps to strengthen maternal and child health services in the First and Second Five Years Plans (1951-56 and 1956-61). The integration of family planning services with maternal and child health services and nutrition services was introduced as a part of the Minimum Needs Programme during the Fifth Five Year Plan (1974-79). The primary objective was to provide basic public health services to vulnerable groups of pregnant women, lactating mothers, and preschool children (Kanitkar, 1979). Since then, the promotion of health of mothers and children has been one of the most important aspects of the Family Welfare Programme in India and has now been further strengthened by introducing the Child Survival and Safe Motherhood Programme (Ministry of Health and Family Welfare, 1992a). The Ministry of Health and Family Welfare has also sponsored special schemes, under the Maternal and Child Health Programme, including the programme of Oral Rehydration Therapy, development of Regional Institutes of Maternal and Child Health in states where infant mortality rates are high, the Universal Immunization Programme, and the Maternal and Child Health Supplemental Programme within the Post-Partum Programme (Ministry of Health and Family Welfare, 1992a).

In the rural areas of India, maternal and child health services are delivered mainly by government-run Primary Health Centres and sub-centres. Services for pregnant women and children can also be obtained from private and public maternity homes or hospitals, as well as from private practitioners. In urban areas, maternal and child health (MCH) services are available mainly through government or municipal hospitals, urban health posts, hospitals and nursing homes operated by non-governmental voluntary organizations, and various private nursing homes or maternity homes.

The Village Health Guide is a link between the community and MCH services in rural areas. The Female Health Worker, who is an Auxiliary Nurse Midwife, renders maternal and child health and family welfare services (Ministry of Health and Family Welfare, 1978). The Female Health Worker is supposed to assist the Medical Officer and Female Health Assistant in providing maternal and child health services. She is responsible for registering pregnant women and assessing their health throughout pregnancy in their homes or in the antenatal clinic. Another responsibility of the Female Health Worker is to refer pregnant women who have symptoms of abnormal pregnancy or labour, or who have gynaecological problems that are beyond her level of competence, to the Primary Health Centre. The basic maternal and child care services offered at Primary Health Centres are antenatal and postnatal care of mothers as well as care of infants and children.

A major objective of the NFHS was to provide information on maternal and child health care practices. The relevant information was collected in the Woman's Questionnaire from the mothers of all children born since 1 January, 1988 for states where the NFHS was initiated in 1992, and 1 January, 1989, where the NFHS was carried out in 1993 (see Table 2.1 for the dates of fieldwork). The information covered matters related to pregnancy and childbirth; infant and child feeding practices, including breastfeeding; immunizations; episodes of illnesses such as acute respiratory infection, fever and diarrhoea, and the treatment received; mothers' knowledge and use of Oral Rehydration Salts (ORS); and the level of child nutrition assessed by measuring the weight and height of children.

This chapter analyzes the data collected on antenatal and delivery care, immunization coverage, prevalence of acute respiratory infection, fever and diarrhoea and their treatment, and mothers' knowledge and use of ORS. Chapter 10 deals with infant feeding and child nutrition.

Although information was obtained for each child born since January 1988/1989, the analysis in this chapter is restricted to children born during the four years before the date each woman was interviewed. If a woman had more than one live birth during this four-year period, information was collected for the three most recent live births; all of these births are used in the current analysis.

9.1 Maternal Care Indicators

Antenatal Care

Antenatal care (ANC) refers to pregnancy-related health care provided by a doctor or a health worker in a medical facility or at home. The Safe Motherhood Initiative proclaims that all pregnant women must receive basic but professional antenatal care (Harrison, 1990). Antenatal care can contribute significantly to the reduction of maternal morbidity and mortality because it also includes advice on the correct diet and the provision of iron and folic acid tablets to pregnant women, besides medical care. Improved nutritional status, coupled with improved antenatal care, can help to reduce the incidence of low birth weight babies and thus reduce perinatal, neonatal, and infant mortality.

A pregnant woman can receive antenatal care by visiting a doctor or other health professional in a medical facility, or by receiving a home visit from a health worker, or both. In the NFHS, each woman who had a live birth during the four years prior to the survey was initially asked whether any health worker visited her at home for an antenatal check-up when she was pregnant and, if so, at which month of pregnancy the first visit was made and how many such visits were made in all. Next she was asked whether she had gone for an antenatal check-up outside the home and whom she saw for the check-up. If she saw more than one person, information was collected on all persons seen. she was asked at which month of pregnancy she first went for an antenatal check-up and how many such visits she made.

Table 9.1 and Figure 9.1 show the percentage distribution of live births in the last four years by the source of antenatal care received during pregnancy, according to selected background characteristics. Although the interviewer was instructed to record all persons if more than one source of antenatal care outside the home was mentioned for the same pregnancy, for the purpose of this tabulation only the provider with the highest qualifications is considered For 62 per cent of births during the last four years, mothers received antenatal care during pregnancy. Allopathic doctors provided antenatal care for 40 per cent of births and other health professionals (such as nurse/midwives, ayurvedic doctors and homoeopathic doctors) provides care for 9 per cent of births. Mothers received antenatal care only at home from a health worker for 13 per cent of births. Note that in this tabulation, those who received antenatal care outside the home, whether or not they also received care at home from a health worker, are classified as "outside home". A sizeable percentage of births (37 per cent) were to mothers who did not receive any

Table 9.1: Antenatal care

Per cent distribution of live births during the four years preceding the survey by source of antenatal care (ANC) during pregnancy, according to selected background characteristics, India, 1992-93

		Antenatal care provider (outside home)[1]						
Background characteristic	ANC only at home from health worker	Doctor	Other health professional	Traditional birth attendant, other[2]	No ANC	Missing	Total percent	Number of births
Mother's age at birth								
<20	13.3	40.8	9.8	0.4	34.6	1.1	100.0	11514
20-34	12.6	40.8	9.4	0.3	36.0	0.9	100.0	35258
35+	13.1	22.5	5.9	0.3	57.2	1.1	100.0	2597
Birth order								
1	10.4	51.9	10.0	0.4	26.2	1.0	100.0	13594
2-3	12.8	42.7	10.0	0.3	33.3	0.9	100.0	20433
4-5	15.4	28.9	8.8	0.4	45.5	1.0	100.0	9542
6+	13.9	19.6	6.2	.0.1	59.4	0.8	100.0	5800
Residence								
Urban	3.9	69.6	7.2	0.4	17.8	1.1	100.0	11242
Rural	15.4	31.1	10.0	0.3	42.4	0.9	100.0	38128
Education								
Illiterate	15.5	25.3	9.2	0.3	48.8	1.0	100.0	32770

Literate, < middle complete	10.1	57.6	11.3	0.3	19.9	0.7	100.0	8190
Middle school complete	6.5	72.1	10.5	0.3	9.8	0.7	100.0	3505
High school and above	3.6	84.2	6.5	0.2	4.2	1.2	100.0	4904
Religion								
Hindu	14.0	38.6	8.9	0.3	37.2	1.0	100.0	39223
Muslim	8.6	41.6	8.5	0.4	40.3	0.6	100.0	7613
Christian	6.5	61.4	7.3	0.2	23.9	0.6	100.0	981
Sikh	3.6	37.2	44.3	0.4	14.3	0.1	100.0	822
Jain	0.6	83.3	8.1	2.4	4.3	1.3	100.0	142
Buddhist	11.6	68.6	5.7	—	14.1	—	100.0	351
Other	15.6	34.9	9.7	0.6	38.5	0.8	100.0	237
Caste/tribe								
Scheduled caste	14.0	29.4	12.8	0.2	42.2	1.4	100.0	6590
Scheduled tribe	18.5	21.0	7.1	0.2	52.3	0 9	100.0	4703
Other	11.9	44.0	9.0	0.3	34.0	0 8	100.0	38076
Total	12.8	39.8	9.3	0.3	36.8	0.9	100.0	49369

Note: Table is based on births in the period 1-47 months prior to the survey. ANC refers to pregnancy related health care provided by a doctor or a health worker in a medical facility or at home.

— Less than 0.05 per cent

1 Includes women who received ANC outside the home, whether or not they also received ANC at home from a health worker. If more than one source of ANC was mentioned, only the provider with the highest qualifications is considered.

2 Includes hakim and "Don't know"

antenatal care.

As expected, utilization of antenatal care services is substantially better in urban than in rural areas; mothers of 81 per cent of births during the four years preceding the survey received antenatal care in urban areas compared with 57 per cent in rural areas. Urban women are more than twice as likely to receive antenatal care from an allopathic doctor as rural women (70 per cent compared with 31 per cent), whereas rural women are more likely to receive antenatal care from a health worker or a health professional who is not a doctor.

The utilization of antenatal care during pregnancy decreases with the age of the mother. The coverage of antenatal care is greatest (64 per cent) among births to young mothers below age 20 and lowest (42 per cent) among births to mothers age 35 and over. A consistent negative relationship is also observed between the birth order and overall utilization of antenatal care services, especially care provided by allopathic doctors. While the mothers of 52 per cent of first order births received antenatal care from allopathic doctors, this percentage is only 20 for births of order six or higher. The proportion of births whose mothers received antenatal care increases steadily with an increase in the educational level of the mother, from 50 per cent for births to illiterate mothers to 90 per cent for births to mothers who completed middle school and to 95 per cent for births to mothers who completed at least high school. This relationship is produced entirely by variations in the antenatal care provided by allopathic doctors; antenatal care only at home from health workers is actually more common among births to illiterate mothers (1 per cent) than among births to mothers with at least a high school education (4 per cent).

Jain, Buddhist, Sikh and Christian mothers are more likely to receive antenatal care, although Sikhs are the only group who are more likely to receive antenatal care from other health professionals (44 per cent) than from allopathic doctors (37 per cent). Hindus are slightly more likely to be covered by antenatal care than Muslims although Muslims are more likely to consult doctors than are Hindus. Mothers from scheduled tribes are less likely to receive antenatal care (47 per cent) than mothers from either scheduled castes (56 per cent) or nonscheduled castes/tribes (65 per cent).

It is encouraging to note that mothers in India receive antenatal care for 62 per cent of births and that a large majority of all births covered by antenatal care were to mothers who received antenatal care from allopathic doctors. However, more efforts are needed to achieve the goal of providing professional antenatal care to all pregnant women. The

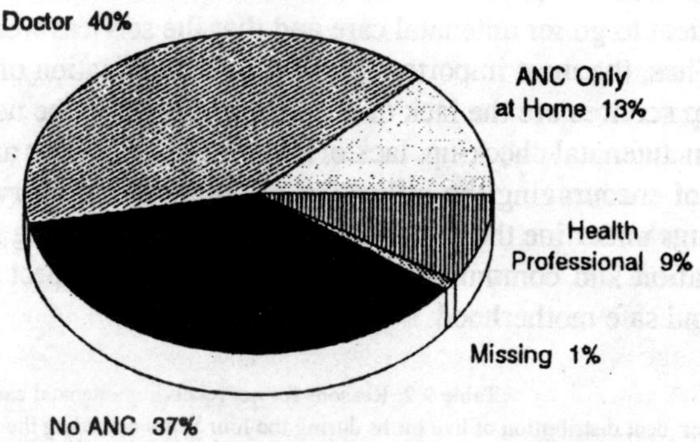

Figure 9.1: Source of Antenatal Care (ANC) During Pregnancy

most pressing need is for the provision of professional antenatal care services in rural areas and the encouragement of pregnant women to avail themselves of the services provided, since 43 per cent of births in rural areas were to mothers who did not receive any antenatal care.

Reasons for Not Seeking Antenatal Care Services

Mothers who had not sought antenatal care outside the home were asked about the main reason for not going for an antenatal check-up. The findings shown in Table 9.2 for women who did not receive any antenatal care are quite revealing. For this group, nearly three-fifths of the births were to mothers who stated that it was not necessary to go for an antenatal checkup. Thus, a large proportion of births are to mothers who do not realize the importance of safe motherhood. It is surprising to note that a higher proportion of urban births (66 per cent) than rural births (58 per cent) were to mothers who felt this way, but it must be remembered that the table includes only women whose births did not involve any antenatal care, a category that is far smaller among urban births (18 per cent) than among rural births (42 per cent). Other major factors contributing to the nonuse of antenatal care were lack of knowledge of antenatal care services (13 per cent) and financial cost (7 per cent). Mothers of 6 per cent of births felt that it is not customary in the community to go for an antenatal check-up. Five per cent of births were to women who had no time to go for antenatal care and another 5 per cent were to women who were not permitted to go for an antenatal check-up. One to 3 per cent of births were to mothers who said it was inconvenient to go for antenatal care and that the services were of poor quality. Thus, the most important barriers to the utilization of antenatal check-up services are the lack of conviction regarding the necessity of having an antenatal check-up, lack of knowledge of services and social customs not encouraging the utilization of antenatal care services. These findings underline the importance of developing a strong information, education and communication programme with respect to antenatal care and safe motherhood.

Table 9.2: Reasons for not receiving antenatal care

Per cent distribution of live births during the four years preceding the survey to mothers who did not receive antenatal care, by main reason for not receiving antenatal care and residence, India, 1992-93

Reason for not receiving antenatal care	Urban	Rural	Total
Lack of knowledge of services	7.6	13.4	12.8
Not necessary	66.4	57.6	58.5
Not customary	4-4	5-7	5.5
Financial cost	7.3	6.8	6.9
Inconvenient	1.7	2.6	2.5
Poor quality service	1.0	1.4	1.3
No time to go	3.0	5.5	5.3
Not permitted to go	5.3	5.2	5.2
Other	2.7	1.6	1.7
Don't know, missing	0.6	0.1	0.2
Totat per cent	100.0	100.0	100.0
Number	1996	16171	18168

Number and Timing of Antenatal Care Visits

The number of antenatal care visits and the timing of the first antenatal check-up are important for the health of the mother and the outcome of the pregnancy. Ideally, for normal cases antenatal care visits after confirmation of pregnancy should be scheduled at intervals of four weeks throughout the first seven months, then every two weeks until the last month and weekly thereafter (MacDonald and Pritchard, 1980). However, working women, particularly those from lower socioeconomic groups, often find it difficult to make frequent visits to an antenatal clinic because they face a loss of wages whenever they attend. Under these circumstances, a minimum of four antenatal visits are recommended during the third, sixth eighth, and ninth months of the pregnancy (Park and Park, 1989). The Child Survival and Satre Motherhood Programme has a slightly more modest goal of providing at least three antenatal check-ups to all pregnant women (Ministry of Health and Family Welfare, 1992b).

Table 9.3 and Figure 9.2 show the percentage distribution of live births in the last foul years by the number and timing of antenatal visits. Among the births for which the mother received any form of antenatal care, the median frequency of antenatal care visits either in the home or elsewhere is 3.7; the median number of home visits is 3.2 and of visits outside the home is 3.6. These medians make it clear that women who receive antenatal care are meeting the recommended minimum of 3 visits during pregnancy but they are far behind the expanded recommendation of 12 visits during a normal pregnancy. The median number of visits is large in urban areas (4.6) than in rural areas (3.5), but even in urban areas the expanded recommendations are not being met. No home visits were made by health workers to the mothers of 79 per cent of births; only 24 per cent of births in rural areas and 10 per cent of birth in urban areas received antenatal care through home visits.

Obstetricians advise that antenatal care should begin, at the latest, six weeks after the last menstrual period. However, studies of the impact of the initial antenatal visit show that, even when antenatal care is initiated as late as the third trimester, there is a substantial reduction in perinatal mortality (Ramachandran, 1992). The median gestational age for the first antenatal visit of either type (home or outside) is 5.0 months. It is 4.2 months in urban areas and 5.1 months in rural areas. The median gestational age in urban areas is higher for home visits (5.2 months) than outside visits (4.2 months). No such difference is observed in rural areas. The proportion of births whose mothers received antenatal care in the first trimester is 39 per cent in urban areas, 20 per cent in rural areas, and 24 per cent in the country as a whole. Thus, both urban and rural areas a substantial majority of mothers who receive antenatal care receive it for the first time at a later gestational age than is recommended.

Tetanus Toxoid Vaccination

Tetanus is an important cause of death among neonates in India. Neonatal tetanus is a particular problem in Madhya Pradesh, Orissa, and Uttar Pradesh, where the proportion of all deaths due to neonatal tetanus is higher than the state's share in the total population of India (Central Bureau of Health Intelligence, 1991).

Table 9.3: Number of antenatal care visits and stage of pregnancy
Per cent distribution of live births during the four years preceding the survey by number of antenatal care (ANC) visits, and by the stage of pregnancy at the time of the first visit, according to residence, India, 1492-93

ANC visits/ months pregnant	Home visits	Outside visits	Any type
1	2	3	4
	URBAN		
Number of ANC visits			
None	89.9	21.6	17.8
1 visit	1.9	4.2	4.1
2-3 visits	5.0	30.4	30.7
4 or more visits	2.7	43.5	46.9
Don't know/missing	0.5	0.3	0.5
Total per cent	100.0	100.0	100.0
Median number of visits (for those with ANC)	3.2	4.5	4.6
Months pregnant at the time of the first ANC visit			
No antenatal care	89.9	21.6	17.8
First trimester	2.9	37.4	39.3
Second trimester	4.7	26.4	28.1
Third trimester	2.0	14.3	14.4
Don't know/missing	0.4	0.3	0.3
Total per cent	100.0	100.0	100.0
Median months pregnant at first visit (for those with ANC)	5.2	4.2	4.2
Number of live births	11242	11242	11242
	RURAL		
Number of AMC visits			
None	75.2	57.8	42.4
1 visit	4.1	5.7	6.7
2-3 visits	13.2	23.0	28.9
4 or more visits	6.6	13.0	21.0
Don't know/missing	0.9	0.5	0.9
Total per cent	100.0	100.0	100.0
Median number of visits (for those with ANC)	3.2	3.3	3.5

{Cont}....

1	2	3	4
Months pregnant at the time of the first ANC visit			
No antenatal care	75.2	57.8	42.4
First trimester	7.0	13.9	19.5
Second trimester	12.4	18.7	26.9
Third trimester	4.7	9.0	10.5
Don't know/missing	0.8	0.5	0.7
Total per cent	100.0	100.0	100.0
Median months pregnant at first visit (for those with ANC)	5.3	5.3	5.1
Number of live births	38128	38128	38128
	TOTAL		
Number of ANC visits			
None	78.6	49.6	36.8
1 visit	3.6	5.3	6.1
2-3 visits	11.3	24.7	29.3
4 or more visits	5.7	19.9	26.9
Don't know/missing	0.8	0.5	0.8
Total per cent	100.0	100.0	100.0
Median number of visits (for those with ANC)	3.2	3.6	3.7
Months pregnant at the time of the first ANC visit			
No antenatal care	78.6	49.6	36.8
First trimester	6.0	19.2	24.0
Second trimester	10.6	20.5	27.2
Third trimester	4.1	10.2	11.4
Don't know/missing	0.7	0.5	0.6
Total per cent	100.0	100.0	100.0
Median months pregnant at first visit (for those with ANC)	5.3	5.0	5.0
Number of live births	49369	49369	49369

Note: Table is based on births in the period 1-47 months prior to the survey.

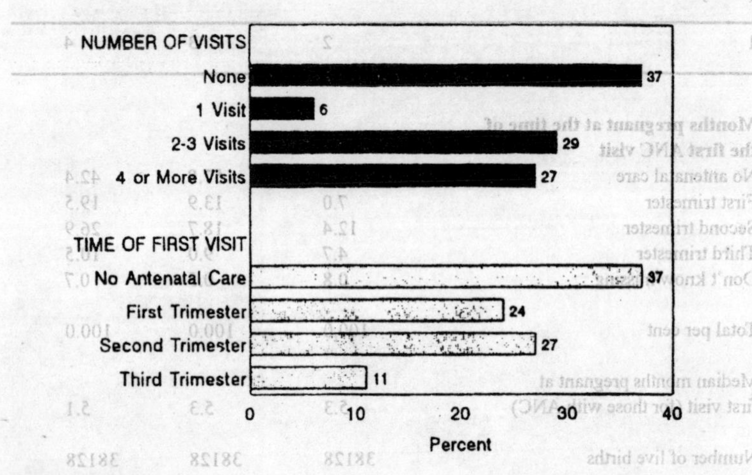

Figure 9.2 Number and Timing of Antenatal Visits

Neonatal tetanus is caused by infection of the newborn (usually at the umbilical stump) with tetanus organisms. Neonatal tetanus is most common when the delivery takes place in an unhygienic environment and nonsterilized instruments are used for cutting the umbilical cord. Tetanus typically develops during the first or second week of life and is fatal in 70 to 90 per cent of cases (Foster, 1984). Where this disease is most common, such as in rural areas of several states, expert medical help is also rarely available, thereby leading to a particularly high fatality rate. Neonatal tetanus is a preventable disease, however. Two doses of tetanus toxoid vaccine given to the pregnant woman one month apart during early pregnancy are nearly 100 per cent effective in preventing tetanus among newborns (and among mothers).

In India, the tetanus immunization programme for expectant mothers was initiated in 1975-76 and was integrated with the Expanded Programme on Immunization (EPI) in 1978 (Ministry of Health and Family Welfare, 1991). In order to hasten implementation of the immunization programme the Government of India started a special programme called the Universal Immunization Programme (UIP) in 1985-86. In 1986, the UIP was recognized as one of the seven Technology Missions. According to the National Immunization Schedule, a pregnant woman should receive two doses of tetanus toxoid injection, the first when she is

16 weeks pregnant and the second when she is 20 weeks pregnant (Central Bureau of Health Intelligence, 1991). Reinoculation is recommended every three years. If the initial doses were received less than three years ago a single booster injection is recommended.

In the NFHS, each mother who had a live birth during the four years prior to the survey was asked whether she was given an injection in the arm to prevent her and her baby from getting tetanus and, if so, how many times she received such an injection. The distribution of births by the number of tetanus toxoid injections given to the mother according to selected background characteristics is shown in Table 9.4. Fifty-four per cent of births were to mothers who had received two or more doses of tetanus toxoid vaccine, 7 per cent were to those who had received one dose, and 39 per cent were to those who did not receive even a single dose.

The receipt of two doses of tetanus toxoid vaccine is significantly higher in urban than in rural areas (74 per cent compared with 48 per cent). For births in the last four years, tetanus toxoid coverage is lower for older mothers and decreases consistently with an increase in birth order. The proportion of births whose mothers received two doses of tetanus toxoid vaccine increases steadily from 40 per cent for illiterate mothers to 84 per cent for mothers who completed middle school and to 92 per cent for mothers with at least a high school education. Vaccination against tetanus is highest among births to Jain mothers (92 per cent?, followed by births to Sikh mothers (80 per cent), Buddhist mothers (76 per cent), and Christian mothers (65 per cent). Vaccination against tetanus is almost the same among births to Muslim mothers (52 per cent) as among birth to Hindu mothers (53 per cent). The coverage is considerably lower among scheduled tribe mothers (34 per cent) than scheduled caste mothers (47 per cent) or non-SC/ST mothers (57 per cent).

Iron and Folic Acid Tablets

The size of a woman's baby, her preparation for lactation, and the iron and folate status of both the mother and the child depends upon the mother's nutritional status at the time of conception as well as her diet during pregnancy (World Health Organization, 1994a). Proper maternal care is important for the healthy intrauterine growth of the baby and may affect the baby's birth weight. Studies in various parts of India have indicated that the percentage of low birth weight babies (weighing less than 2,500 grams) ranged from 15 in Trivandrum to 46 in Baroda (Nutrition Foundation of India, 1993). Improved nutrition (coupled with

Table 9.4 Tetanus toxoid vaccinations

Per cent distribution of live births during the four years preceding the survey by number of tetanus toxoid injections and whether the respondent was given Iron folic tablets during pregnancy, according to selected background characteristics, India, 1992-93

Backgound Characteristic	Number of tetanus toxoid injections				Total per cent	Per cent given iron/ folic tablets	Number of births
	None	One dose	Two doses[1]	Don't know/ missing			
Mother's age at birth							
< 20	37.0	7.7	55.1	0.1	100.0	51.8	11514
20-34	37.8	6.9	55.1	0.2	100.0	51.5	35258
35+	62.8	6.8	30.3	0.1	100.0	30.3	2597
Birth order							
1	28.1	6.2	65.5	0.2	100.0	60.6	13594
2	32.2	7.3	60.4	0.2	100.0	56.7	11794
3	38.5	7.6	53.7	0.2	100.0	50.6	8639
4	45.8	7.8	46.4	0.1	100.0	43.3	5797
5	50.6	8.5	40.7	0.1	100.0	38.9	3745
6+	64.6	6.6	28.8	0.1	100.0	28.5	5800
Residence							
Urban	19.4	6.0	74.4	0.3	100.0	68.7	11242
Rural	44.7	7.4	47.7	0.1	100.0	45.1	38128
Education							
Illiterate	51.7	7.8	40.3	0.1	100.0	38.3	32770
Literate, < middle complete	20.9	7.0	71.9	0.2	100.0	66.6	8190
Middle school complete	10.0	5.3	84.3	0.3	100.0	77.2	3505

High school and above	4.4	4.0	91.5	0.2	100.0	85.6	4904N2
Religion							
Hindu	39.6	7.2	53.0	0.2	100.0	50.5	39223
Muslim	41.2	6.8	51.8	0.2	100.0	44.3	7613
Christian	27.4	7.1	65.0	0.5	100.0	65.0	981'
Sikh	15.1	4.7	80.2	—	100.0	71.0	8222
Jain	6.4	1.0	91.8	0.8	100.0	89.7	142
Buddhist	14.7	9.5	75.6	0.1	100.0	74.5	351
Other	42.0	9.8	47.8	0.4	100.0	49.0	237
Caste/tribe							
Scheduled caste	45.4	7.0	47.4	0.2	100.0	44.2	6590
Scheduled tribe	56.2	9.4	34.1	0.3	100.0	40.2	4703
Other	35.7	6.8	57.3	0.2	100.0	52.8	38076
Total	39.0	7.1	53.8	0.2	100.0	50.5	49369

Note: Table is based on births in the period 1-47 months prior to the survey.
— Less than 0.05 percent.
Includes women who received more than two doses.

improved health care in pregnancy) has, however, substantially improved birth weights in India (Ramachandran, 1992). The provision of iron and folic acid tablets as a prophylaxis against nutritional anaemia among pregnant women forms an integral part of the MCH activities of the Indian Family Welfare Programme (Ministry of Health and Family Welfare, 1991). It is recommended that a pregnant woman take 100 tablets of iron and folic acid during her pregnancy, and health workers are instructed accordingly.

In the NFHS, information was collected on whether the mother received iron and folic acid tablets during each pregnancy resulting in a live birth during the last four years. This information is presented in Table 9.4. Fifty-one per cent of births were to mothers who had received iron and folic acid tablets. Because nearly one-third of new babies in India are of low birth weight (WHO-UNICEF, 1992), the performance with regard to the intake of iron and folic acid tablets by pregnant women is very inadequate. As expected, the receipt of iron and folic acid tablets is higher in urban areas (69 per cent) than in rural areas (45 per cent). The differentials in the distribution of iron and folic acid tablets by other background characteristics are almost the same as those for tetanus toxoid injections.

Place of Delivery and Assistance During Delivery

From the standpoint of child survival and health of the mother, the first priority for delivery care is that it is safe and clean (World Health Organization, 1994). The majority of maternal deaths and much of the chronic morbidity resulting from childbirth are due to the failure to get timely help for complications at delivery. It is essential that delivery be conducted under proper hygienic conditions with the assistance of a trained medical practitioner. Table 9.5 and Figure 9.3 present the per cent distribution of live births occurring during the four years preceding the survey according to place of delivery and selected background characteristics. Only one-quarter of births during the last four years occurred in medical institutions, with 15 per cent in public institutions and 11 per cent in private health facilities. Overall, 74 per cent of births in India took place at home—62 per cent in the woman's own home and 12 per cent in the parents' home. The percentage of births that took place in medical institutions is three and a half times as high in urban areas (58 per cent) as in rural areas (16 per cent). Information on the per cent distribution of births by place of delivery and type of attendance at birth (for home deliveries) is also available from the Sample Registration System (SRS) (Office of the Registrar General, 1993a, 1993b). The SRS information for 1990-91 (averaged) puts the percentage of births in India occurring in medical institutions at 24 per cent (53 per cent in urban areas and 17 per cent in rural areas) The estimates from the NFHS and SRS for India as a whole are quite close. The estimates for urban areas differ by less than 5 percentage points and the estimates for rural areas are almost identical.

The proportion of births taking place in medical institutions is lower among births to older women than among births to younger women and is likewise lower among higher order births than among lower order births. As is the case for antenatal visits, tetanus vaccination, and iron and folic acid supplements, institutional deliveries are also more common among births to well educated women than among births to poorly educated women. For example, only 12 per cent of births to illiterate women occurred in medical institutions, compared to 75 per cent of births to women with at least a high school education. Institutional births are most common among Jain women (81 per cent), followed by Buddhist women (53 per cent), Christian women (49 per cent) and Sikh women (29 per cent). There is not much difference in the proportion of institutional deliveries between Hindu and Muslim women. Institutional deliveries are less common among births to scheduled tribe women (9 per cent) than among births to scheduled caste women (16 per cent) or non-SC/ST women (29 per cent).

In India, delivery in a medical institution (26 per cent) is less common than antenatal care (62 per cent), but the two are related. The percentage of institutional births is higher among women who had four or more antenatal visits (58 per cent) than among women who had fewer than four antenatal visits (23 per cent) or none (4 per cent). This could be due to the availability of both antenatal and delivery care services in the same setting. It might also reflect complications during pregnancy which often lead women to seek antenatal care and to deliver in an institutional setting. It is also possible that pregnant women receiving antenatal care are encouraged by the antenatal care provider to have medical assistance during delivery.

Table 9.6 and Figure 9.3 present information on assistance during delivery according to. selected background characteristics. As in the case of antenatal care, the interviewer was instructed to record all responses if more than one person was reported to have assisted during delivery. In Table 9.6 and Figure 9.3, however, only the most highly qualified attendant is considered if there is more than one attendant. In all, slightly more than one-fifth of all birth were attended by a doctor (22 per cent) and 13 per cent were attended by a nurse/midwife. Only 34 per

Table 9.5 : Place of delivery

Per cent distribution of live births during the four years preceding the survey by place of delivery, according to selected background characteristics, India, 1992-93

	Place of delivery							
	Health facility/ institution		Home					
Background characteristic	Public	Private	Own home	Parents[1] home	Other	Don't know/ missing	Total per cent	Number of live births
Mother's age at birth								
< 20	15.2	8.8	54.1	20.7	0.6	0.7	100.0	11514
20-34	15.0	12.0	62.3	9.8	0.5	0.4	100.0	35258
35+	7.2	5.3	84.2	1.9	0.6	0.8	100.0	2597
Birth order								
1	21.1	17.1	42.7	18.1	0.5	0.5	100.0	13594
2-3	15.3	11.6	59.6	12.5	0.5	0.4	100.0	20433
4-5	9.3	5.2	77.1	7.2	0.6	0.6	100.0	9542
6+	5.9	3.0	87.1	3.0	0.5	0.5	100.0	5800
Residence								
Urban	30.2	27.4	34.6	6.9	0.5	0.4	100.0	11242
Rural	10.0	6.0	69.5	13.4	0.5	0.5	100.0	38128
Education								
Illiterate	8.6	3.2	74.5	12.7	0.5	0.6	100.0	32770
Lit., < middle complete	23.1	14.7	48.1	13.1	0.7	0.3	100.0	8190
Middle school complete	30.9	24.5	34.5	9.3	0.7	0.1	100.0	3505
High school and above	29.3	46.0	17.2	7.0	0.2	0.3	100.0	4904

Religion								
Hindu	14.8	10.0	62.0	12.1	0.5	0.5	100.0	39223
Muslim	11.9	11.8	64.8	10.8	0.5	0.2	100.0	7613
Christian	22.3	26.2	43.5	7.4	0.4	0.2	100.0	981
Sikh	12.9	16.1	54.9	15.7	0.5	—	100.0	822
Jain	21.3	59.8	8.8	10.1	—	—	100.0	142
Buddhist	40.2	12.9	30.4	15.9	0.6	—	100.0	351
Other	10.2	7.7	69.5	12.4	—	0.2	100.0	237
Caste/tribe								
Scheduled caste	10.9	5.1	71.5	11.2	0.6	0.8	100.0	6590
Scheduled tribe	6.7	2.4	77.9	11.7	0.6	0.8	100.0	4703
Other	16.3	12.9	57.8	12.1	0.5	0.4	100.0	38076
Antenatal care visits								
None	3.0	1.2	84.8	10.5	0.5	—	100.0	18168
1-3 visits	16.2	7.2	61.9	14.1	0.5	—	100.0	17513
4+ visits	28.8	29.2	30.2	11.2	0.6	0.1	100.0	13279
Don't kno"/missing	4.4	1.8	33.9	6.2	—	53.7	100.0	410
Total	14.6	10.9	61.6	11.9	0.5	0.5	100.0	49369

Note: Table is based on births in the period 1-47 months prior to the survey. — Less-than 0.05 per cent.

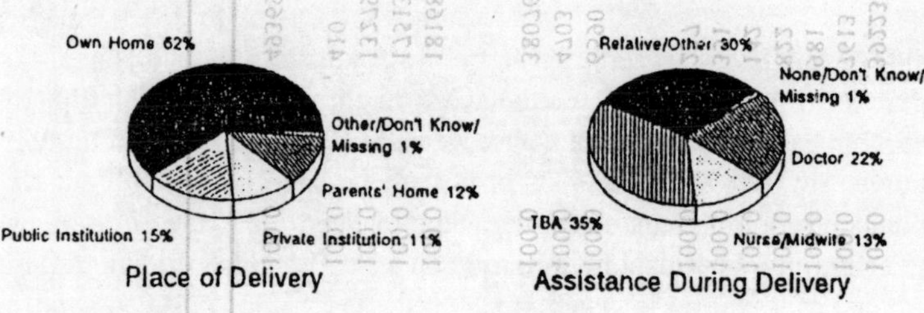

Figure 9.3 : Place of Delivery and Assistance During Delivery

cent of births were attended by trained medical persons. Another 35 per cent of deliveries were attended by traditional birth attendants, and 30 per cent were attended only by relatively friends or neighbours.

As one would expect, the proportion of deliveries attended by doctors is higher in urba areas (48 per cent) than in rural areas (14 per cent). Birth attendance by a nurse/midwife is als more common in urban areas (18 per cent) than in rural areas (11 per cent). Attendance by trained medical person increases steadily with an increase in the educational attainment of women. The proportion of births delivered by a trained medical person is 20 per cent among births to illiterate mothers, 65 per cent among births to mothers who completed middle scho, and 83 per cent among births to mothers who completed at least high school. Attendance durir delivery by a trained medical person is most common among Jains (93 per cent), Buddhists (60 per cent), and Christians (56 per cent). Fifty per cent of births to Sikh mothers were attended by trained medical persons. However, the proportion of births delivered by traditional bir attendant is 45 per cent among Sikh mothers (higher than any other religion). One-third of the births to Hindu women received assistance from a trained medical person, as did 30 per cent of births to Muslim women. Attendance at birth by a trained medical person is less common among births to mothers of scheduled tribes (18 per cent) and scheduled castes (25 per cent) than among births to women in the non-SC/ST category (38 per cent). Trained medical assistance during a birth is strongly related to the number of antenatal visits.

The type of assistance during delivery also varies according to the place of delivery Among deliveries that occurred in private medical facilities, 86 per cent were attended by a) doctor and 13 per cent by a nurse/midwife, whereas among deliveries in public health facilities 67 per cent were attended by a doctor and 31 per cent by a nurse/midwife. Among deliveries taking place in the woman's home, 48 per cent were attended by a traditional birth attendant, 40 per cent by relatives or others, less than 3 per cent by a doctor, and 8 per cent by a nurse/midwife Because nearly three-quarters of births take place at home, it is not surprising to find that traditional birth attendants, relatives, friends and neighbours play a major role in assisti deliveries in India.

Because only one-quarter of deliveries in India take place in medical institutions and two thirds of deliveries are unattended by a trained medical professional, a large majority of deliveries are likely to take place without proper hygienic care and timely professional help when complications develop. The situation is particularly serious in rural areas where five out of every six births take place at home and medical assistance is not available for three-quarters births.

Maternal Care Indicators by State

Table 9.7 provides information on several important maternal care indicators for Indian states. Interstate variations are substantial on each of the indicators of maternal care. The percentage of births for which mothers received antenatal care is highest in Kerala (97 per cent), followed by Goa (95 per cent), and Tamil Nadu (94 per cent). Among the major states (states with more than 5 million population in 1991), Punjab, Andhra Pradesh, Karnataka, Maharashtra and Delhi have also achieved antenatal coverage for more than 80 per cent of births. Among the smaller states, Mizoram and Jammu stand out with coverage rates of 89 and 80 per cent, respectively. Utilization of antenatal care services is lowest in Rajasthan (only 31 per cent of births during the last four years were to mothers who received antenatal care). The percentage of births for which mothers received antenatal care is also low in Bihar (37 per cent), Uttar Pradesh (45 per cent), Assam (49 per cent), Madhya Pradesh (52 per cent) and Orissa (62 per cent). In the six small states in the northeastern region, there is substantial variation in the coverage of antenatal care, ranging from 39 per cent in Nagaland to more than 60 per cent in Mizoram, Tripura and Manipur.

Because tetanus toxoid vaccinations and iron/folic acid tablets are often given during antenatal check-ups, it is not surprising that the interstate variations in these two maternal care indicators are similar to the variations observed in the utilization of antenatal care services. The

Table 9.6: Assistance during delivery

Per cent distribution of live births during the four years preceding the survey by type of assistance during delivery, according to selected background characteristics, India, 1992-93

Background characteristic	Attendant assisting during delivery[1]							
	Doctor	Nurse/ midwife	Traditional birth attendant	Relative/ other	None	Don't know/ missing	Total per cent	Number of live births
Mother's age at birth								
< 20	20.8	13.5	35.1	29.7	0.4	0.5	100.0	11514
20-34	22.6	12.6	34.8	28.8	0.6	0.5	100.0	35258
35+	10.3	8.8	41.3	37.6	1.0	1.0	100.0	2597
Birth order								
1	33.6	14.4	28.9	22.3	0.2	0.4	100.0	13594
2-3	22.3	13.6	34.4	28.8	0.5	0.4	100.0	20433
4-5	11.7	10.7	41.0	35.1	0.9	0.6	100.0	9542
6+	6.9	8.0	43.7	39.5	1.2	0.7	100.0	5800
Residence								
Urban	47.6	17.7	22.0	12.0	0.4	0.3	100.0	11242
Rural	13.9	11.1	39.1	34.6	0.6	0.6	100.0	38128
Mother's education								
Illiterate	9.9	10.1	41.8	36.8	0.7	0.7	100.0	32770
Lit., < middle complete	29.6	18.9	30.2	20.6	0.5	0.2	100.0	8190
Middle school complete	45.5	19.3	20.4	14.5	0.1	0.2	100.0	3505
High school and above	68.7	14.5	10.5	5.9	0.2	0.2	100.0	4904

Religion								
Hindu	21.0	12.6	35.3	29.9	0.6	0.6	100.0	39223
Muslim	19.6	10.6	37.4	31.5	0.6	0.3	100.0	7613
Christian	41.7	14.3	18.7	24.3	0.8	0.2	100.0	981
Sikh	27.0	22.9	45.1	5.0	—	—	100.0	822
Jain	80.9	12.1	4.7	2.3	—	—	100.0	142
Buddhist	32.6	27.8	17.8	21.2	0.6	—	100.0	351
Other	15.9	10.4	40.7	31.7	1.4	—	100.0	237
Caste/tribe								
Scheduled caste	13.7	11.4	39.5	33.9	0.7	0.9	100.0	6590
Scheduled tribe	7.4	10.1	41.8	39.2	0.9	0.7	100.0	4703
Other	24.7	13.2	33.7	27.5	0.5	0.4	100.0	38076
Antenatal care								
None	3.9	5.2	45.6	44.3	0.7	0.2	100.0	18168
1-3 visits	18.5	15.7	36.6	28.6	0.6	0.1	100.0	17513
4+ visits	50.3	18.8	20.1	10.6	0.2	—	100.0	13279
Don't know/missing	5.8	6.0	14.1	22.6	4.8	46.7	100.0	410
Place of delivery								
Public health facility	67.1	31.1	0.9	0.7	0.1	—	100.0	7226
Private health facility	86.2	12.9	0.4	0.5	—	—	100.0	5368
Own home	2.5	8.2	48.1	40.3	0.7	0.2	100.0	30397
Parents' home	6.3	13.0	43.8	36.3	0.5	0.1	100.0	5887
Other	11.0	15.1	40.9	31.4	1.7	—	100.0	258
Don't know/missing	5.3	—	1.1	3.9	8.5	81.2	100.0	234
Total	21.6	12.6	35.2	29.5	0.6	0.5	100.0	49369

Note: Table is based on births in the period 1-47 months prior to the survey.

— Less than 0.05 percent. 1 If the respondent mentioned more than one attendant, only the most qualified attendant is considered.

Table 9.7: Maternal care indicators by state

Percentage of live births during the four years preceding the survey by various maternal care indicators and state, India, 1992-93

State	Percentage receiving antenatal care	Percentage receiving two doses of tetanus toxoid vaccine[1]	Percentage receiving iron/ folic tablets	Percentage of births delivered in medical institutions	Percentage of deliveries assisted by health professionals[2]
India	62.3	53.8	50.5	25.5	34.2
North					
Delhi	82.4	72.5	74.9	44.3	53.0
Haryana	72.7	63.3	59.9	16.7	30.3
Himachal Pradesh	76.0	47.4	71.7	16.0	25.6
Jammu Region of J & K	79.5	68.9	70.7	21.9	31.2
Punjab	87.9	82.7	73 .6	24.8	48.3
Rajasthan	31.2	28.3	29.2	11.6	21.8
Central					
Madhya Pradesh	52.1	42.8	44.3	15.9	30.0
Uttar Pradesh	44.7	37.4	29.5	11.2	17.2
East					
Bihar	36.8	30.7	21.4	12.1	19.0
Orissa	61.6	53.8	49.9	14.1	20.5
West Bengal	75.3	70.4	56.3	31.5	33.0
Northeast					
Arunachal Pradesh	48.9	31.9	44.7	19.9	21.3

Assam	49 3	34 9	39 4	11.1	17.9
Manipur	63.4	48.0	35.5	23.0	40.4
Meghalaya	51.8	30.0	49.6	29.6	36.9
Mizoram	88.9	42.5	63.7	48.9	61.5
Nagaland	39.3	33.0	23.9	6.0	22.2
Tripura	64.9	58.7	53.2	30.7	33.5
West					
Goa	95.4	83.4	89.3	86.8	88.4
Gujarat	75.7	62.7	69.3	35.6	42.5
Maharashtra	82.7	71.0	70.6	43.9	53.2
South					
Andhra Pradesh	86.3	74.8	76.4	32.8	49.3
Karnataka	83.5	69.8	74.9	37.5	50.9
Kerala	97.3	89.8	91.2	87.8	89.7
Tamil Nadu	94.2	90.1	84.1	63.4	71.2

Note: Table is based on births in the period 1-47 months prior to the survey.

1 Includes women who received more than two doses.

2 Allopathic doctor or nurse/midwife.

states which have a higher percentage of births covered by antenatal care also have higher percentages of births whose mothers received two doses of anti-tetanus injections and iron and folic acid tablets during pregnancy.

There are also large interstate variations in the proportion of institutional deliveries, ranging from 87-88 per cent in Kerala and Goa to 11-12 per cent in Rajasthan, Assam, Bihar and Uttar Pradesh. Only 6 per cent of births in Nagaland are reported to have occurred in a health facility. Apart from Kerala and Goa, the only other state where more than half of all births take place in institutions is Tamil Nadu. It is surprising to note that in Punjab, which has achieved a strong performance in the provision of antenatal care services, only 25 per cent of births are institutional. Between 13 and 17 per cent of births take place in health facilities in Orissa, Madhya Pradesh, Himachal Pradesh and Haryana. Even in the predominantly urban state of Delhi, only 44 per cent of births occur in institutions. In every state, more births are assisted by health professionals than take place in a medical institution, but the pattern of variations among the states is similar for these two indicators.

In sum, the provision of antenatal and delivery care services is better than average in all of the southern and western states in India. The northern states (with the major exception of Rajasthan) perform relatively well on the antenatal care indicators, but the situation with respect to delivery care is quite mixed. Maternal care is poor across the board in Rajasthan, Bihar, Uttar Pradesh, Assam and Nagaland. Renewed efforts to improve maternal care in these states should be a top priority.

Delivery Characteristics

Table 9.8 presents findings on complications during delivery, prematurity, birth weight and the mother's estimates of the baby's size at birth for live births in the four years preceding the survey. As reported by mothers, 88 per cent of the deliveries had no complications, 6 per cent were characterized by a long period of labour, 2 per cent were accompanied by excessive bleeding, and 3 per cent required a Caesarian section (C-section). Forceps were used for less than one per cent of births and a similar proportion had the delayed delivery of the placenta. Csection deliveries were three and a half times as prevalent in urban areas (where institutional deliveries are more common) as in rural areas; otherwise, urban-rural differences in delivery complications are minor. A very small proportion of live births (3 per cent) are reported as premature.

Table 9.8: Delivery characteristics

Per cent distribution of live births during the four years preceding the survey by whether the delivery had complications, whether premature, and by birth weight and the mother's estimate of the baby's size at birth, according to residence, India, 1992-93

Delivery characteristic	Urban	Rural	Total
Complications at delivery[1]			
No complications	84.7	88.8	87.9
Caesarian section	5.7	1.6	2.5
Use of forceps	1.6	0.7	0.9
Excessive bleeding	1.6	1.8	1.8
Long period of labour	5.1	6.5	6.2
Delayed delivery of placenta	0.9	1.0	0.9
Other	1.4	0.7	0.9
Premature birth			
Yes	3.9	3.0	3.2
No	95.6	96.0	95.9
Don't know/missing	0.5	1.0	0.9
Total per cent	100.0	100.0	100.0
Birth weight			
Less than 2.5 kg	10.0	1.9	3.8
2.5 kg or more	28.0	5.8	10.8
Don't know/missing	12.3	4.5	6.3
Not weighed	49.7	87.8	79.1
Total per cent	100.0	100.0	100.0
Size at birth			
Large	15.3	13.4	13.8
Average	63.8	63.5	63.6
Small	20.0	21.4	21.1
Don't know/missing	0.9	1.6	1.5
Total per cent	100.0	100.0	100.0
Number of births	11242	38128	49369

Note: Table is based on births in the period 1-47 months prior to the survey.

1 All complications were recorded if there was more than one complication. Births with missing information on complications are not included.

A large majority of children (79 per cent) were not weighed at birth. Fifty per cent of children born in urban areas and 88 per cent in rural areas were not weighed at birth, which is to be expected because of the large proportion of deliveries that take place at home, where scales for weighing babies are rarely available. Moreover, for 12 per cent of births in urban areas and 5 per cent in rural areas, the baby was weighed

Table 9.9: Delivery characteristics by background characteristics

Per cent distribution of live births during the four years preceding the survey by whether the delivery had complications whether premature and by birth weight and the mother's estimate of the baby's size at birth[1] according to antenatal care birth interval and mother's age India, 1992-93.

Delivery characteristic	Antenatal care			Previous birth interval				Age of mother at birth		
	None	1-3 visits	4+ visits	Under 2 years	2-3 years	4+ years	First birth	<20	20-34	35+
Complications at delivery										
No complications	91.8	88.4	81.6	90.5	90.5	88.5	82.1	86.7	88.1	90.6
Caesarian section	0.3	1.4	7.0	1.2	1.4	2.2	5.2	2.1	2.7	1.4
Use of forceps	0.1	0.7	2.3	0.6	0.4	0.6	2.0	1.3	0.8	0.1
Excessive bleeding	1.9	1.7	1.7	1.9	1.8	1.5	1.9	1.8	1.8	2.2
Long period of labour	5.6	6.7	6.3	5.1	5.3	6.4	8.0	7.3	5.8	5.6
Delayed delivery of placenta	0.8	1.0	1.1	0.8	0.8	1.2	1.1	1.1	0.9	0.4
Other	0.6	1.0	1.2	0.9	0.7	0.9	1.1	1.0	0.9	0.4
Premature birth										
Yes	2.9	3.1	3.8	3.4	2.2	2.4	4.8	4.6	2.8	2.5
No	96.3	96.5	96.1	95.5	97.0	96.7	94.2	94.2	96.5	96.2
Don t know/missing	0.8	0.4	0.2	1.0	0.9	0.9	0.9	1.2	0.8	1.3
Total per cent	100.0	100.0	100.0	100.0	100.0	100.0	100.0	100.0	100.0	100.0
Birth weight										
Less than 2.5 kg	0.4	3.3	9.1	3.2	2.4	2.9	6.6	3.8	3.9	1.4
2.5 kg or more	0.7	7.7	29.1	9.3	7.3	11.1	16.7	8.5	12.0	4.7
Don t know/missing	1.1	5.7	12.6	6.0	5.3	5.4	8.3	6.6	6.3	3.9

Not weighed	97.8	83.4	49.2	81.5	85.0	80.6	68.3	81.1	77.7	90.0
Total per cent	100.0	100.0	100.0	100.0	100.0	100.0	100.0	100.0	100.0	100.0
Size at birth										
Large	11.8	13.0	18.0	13.9	13.3	14.7	14.0	14.6	13.8	10.9
Average	65.1	64.4	61.5	63.6	65.1	64.5	61.0	59.1	64.9	65.3
Small	21.6	21.8	19.9	20.6	20.2	19.5	23.6	24.5	19.9	22.1
Don t know/missing	1.5	0.8	0.6	1.9	1.4	1.3	1.3	1.8	1.3	1.7
Total per cent	100.0	100.0	100.0	100.0	100.0	100.0	100.0	100.0	100.0	100.0
Number of births	18168	17513	13279	8912	19776	7012	13670	11514	35258	2597

Note: Table is based on births in the period 1-47 months prior to the survey. Cases with missing information on antenatal care visits are not shown separately.

1 All complications were recorded if there was more than one complication. Births with missing information on complications are not included.

but the mother could not provide information on the birth weight at the time of the interview. Thus, the resulting sample of birth weights is small and subject to substantial selection bias. Twenty-six per cent of babies whose weight at birth was known had a low birth weight (less than 2.5 kg.). The proportion of low birth weight babies is almost the same in urban and rural areas. The proportion of low birth weight babies observed in the NFHS is slightly smaller than observed in several previous studies conducted in India, according to which around 30 per cent of babies have a low birth weight (WHO- UNICEF, 1992).

Because of the difficulty of weighing newborns in India due to the fact that most deliveries take place at home, a question on the size of the baby at the time of birth (small, average or large) was asked in the NFHS. Experience has shown that mothers can give useful information about the size of their newborns. Slightly more than one-fifth of newborns were reported by mothers to be small in size. As previously noted in Chapter 8, these children have a much higher risk of dying than children who are at least of average size at the time of birth.

Table 9.9 shows differentials in delivery characteristics by the type of antenatal care, length of the previous birth interval and the mother's age at birth. Complications and premature births were more common for births to mothers who had four or more antenatal visits. This suggests that there is a tendency among pregnant women having complications to obtain antenatal care. Not surprisingly, antenatal care is also related to newborns being weighed. The proportion of newborns who were weighed was 2 per cent for those whose mothers did not receive antenatal care, 17 per cent for those whose mothers had 1-3 antenatal check-ups and 51 per cent for those whose mothers had 4 or more antenatal visits. As indicated in Table 9.5, 58 per cent of births to mothers who had four or more antenatal visits were delivered in institutions, where the probability of weighing children is very high.

There is little relationship between the previous birth interval and complications at delivery, but first births have a slightly higher complication rate, especially with respect to the period of labour. Perhaps because of the long period of labour, C-sections were carried out for 5 per cent of first births compared with 1-2 per cent of other births. First births are also slightly more likely to be premature (5 per cent compared with 2-3 per cent for other births), to have a low birth weight, and to be smaller than average at the time of birth. Births to mothers less than 20 years of age at the time of delivery are also more likely than other births to be premature, small in size and underweight.

9.2 Child Care Indicators

Immununization of Children

The immunization of children against six serious but preventable diseases (namely, tuberculosis, diphtheria, pertussis, tetanus, poliomyelitis and measles) has been a cornerstone of the child health care system in India. As part of the National Health Policy, the National Immunization Programme is being implemented in India on a priority basis (Gupta and Murli 1989). The Expanded Programme on Immunization (EPI) was started by the Government of India in 1978 with the objective of reducing morbidity, mortality, and disabilities due to these six diseases by making free vaccinations easily available to all eligible children. Immunization against polio was introduced to the programme in 1979-80 and tetanus toxoid for school children was added in 1980-81. BCG was brought under the EPI in 1981-82. The latest addition to the Programme is vaccination against measles, introduced in 1985-86 (Ministry of Health anz Family Welfare, 1991).

In order to accelerate implementation of the immunization scheme, the Government a India started a special programme called the Universal Immunization Programme (UIP) in 1985-86. The UIP was designated as one of the seven Technology Missions and was charged wit two objectives: (i) to vaccinate at least 85 per cent of all infants by 1990 against the six vaccine preventable diseases; and (ii) to achieve self-sufficiency in vaccine production and the manufacture of cold chain equipment (Ministry of Health and Family Welfare, 1991).

The standard immunization schedule developed for the immunization programme for children contains the age at which each vaccine is to be administered, the number of doses to be given, and the route of vaccination (intramuscular, oral or subcutaneous). Vaccinations received by infants and children are usually recorded on a vaccination card, which is given to the mother of each child.

In the NFHS, every mother was asked whether she had a vaccination card for each child born since 1 January 1988 for surveys that started in 1992 and 1 January 1989 for surveys that started in 1993. If a card was available, the interviewer was required to copy carefully the dates on which the child received vaccinations against each disease. When the mother could not produce the vaccination card, she was asked whether the child had received a vaccination against tuberculosis (BCG); diphtheria, whooping cough (pertussis) and tetanus (DPT); poliomyelitis (polio) and measles. For DPT and polio, information was obtained on the number of injections or oral doses given. The date of vaccination was not asked of the mother.

Table 9.10 presents the percentage of children age 12-23 months who received each vaccine at any time before the interview and the percentage who received each vaccine before 12 months of age, according to whether a written vaccination record was shown to the interviewer or the mother was the source of all vaccination information. The proportion receiving vaccinations before 12 months is chosen for analysis because international guidelines specify that children should be fully immunized by the time they complete their first year of life. The denominator for any given row in each part of the table is the number of children age 12-23 months whose vaccination status was recorded from a card (Row 1), reported by the mother (Row 2), or determined from either source (Rows 3 and 4). The numerator of each entry in the row labelled "Vaccination card" is the number of children who received the specific vaccination or dose any time prior to the survey, as indicated in the vaccination card seen by the interviewer. The numerator for this row also includes those cases where a card was shown and (1) there was an indication on the card that the vaccination was given but the actual date was either missing or inconsistent, or (2) there was no record of receipt of the vaccination on the card, but the mother reported that the vaccination was given. The numerator for each entry in the row labelled "Mother's report" is the number of children whose mothers did not show a card to the interviewer but reported that the child had received the vaccination. The numerator for each entry in the row labelled "Either source" is the sum of the numerators in the preceding two rows for the vaccination under consideration. The numerator for each entry in the fourth row, "Vaccinated by 12 months of age", is derived from the numerators of the preceding two rows. Because the date of vaccination was not asked of the mother if she could not show the card, the proportion of vaccinations given during the first year of life among children whose information is based on the mother's report is assumed to be the same as the proportion of vaccinations given during the first year of life among children with an exact date of vaccination on the card.

Of the 11,853 children age 12-23 months, vaccination cards were seen by the interviewers for only 31 per cent. The percentage producing cards was 38 for urban areas and 29 for rural areas. As expected, the percentages vaccinated are much higher for children whose vaccination cards were seen by the interviewer than for children who either did not have a card or whose card was not seen.

Based on the information either recorded on cards or reported by the mother, only 35 per cent of children in India are fully vaccinated.[1]

Another 35 per cent have received some vaccinations and 30 per cent have not received any vaccinations. Thus, India has a long was go to achieve the goal of the universal immunization of children.

Analysis of vaccine-specific data shows that more than three-fifths (62 per cent of children have received BCG vaccine, and two-thirds have received the first dose of DPT 66 per cent) and the first dose of polio vaccine (67 per cent). The coverage of three doses of DPT and three doses of polio vaccine is 52 and 53 per cent, respectively. The DPT and p coverage rates are about the same because both vaccines are normally administ simultaneously. The continuation rate from the first to the third dose of the DPT and polio vaccines indicates considerable drop-out (22 per cent in the case of DPT and 20 per cent in case of polio). Only 42 per cent of children age 12-23 months have been vaccinated against measles. The low rate of measles vaccination is responsible for lowering the percentage of children fully vaccinated.

The urban-rural differences in coverage rates are substantial. More than half (51 per cent) of children in urban areas have received all the vaccines compared to 31 per cent in rural areas. The urban-rural difference is also marked for individual vaccines, with the urban coverage rates for BCG, three doses of DPT and polio, and measles being higher than the rural coverage rates by 20-22 percentage points.

According to the immunization schedule, all primary vaccinations, (including measles) should be completed by the time a child is 12 months old. The data presented in Table 9.10 indicate that most vaccinations that are given are administered within the first year of life. For example, 28 per cent of children were fully vaccinated by age 12 months compared with 35 per cent who were fully vaccinated by the time of the survey. Thus, 78 per cent of children who were fully vaccinated received all vaccinations before their first birthday. The gap between ontime and late vaccination is particularly wide for measles. Only 77 per cent of children who were vaccinated against measles by the time of the survey had received the measles vaccination before their first birthday. This contrasts with on-time rates of 94 per cent for BCG, 91 per cent for the third dose of DPT and 90 per cent for the third dose of polio.

Table 9.11 and Figure 9.4 present vaccination coverage rates among children age 12-23 months by selected background characteristics. The proportion of children for whom the mother showed a vaccination card varies by background characteristics. Vaccination cards were seen for a higher percentage of male children, lower order births, children in urban areas, children of mothers with at least a middle school education, and Jain, Buddhist and Sikh and non-SC/ST children. There

Table 9.10: Vaccinations by source of information

Among children age 12-23 months, the percentage who have received each vaccine at any time before the interview and before 12 months of age, according to whether the information is from the vaccination card or from the mother, India, 1992-93.

Source of information	Percentage vaccinated among children age 12-23 months											Number of children
	BCG	Polio 0	DPT 1	DPT 2	DPT 3	Polio 1	Polio 2	Polio 3	Measles	All[1]	None	
					URBAN							
Vaccinated at any time before interview												
Vaccination card	93.4	8.0	99.1	95.7	89.3	99.0	96.1	89.1	72.8	67.5	—	1027
Mother's report	68.0	7.7	69.0	62.7	56.3	69.8	65.1	58.8	48.2	40.5	26.4	1688
Either source	77.6	7.8	80.4	75.2	68.8	80.8	76.8	70.2	57.5	50.7	16.4	2715
Vaccinated by 12 months of age[2]	74.8	7.8	77.3	72.1	64.2	78.0	73.0	65.8	46.3	41.5	19.5	2715
					RURAL							
Vaccinated at any time before interview												
Vaccination card	89.4	4.2	98.8	91.3	82.3	98.3	91.2	82.8	64.4	57.9	0.1	2603
Mother's report	45.0	3.4	47.5	39.9	32.4	48.8	42.7	34.7	27.0	20.1	47.5	6535
Either source	57.6	3.6	62.1	54.5	46.6	62.9	56.5	48.4	37.7	30.9	34.0	9134
Vaccinated by 12 months of age[2]	54.0	3.6	58.0	50.3	41.8	58.8	52.1	43.2	28.7	23.4	38.0	9138

TOTAL												
Vaccinated at ary time before interview												
Vaccination card	90.5	5.3	98.9	92.5	84.3	98.5	92.6	84.6	66.8	60.6	—	3630
Mother's report	49.7	4.3	51.9	44.6	37.3	53.1	47.3	39.6	31.3	24.3	43.2	8223
Either source	62.2	4.6	66.3	59.2	51.7	67.0	61.2	53.4	42.2	35.4	30.0	11853
Vaccinated by												
12 months of age[2]	58.7	4.6	62.4	55.3	46.9	63.2	56.9	48.3	32.7	27.5	33.7	11853

— Less than 0.05 per cent.

1 Children who are fully vaccinated, i.e., those who have received BCG, measles and three doses of DPT and polio vaccine (excluding polio 0).

2 For children whose information was based on the mother's report, the proportion of vaccinations given during the first year of life was assumed to be the same as for children with a written record of vaccination.

are marked differences in vaccination coverage by these characteristics as well. For every type of vaccination except polio 0, coverage is higher among male than among female children, although by only a relatively small amount. The difference in coverage rates for male and female children ranges from 3 percentage points for measles to 5 per centage points for polio 2. Thus, while there appears to be discrimination against female children with regard to immunizations, the level of this discrimination is relatively modest. Sex differentials in immunizations might nevertheless be an important factor underlying higher female than male mortality in childhood, as observed in Chapter 8.

The relationship between vaccination coverage and birth order is consistently negative for all vaccinations. The majority of first order births occur to younger women who have been observed to have a higher degree of utilization of health care services, such as antenatal and natal services. As in the case of utilization of maternal health care services, there is a consistent positive relationship between the educational level of the mother and utilization of immunization services. The per centage of children who are fully vaccinated increases from 24 per cent for children whose mothers are illiterate to 70 per cent for children whose mothers have completed high school.

The coverage rate for all vaccinations is highest among Jain children (74 per cent) followed by Buddhist (68 per cent), Sikh (60 per cent) and Christian children (42 per cent). Hindu children are much more likely to be fully vaccinated (36 per cent) than Muslim children (26 per cent), despite the fact that Muslim children are more concentrated in urban areas where vaccination rates are relatively high. Children from scheduled castes and scheduled tribes are much less likely to be fully vaccinated than non-SC/ST children.

Table 9.12 and Figure 9.5 show vaccination coverage rates for each type of vaccination and the per centage with a vaccination card among children age 12-23 months for each state. There is a considerable interstate variation in the coverage rates for different vaccinations and for children receiving all vaccinations. The percentage of children who are fully vaccinated ranges from 4 per cent in Nagaland to 75 per cent in Goa. Among the major states, the percentage of children who are fully vaccinated ranges from 11 per cent for Bihar to 65 per cent for Tamil Nadu. Bihar (11 per cent), Assam (19 per cent), Uttar Pradesh (20 per cent), Rajasthan (21 per cent), and Madhya Pradesh (29 per cent) stand out as having a much lower percentage of children fully vaccinated than the national average of 35 per cent. As these states account for more than 40 per cent of the total population of the country, their low coverage

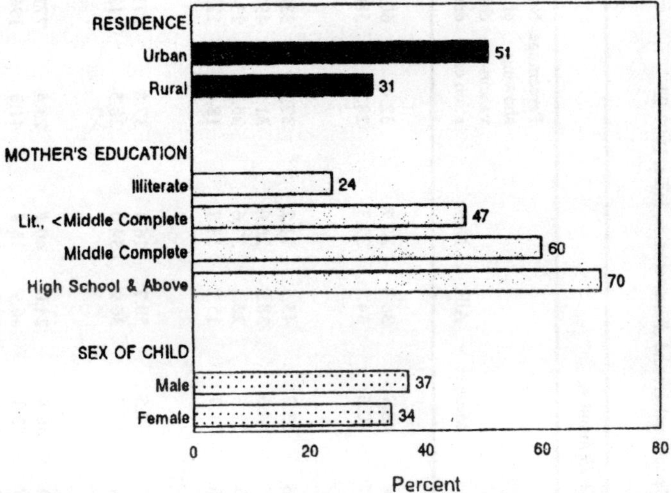

Figure 9.4: Percentage of Children Age 12-23 Months Who have Received All Vaccinations

for vaccination pulls down the coverage rate of the country as a whole. Generally, the northern states of Jammu, Himachal Pradesh, Punjab, Delhi and Haryana have fared well with regard to full coverage of vaccinations. Similarly, all of the western states and southern states have done relatively well with respect to full coverage of immunizations. All the northeastern states except Mizoram have a poor vaccination performance. With respect to individual vaccinations, a similar picture emerges for the various states in India. In the case of BCG, and three doses of DPT and polio, Goa and Tamil Nadu are the only states to attain the national goal of at least 85 per cent immunization, although neither state has attained this goal for all of the recommended vaccinations. In every state, fewer children have received measles vaccine than any of the other vaccinations. The relatively low levels of coverage for measles is a major factor in the failure to achieve full immunization. However, even if the measles vaccine were not required to achieve full immunization every state except Goa and Tamil Nadu would still fall short of the national immunization goal.

Table 9.13 shows the percentage of children age 1-3 years with vaccination cards shown to the interviewer and the percentage receiving various vaccinations in the first year of life, according to the current age of the child and the place of residence. The table illustrates changes in

Table 9.11: Vaccinations by background characteristics

Among Children age 12-23 months, the percentage who had received each vaccine by the time of the survey (according to the vaccination card or the mother) and the percentage with a vaccination card which was shown to the interviewer, by selected background characteristics, India, 1992-93

Background Characterisitc	Percentage vaccinated among children age 12-23 months											Percentage showing vaccin-ation card	Number of chil-dren
			DPT			Polio							
	BCG	Polio 0	1	2	3	1	2	3	Measles	All[1]	None		
Sex													
Male	64.0	4.6	68.2	61.3	53.5	69.1	63.4	55.0	43.7	36.7	27.8	32.4	6053
Female	60.3	4.6	64.4	57.1	49.8	64.8	58.9	51.7	40.6	34.1	32.3	28.7	5800
Birth order													
1	71.3	6.2	75.8	69.2	61.6	76.6	70.8	63.6	53.2	45.5	21.2	37.3	3312
2-3	66.4	5.0	69.5	63.2	56.3	70.5	65.3	57.3	44.6	38.3	26.6	31.8	4924
4-5	53.4	3.0	58.6	50.2	42.2	58.7	52.1	44.2	32.6	26.1	37.6	25.3	2342
6+	38.6	1.8	43.2	34.5	26.0	43.8	36.7	28.9	21.9	15.2	51.7	18.6	1275
Residence													
Urban	77.6	7.8	80.4	75.2	68.8	80.8	76.8	70.2	57.5	50.7	16.4	37.8	2715
Rural	57.6	3.6	62.1	54.5	46.6	62.9	56.5	48.4	37.7	30.9	34.0	28.5	9138
Mother's education													
Illiterate	50.8	2.9	55.4	47.5	39.0	56.4	49.5	41.0	30.8	24.0	40.1	23.4	7726
Lit., <middle complete	75.9	5.4	80.3	73.7	66.7	81.0	76.0	68.7	53.3	46.9	16.9	41.3	1965
Middie school complete	87.1	9.0	90.0	84.8	79.3	88.7	85.4	78.7	67.4	60.3	8.2	47.5	901

High school and above	92.8	10.4	94.2	90.5	86.3	94.6	91.9	87.7	76.7	70.0	4.2	46.1	1261
Religion													
Hindu	63.3	4.6	67.6	60.5	53.1	68.3	62.4	54.6	42.9	36.0	28.6	30.9	9467
Muslim	51.2	3.4	54.9	47.0	38.6	55.9	49.6	41.5	32.3	26.3	41.1	25.4	1769
Christian	70.7	13.4	72.3	66.9	60.3	72.9	67.7	60.6	50.0	42.4	23.4	39.1	229
Sikh	79.8	2.9	82.3	79.3	72.0	83.0	79.5	73.2	64.7	60.4	16.6	43.3	209
Jain	(99.7)	(14.9)	(99.7)	(99.7)	(92.5)	(99.7)	(98.1)	(90.9)	(81.8)	(73.7)	(0.3)	(48.9)	42
Buddhist	82.6	8.6	85.5	82.4	78.5	82.6	82.3	78.5	74.9	68.1	14.4	58.3	72
Other	67.8	0.8	69.1	64.6	49.9	73.1	68.9	57.6	42.9	36.4	23.6	19.3	66
Caste/tribe													
Scheduled caste	52.9	3.5	58.7	51.4	43.3	60.2	53.0	44.4	33.9	26.8	36.9	25.3	1565
Scheduled tribe	50.2	2.7	52.9	45.4	36.5	54.7	47.6	37.6	32.7	24.8	41.8	21.2	1104
Other	65.2	5.0	69.2	62.2	55.0	69.6	64.2	56.8	44.7	38.2	27.4	32.7	9184
Total	62.2	4.6	66.3	59.2	51.7	67.0	61.2	53.4	42.2	35.4	30.0	30.6	11853

( ) Based on 25-49 unweighted cases.

1 Children who are fully vaccinated, i.e., those who have received BCG, measles and three doses of DPT and polio vaccine (excluding polio 0).

Table 9.12: Vaccinations by state

Among Children age 12-23 months, the percentage who have received each vaccine at any time before the interview and the percentage with a vaccination card which was shown to the interviewer, by state, India, 1992-93

	Percentage vaccinated among children age 12-23 months											
		Polio	DPT			Polio						Percentage showing vaccin-ation card
State	BCG	0	1	2	3	1	2	3	Measles	All[1]	None	
India	62.2	4.6	66.3	59.2	51.7	67.0	61.2	53.4	42.2	35.4	30.0	30.6
North												
Delhi	90.1	12.3	89.0	81.9	71.6	88.8	85.1	75.0	69.6	57.8	6.7	45.5
Haryana	77.4	2.1	80.5	75.0	66.8	80.5	75.4	67.7	60.9	53.5	17.5	31.3
Himachal Pradesh	84.5	2.2	90.1	83.8	78.2	90.1	85.9	77.7	71.5	62.9	8.7	53.6
Jammu Region of J & K	81.3	1.7	83.7	82.3	77.8	83.8	82.4	77.1	69.1	65.7	16.2	47.9
Punjab	77.4	1.7	81.9	78.5	73.6	82.2	78.2	73 .4	64.8	61.9	17.5	37.8
Rajasthan	45.7	11.4	47.8	38.6	29.7	48.8	41.2	32.8	31 2	21.1	48.5	16.3
Central												
Madhya Pradesh	56.8	4.3	60.8	53.5	43.7	62.8	56.7	46.6	40.7	29.2	34.4	21.8
Uttar Pradesh	48.9	1.5	52.2	41.8	34.1	51.8	44.7	37.1	26.3	19.8	43.3	23.0
East												
Bihar	33.9	2.8	42.8	37.0	29.1	45.0	40.6	31.6	14.6	10.7	53.5	16.7
Orissa	63.3	3.1	69.0	63.6	56.3	70.3	64.8	56.7	40.2	36.1	28.0	41.7
West Bengal	63.1	0.9	73 .7	62.9	51.9	75.2	66.6	56.0	42.5	34.2	22.4	47.7

Northeast												
Arunachal Pradesh	46.3	2.5	50.0	45.6	38.8	48.1	44.4	38.8	27.5	22.5	47.5	37.5
Assam	48.2	1.2	53.4	42.2	31.0	54.2	42.9	32.7	25.8	19.4	43.6	39.5
Manipur	63.8	3.1	66.1	55.9	43.3	63.8	51.2	39.4	37.0	29.1	32.3	42.5
Meghalaya	43.8	1.4	36.8	30.6	22.9	36.1	31.9	23.6	13.2	9.7	54.9	15.3
Mizoram	77.3	4.5	83.6	80.0	71.8	80.9	76.4	69.1	65.5	56.4	14.5	38.2
Nagaland	19.4	3.1	21.3	16.9	12.5	21.9	18.8	15.0	10.0	3.8	75.0	11.9
Tripura	39.7	0.8	57.0	43.8	32.2	57.0	43.0	32.2	28.9	19.0	42.1	43.0
West												
Goa	93.5	14.0	93.9	90.0	86.7	94.3	90.7	87.1	77.8	74.9	5.4	74.9
Gujarat	77.1	4.4	77.8	71.4	63.8	77.8	71.2	62.9	55.9	49.8	18.9	32.0
Maharashtra	86.9	5.9	90.0	85.9	83.1	90.2	85.5	81.6	70.2	64.1	7.5	39.2
South												
Andhra Pradesh	73.9	3.3	77.3	72.3	66.1	78.9	74.6	68.0	53.8	45.0	17.5	35.3
Karnataka	81.7	5.3	80.6	76.6	70.7	81.9	77.7	71.4	54.9	52.2	15.2	34.4
Kerala	86.1	11.9	84.8	81.5	73.7	85.1	82.3	75.2	60.5	54.4	11.4	56.2
Tamil Nadu	91.7	19.4	95.0	92.2	86.5	94.1	91.0	85.3	71.6	64.9	3.3	38.2

1 Children who are fully vaccinated, i.e., those who have received BCG, measles and three doses of DPT and polio vaccine (excluding polio 0).

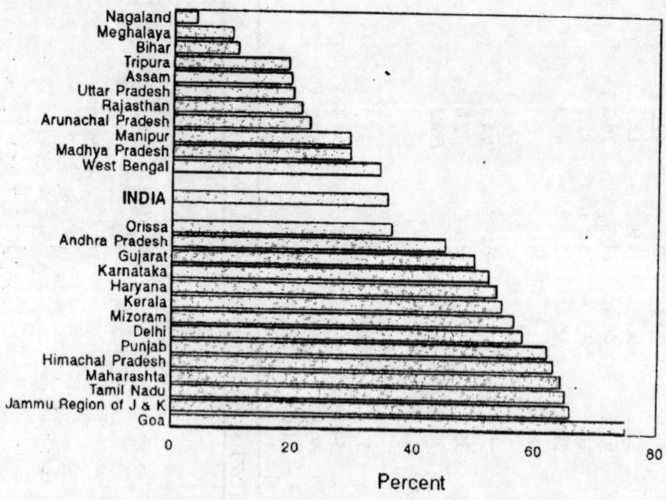

Figure 9.5: Percentage of Children Age 12-23 Months who have Received all VAccinations by State

vaccination coverage over time. The method of estimating vaccination coverage is the same as that used in Table 9.10. Among children without a vaccination card the proportion vaccinated during the first year of life is estimated separately for children in each age group. The row "No vaccinations" indicates the percentage of children who have not received any vaccination by 12 months of age. In all cases, the percentage of children whose vaccination status was determined by seeing a vaccination card declines with age of the child. This may be a reflection of the increased use of vaccination cards in recent years as well as the increased overall coverage of vaccinations. In addition, in many cases the vaccination cards of older children are discarded once they have completed their vaccinations or the cards are lost.

The highest level of vaccination coverage for each vaccination except polio 0 is observed at age 12-23 months. The coverage then progressively declines with an increase in age in both urban and rural areas. The degree of progress has been substantial over this short period of time, but progress must be further accelerated if India's immunization goal is to be achieved in the near future.

Child Morbidity and Treatment Patterns

Because the two major causes of death among infants and children in India are acute respiratory infection and diarrhoea (Central Bureau of Health Intelligence, 1991), the NFHS collected information on the occurrence of the symptoms of these diseases. Information was also collected on recent episodes of fever. Acute respiratory tract infection (ARI), primarily pneumonia, is a common cause of illness and death in infancy and childhood. Early diagnosis and treatment with antibiotics can prevent a large proportion of these deaths. Fever is a major manifestation of malaria, although it also accompanies various other illnesses. The prevention of diarrhoea and its treatment with oral rehydration therapy are also necessary to improve the chances of survival of children and their quality of life. The goals of the National Child Survival and Safe Motherhood Programme are to prevent 70 per cent of deaths due to diarrhoea and 25 per cent of diarrhoea cases by 2000 and to prevent 40 per cent of ARI deaths by the same year (Ministry of Health and Family Welfare, 1992b).

In the NFHS the mothers of children born during the past four years were asked a series of questions on the incidence of cough, fever and diarrhoea during the last two weeks and the type of treatment given to the child. Table 9.14 shows the per centage of children with cough accompanied by rapid breathing (symptoms of acute respiratory infection), fever and diarrhoea during the two weeks prior to the survey and the percentage with diarrhoea in the 24 hours before the survey by selected background characteristics. Fever was the most common of the three conditions examined, with 20 per cent of children suffering from this problem during the two weeks prior to the survey. Children age 6-23 months were somewhat more prone to fever than were other children. Male children, Muslim and Christian children and children residing in rural areas also have slightly higher prevalence rates. Education generally makes little difference for the prevalence of fever.

Seven per cent of children suffered from the symptoms of ARI during the two weeks preceding the survey. The highest prevalence occurs among children age 6-11 months (8 per cent). Small differences are observed according to the gender and birth order of the child, residence and educational level of the mother. Sikh and Jain children are least likely to have suffered from ARI during the two weeks preceding the survey.

Table 9.14 also provides two types of prevalence estimates for diarrhoea: (1) a period prevalence measure, namely the percentage of children under age four whose mothers reported that they had diarrhoea in the two-week period before the interview and (2) a point prevalence measure, namely the percentage of children under four years of age whose mothers reported that they had diarrhoea in the 24-hour period before the interview. Both of these measures are affected by the reliability of the mother's recall of when the diarrhoeal episode occurred. In addition, the NFHS questions allow estimation of the proportion of children under four years who had bloody diarrhoea, a symptom of dysentery, during the two weeks preceding the survey.

Table 9.13: Vaccinations in the first year of life by current age

Among Children one to three years of age, the percentage with a vaccination card which was shown to the interviewer and the percentage who have received each vaccine during the first year of life, according to the current age of the child and residence, India, 1992-93

Vaccination status	Current age of child in months			
	12-23	24-35	36-47	Total
	URBAN			
Vaccination card shown to interviewer	37.8	27.4	17.7	27.7
Per cent vaccinated at 0-11 months				
BCG	74.8	70.2	68.2	71.1
Polio 0	7.8	9.5	7.2	8.1
DPT				
1	77.3	73.6	67.6	72.8
2	72.1	68.8	63.5	68.1
3	64.2	61.4	57.4	61.0
Polio				
1	78.0	73.9	68.6	73.5
2	73.0	70.7	65.7	69.8
3	65.8	63.0	60.5	63.1
Measles	46.3	43.7	39.4	43.1
All vaccinations[2]	41.5	37.0	33.2	37.2
No vaccinations	19.5	23.3	28.8	23.9
Number of children	2715	2531	2704	7949
	RURAL			
Vaccination card shown to interviewer	28.5	19.8	11.7	20.2
Per cent vaccinated at 0-11 months[1]				
BCG	54.0	46.9	36.6	46.0

{Cont.}.........				
Polio 0	3.6	3.9	3.6	3.7
DPT				
1	58.0	49.9	39.1	49.2
2	50.3	44.6	34.2	43.1
3	41.8	37.3	29.3	36.2
Polio				
1	58.8	50.6	40.2	50.0
2	52.1	46.1	35.9	44.8
3	43.2	38.8	30.3	37.5
Measles	28.7	24.7	19.2	24.3
All vaccinations[2]	23.4	20.3	15.4	19.8
No vaccinations	38.0	46.4	56.9	46.9
Number of children	9138	8116	8639	25892
		TOTAL		
Vaccination card shown to interviewer	30.6	21.6	13.2	21.9
Per cent vaccinated at 0-11 months[1]				
BCG	58.7	52.4	44.0	51.8
Polio 0	4.6	5.2	4.4	4.7
DPT				
1	62.4	55.6	46.1	54.8
2	55.3	50.4	41.3	49.0
3	46 9	43.0	36.1	42.1
Polio				
1	63.2	56.3	47.1	55.6
2	56.9	52.0	43.1	50.8
3	48.3	44.6	37.6	43.6
Measles	32.7	29.3	24.1	28.7
All vaccinations[2]	27.5	24.2	19.5	23.8
No vaccinations	33.7	40.8	50.0	41.4
Number of children	11853	10646	11342	33841

1 Information was obtained either from the vaccination card or from the mother if there was no written record. For children whose information was based on the mother's report, the proportion of vaccinations given during the first year of life was assumed to be the same as for children with a written record of vaccinations.

2 Children who have received BCG, measles and three doses of DPT and polio vaccines (excluding polio 0).

Table 9.14: Prevalence of acute respiratory infection, fever and diarrhoea

Among all children under four years of age, the percentage who were ill with a cough accompanied by fast breathing, fever and diarrhoea during the two weeks before the survey, and the percentage with diarrhoea in the 24 hours before the survey, according to selected background characteristics, India, 1992-93

Background characteristic	Percentage of children suffering in previous two weeks from:				Any diarrhoea in previous 24 hours[2]	Number of children
	Cough accompanied by fast breathing	Fever	Diarrhoea[1] Any[2]	Diarrhoea[1] Bloody		
Child's age						
<6 months	5.6	15.1	10.9	0.6	7.0	5641
6-11 months	8.4	25.9	16.3	1.1	8.6	5881
12-23 months	7.7	25.0	12.8	1.6	5.6	11853
24-35 months	6.0	18.7	8.4	1.6	3.5	10646
36-47 months	5.1	16.3	5.1	1.1	2.1	11342
Sex						
Male	7.1	21.1	10.3	1.4	5.0	23170
Female	5.9	19.4	9.8	1.2	4.6	22193
Birth order						
1	6.3	20.6	10.2	1.1	4.9	12369
2-3	6.5	19.7	9.7	1.2	4.7	19030
4-5	6.6	20.7	10.5	1.4	5.1	8756
6+	6.8	20.6	10.0	1.7	4.6	5208
Residence						
Urban	5.1	18.7	8.8	0.9	4.0	10611

Rural	6.9	20.7	10.4	1.4	5.0	34752
Mother's education						
Illiterate	6.5	19.9	10.3	1.5	4.9	29631
Lit., < middle complete	7.7	23.2	10.4	1.2	5.0	7680
Middle school complete	5.9	20.5	9.6	0.7	4.6	3328
High school and above	4.6	17.4	8.3	0.7	3.9	4724
Religion						
Hindu	6.4	19.4	10.3	1.3	4.9	35937
Muslim	7.3	24.0	8.9	1.3	4.3	7029
Christian	7.7	23.6	8.6	1.1	4.3	928
Sikh	3.8	20.9	10.1	1.2	3.9	784
Jain	1.2	9.5	5.0	—	0.4	140
Buddhist	6.5	22.7	13.2	1.9	8.4	326
Other	6.1	22.4	11.8	0.3	5.2	219
Caste/tribe						
Scheduled caste	6.8	19.0	11.4	1.8	5.5	5983
Scheduled tribe	6.1	20.2	9.9	1.7	4.7	4310
Other	6.5	20.4	9.8	1.1	4.7	35071
Source of drinking water						
Piped water	U	U	9.6	1.0	4.8	13079
Ground water	U	U	9.8	1.3	4.6	17442
Well water	U	U	10.3	1.5	5.0	12180
Surface water	U	U	12.9	1.5	5.9	1759
Other	U	U	11.2	1.7	4.0	905
Total	6.5	20.2	10.0	1.3	4.8	45363

Note: Table is based on children born in the period 1-47 months prior to the survey. U: Not available. --Less than 0.05 per cent.

1. Includes diarrhoea in the past 24 hours. 2. Includes diarrhoea with blood

Before initiating the discussion on the incidence of diarrhoea during the two weeks preceding the survey, it should be noted that the NFHS was not undertaken synchronously (at one point of time) in all states in India and, hence, the calendar dates of the reference period (whether the past 24 hours or the past two weeks) for the assessment of the prevalence of diarrhoea vary from state to state. Since there is seasonal variation in the incidence of diarrhoea, the prevalence rates of diarrhoea for any state cannot be assumed to reflect the situation throughout the year in that state. However, the data collection was conducted in three phases throughout the year, and hence the prevalence rate for total India may be taken as more representative of the situation throughout the year.

During the two weeks before the survey, 10 per cent of children suffered from any type of diarrhoea and less than 2 per cent from bloody diarrhoea. Five per cent of children had diarrhoea during the preceding 24 hours. The incidence of diarrhoea was the highest among children age 6-11 months after which it declines with increasing age. There is little difference in the prevalence of diarrhoea between male and female children and between urban and rural children. The prevalence of diarrhoea is slightly lower among children whose mothers completed high school (8 per cent) than among those with less education (10 per cent). The prevalence of diarrhoea is highest among Buddhist children (13 per cent).

Surprisingly, the source of drinking water makes only a small difference in the prevalence of diarrhoea. As one would expect, the prevalence is highest among those using surface water (13 per cent). There is little difference in the prevalence of diarrhoea among those obtaining drinking water from other sources. In fact, the prevalence of all three conditions varies very little except by the age of the child. These childhood diseases are almost equally likely to strike children in any of the groups examined.

Table 9.15 presents information on the incidence of acute respiratory infection, fever and diarrhoea by state.. There is a considerable variation with respect to the incidence rate of all three illnesses among children. The difference among states may reflect differences in the prevalence of these conditions as well as differences in the timing of fieldwork in each state. The reported prevalence levels may also reflect differences in the way mothers in various states perceive diseases among their children. The highest prevalence rate for ARI is in Tripura (23 per cent) and the lowest is in Punjab and Karnataka (3 per cent each). The prevalence of fever is again highest in Tripura (36 per cent) followed by Kerala (35 per cent), Orissa (32 per cent) and West Bengal (29 per cent). Relatively low prevalence rates for fever are observed in Delhi and Rajasthan (11 per cent each). The prevalence of diarrhoea with blood during the two weeks prior to the survey is low in all states, however Mizoram, Jammu and Himachal Pradesh (all small states) experienced relatively high prevalence rates (3 to 5 per cent). A little more than 1 in 10 children experienced diarrhoea during the 24 hours before the survey in Mizoram (13 per cent) and Arunachal Pradesh (11 per cent). In addition to these two states, diarrhoea during the two weeks prior to the survey was relatively common in Jammu, Himachal Pradesh and Orissa. In each state, fever is the most prevalent of the three conditions examined, except for Jammu where the prevalence rates for fever and diarrhoea are almost the same.

Treatment of Acute Respiratory Infection (ARI)

Table 9.16 presents information on the type of treatment received by children suffering from symptoms of ARI by selected background characteristics. A sizeable majority of children (two-thirds) who suffered from ARI during the past two weeks were taken to a health facility for treatment or were treated by a doctor or other health professional. A little less than one-fifth did not receive any treatment. Sick children were most often treated with oral antibiotics, injections or cough syrups. Home remedies or herbal medicines were used for only 7 per cent of the children. One-third of children received other types of treatment, which include nonantibiotic oral medicine or oral medicine which the respondent could not identify.

Children age less than 6 months or more than 23 months are slightly less likely to receive treatment for ARI from health professionals (60-64 per cent) than children age 6 to 23 months (70 per cent). The percentage of children taken for treatment to health professionals is much higher for boys (71 per cent) than for girls (61 per cent). Twenty-two per cent of girls and 17 per cent of boys did not receive any treatment. Thus, with respect to the provision and use of health care facilities for children suffering from ARI, discrimination against girls is observed. T his finding is consistent with the results of previous studies, which have demonstrated that sons are often treated preferentially in receiving medical care (Jejeebhoy, 1991; Deolalikar and Vashishta, 1992; Miller, 1981). There is a negative relationship between birth order and the treatment received from a health professional. Three-quarters of first-born children suffering from ARI were taken to a health facility or treated by a doctor or a health professional, whereas only 56 per cent of sixth or higher birth order children received treatment from a health professional.

Table 9.15: Prevalence of acute respiratory infection, fever and diarrhoea by state
Among all children under four years of age, the percentage who were ill with a cough accompanied by fast breathing, fever and diarrhoea during the two weeks before the survey, and the percentage with diarrhoea in the 24 hours before the survey, according to state, India, 1992-93

	Percentage of children suffering in previous two weeks from:				
State	Cough accompanied by fast breathing	Fever	Diarrhoea[1] Any[2]	Diarrhoea[1] Bloody	Any diarrhoea in previous 24 hours[2]
India	6.5	20.2	10.0	1.3	4.8
North					
Delhi	4.8	11.4	9.8	0.6	4.5
Haryana	5.4	18.6	12.0	0.9	5.9
Himachal Pradesh	6.4	19.9	19.6	3.2	7.7
Jammu Region of J & K	4.4	21.6	22.3	3.3	9.2
Punjab	3.1	19.9	11.0	1.1	4.4
Rajasthan	4.9,	10.7	5.7	0.7	3.7
Central					
Madhya Pradesh	4.7	15.8	8.6	1.2	3.9
Uttar Pradesh	7.2	19.1	8.9	1.5	4.6
East					
Bihar	4.3	21.1	13.7	1.4	6.3
Orissa	10.4	32.1	21.4	2.7	9.3
West Bengal	110.2	29.4	2.5	0.3	0.4
Northeast					
Arunachal Pradesh	8.7	20.1	17.6	2.0	10.5
Assam	11.3	24.6	6.3	1.3	2.4
Manipur	14.5	25.3	12.4	1.7	7.6
Meghalaya	5.9	15.8	8.3	0.5	5.9
Mizoram	4.1	26.6	22.3	5.0	12.5
Nagaland	6.1	15.9	11.2	2.4	3.6
Tripura	22.8	35.5	3.6	0.6	1.2
West					
Goa	5.6	21.4	7.8	0.8	2.3
Gujarat	5.8	18.5	12.6	1.5	6.5
Maharashtra	5.9	21.7	9.7	1.0	5.1
South					
Andhra Pradesh	4.9	16.5	11.7	1.2	6.0
Karnataka	3.4	16.9	9.7	1.2	5.1
Kerala	9.7	35.4	9.2	1.5	3.4
Tamil Nadu	8.6	17.7	12.7	1.3	5.2

Note: Table is based on children born in the period 1-47 months prior to the survey.

1. Includes diarrhoea in the past 24 hours. 2. Includes diarrhoea with blood.

As expected, sick children in urban areas were more likely to receive treatment from health professionals than those in rural areas. A higher percentage of rural children (8 per cent) than urban children (3 per cent) received home remedies when suffering from ARI. The relationship between a mother's educational level and the treatment given to children by health professionals is consistently positive, with 62 per cent of children of illiterate mothers receiving treatment from health professionals as against 85 per cent of mothers with at least a high school education. Not much difference is observed between the children of Hindu mothers (66 per cent) and Muslim mothers (67 per cent). The children of scheduled tribe mothers are least likely to receive any treatment for ARI.

Treatment of Fever

Table 9.17 presents treatment patterns for children suffering from fever during the two weeks before the survey. A sizeable majority of children (67 per cent) suffering from fever were taken to a health facility or received treatment from a doctor or other health professional. Eight per cent of children were given antimalarial medication, 34 per cent were treated with oral antibiotics, 22 per cent were given injections and 5 per cent were treated with home remedies. The patterns of differentials in the treatment of fever are very similar to those observed earlier for the treatment of ARI. Children age 6-23 months, male children, children of lower birth orders, children from urban areas, children of educated mothers, children of Sikh and Buddhist mothers, and children of non-SC/ST mothers are more likely than other children to receive treatment from health professionals.

Treatment of Diarrhoea

Deaths from acute diarrhoea are most often due to the dehydration that results from the loss of water and electrolytes (Black, 1984). For this reason, nearly all diarrhoeal deaths can be prevented by prompt administration of rehydration solutions. Because deaths due to diarrhoea are a significant proportion of deaths to children in India, the government has launched the Oral Rehydration Therapy Programme as one of its priority activities for child survival. A major purpose of this programme is to increase awareness among women and in the community about the causes and treatment of diarrhoea. Mothers are instructed how to manage diarrhoea by using Oral Rehydration Salt (ORS) packets, which are made widely available. The programme also promotes use of a home made solution made from sugar, salt and water, which is referred to here as a Recommended Home Solution (RHS). This instruction is provided

Table 9.16: Treatment of acute respiratory infection

Among all children under four years of age who had a cough accompanied by fast breathing during the two weeks before the survey, the percentage taken to a health facility or provider and the type of treatment given according to selected background characteristics, India. 1992-93

	Among children with cough and fast breathing								
		Percentage treated with							
Background characteristic	Percentage taken to a health facility or providers[1]	Anti-biotic pill or syrup	Injec-tion	Cough syrup	Home remedy/ herbal medicine	Other	None	Don't know/ missing	Number of Children
Child's age									
<6 months	60.2	32.1	22.9	19.1	10.4	30.5	17.5	—	313
6-11 months	69.6	34.4	24.8	23.6	7.7	31.2	19.3	—	495
12-23 months	70.4	35.3	23.6	21.1	7.0	32.7	17.0	0.2	911
24-35 months	64.1	31.6	23.1	22.1	6.0	34.0	20.7	0.4	640
36-47 months	62.9	32.0	21.2	24.0	6.1	34.5	22.0	0.4	583
Sex									
Male	70.8	34.2	24.8	22.6	6.8	33.8	17.0	0.2	1636
Female	60.8	32.3	21.1	21.4	7.5	31.7	22.0	0.3	1307
Birth order									
1	74.6	36.4	26.3	25.1	5.4	30.3	17.1	0.6	778
2-3	64.5	34.0	21.3	21.7	7.6	33.2	18.8	0.1	1238
4-5	65.6	29.8	22.3	22.8	6.4	35.9	20.9	—	574
6+	56.0	30.4	24.0	15.8	10.2	32.4	22.7	—	352

Residence									
Urban	77.1	37.4	23.1	29.1	3.4	35.5	13.9	—	544
Rural	63.9	32.5	23.1	20.5	7.9	32.3	20.4	0.3	2399
Mother's education									
Illiterate	62.4	32.2	24.5	18.9	7.6	31.5	22.1	0.2	1937
Lit., < middle complete	70.4	31.5	19.8	26.1	7.3	37.7	16.1	0.5	592
Middle school complete	72.0	38.2	23.1	23.7	3.1	34.9	14.4	—	196
High school and above	84.9	44.2	20.1	38.5	5.2	30.1	6.5	—	218
Religion									
Hindu	65.8	34.0	24.8	20.0	7.0	33.2	18.9	0.2	2296
Muslim	66.7	32.3	17.5	26.9	7.9	31.8	20.0	0.5	510
Christian	70.8	28.5	16.8	42.4	5.9	20.8	25.7	—	71
Sikh	(82.8)	(12.2)	(27.4)	(34.0)	(7.1)	(59.7)	(6.1)	(—)	30
Other	(64.3)	(16.7)	(4.4)	(51.4)	(—)	(28.9)	(27.5)	(—)	13
Caste/tribe									
Scheduled caste	64.0	29.7	26.1	15.7	8.1	36.6	22.1	—	410
Scheduled tribe	59.1	27.3	25.1	16.0	6.4	34.1	24.8	0.2	265
Other	67.6	34.7	22.4	23.9	7.0	32.1	18.0	0.3	2269
Total	66.3	33.4	23.1	22.1	7.1	32.9	19.2	0.2	2943

Note: Table is based on children born 1-47 months prior to the survey. Total includes 2 Jain children and 21 Buddhist Children who are not shown separately.

() Based on 25-49 unweighted cases.

— Less than 0.05 per cent .

1. Includes government/municipal hospital, private hospital/clinic, Primary Health Centre, sub-centre, doctor or other health professional.

Table 9.17: Treatment of fever

Among all children under four years of age suffering from fever during the two weeks before the survey, the percentage taken to a health facility or provider and the type of treatment given, according to selected background characteristics, India, 1992-93

	Among children with fever								
		Percentage treated with							
Background characteristic	Percentage taken to a health facility or provider[1]	Anti-malarial	Antibiotic pill or syrup	Injection	Home remedy/ herbal medicine	Other	None	Don't know/ missing	Number of children
Child's age									
<6 months	60.4	6.6	30.7	17.7	6.7	35.7	25.0	0.7	854
6-11 months	68.6	7.3	35.2	21.7	7.5	39.3	18.1	0.4	1521
12-23 months	69.4	8.6	36.2	23.1	4.8	39.4	17.8	0.5	2967
24-35 months	66.5	8.9	32.5	24.4	4.0	39.6	19.9	0.7	1988
36-47 months	64.5	8.1	34.8	21.6	5.4	36.8	21.9	0.6	1849
Sex									
Male	70.1	8.4	36.1	23.5	5.0	39.5	17.8	0.4	4881
Female	63.1	7.9	32.6	21.1	5.7	37.4	22.0	0.7	4298
Birth order									
1	72.8	8.2	34.8	22.0	5.2	42.8	15.9	0.5	2543
2-3	66.8	8.2	34.8	22.0	4.8	39.5	19.2	0.6	3752
4-5	62.9	8.7	32.9	23.1	5.3	35.0	23.2	0.7	1813
6+	59.3	7.0	34.8	23.0	7.9	31.0	25.4	0.5	1071

Residence									
Urban	79.4	9.0	35.8	20.3	4.0	49.4	10.0	0.6	1986
Rural	63.4	7.9	34.1	22.9	5.7	35.6	22.5	0.6	7193
Mother's education									
Illiterate	62.9	7.9	34.6	24.2	5.5	34.3	23.8	0.5	5890
Lit., < middle complete	69.9	8.2	30.1	19.4	6.6	44.5	16.3	1.0	1784
Middle school complete	78.8	9.1	39.3	22.1	2.7	45.8	9.4	0.3	681
High school and above	78.4	9.5	38.7	15.3	4.1	50.0	7.6	0.5	824
Religion									
Hindu	66.7	7.9	35.6	24.0	5.4	37.0	20.0	0.7	6971
Muslim	65.8	9.4	31.7	17.1	5.9	39.3	21.2	0.3	1688
Christian	63.9	6.8	31.1	13.2	4.2	53.7	17.3	0.1	219
Sikh	87.3	12.0	15.5	25.2	3.5	67.0	6.1	—	164
Buddhist	74.9	—	39.0	17.2	—	57.1	16.3	—	75
Other	56.0	12.9	30.1	13.0	6.6	44.6	15.2	—	49
Caste/tribe									
Scheduled caste	67.7	7.8	35.0	27.0	5.7	36.2	20.5	0.8	1139
Scheduled tribe	55.0	6.4	31.2	21.2	5.6	31.8	27.2	0.9	871
Other	68.2	8.4	34.8	21.8	5.3	39.7	18.8	0.5	7169
Total	66.8	8.2	34.4	22.3	5.4	38.5	19.8	0.6	9179

Note: Table is based on children born 1-47 months prior to the survey. Total includes 13 Jain children, who are not shown separately.

— Less than 0.05 per cent.

1 Includes government/municipal hospital, private hospital/clinic, Primary Health Centre, sub-centre, doctor, or other health professional.

mostly through the electronic and print media and in adult literacy classes. Documentaries on diarrhoea among children and the use of ORS and preparation of RHS are regularly shown in cinema theatres. Spot announcements are also shown on Doordarshan, and All India Radio frequently airs messages on ORS and RHS. All the messages are in languages used in the states, with appropriate local terms for ORS and RHS.

In order to gauge the extent of knowledge and use of oral rehydration, the NFHS asked mothers of children born during the last four years a series of questions regarding the knowledge and use of ORS and RHS. Table 9.18 shows that only 43 per cent of mothers in India know about ORS and an even smaller per cent (26 per cent) have used ORS packets at some time in the past. The differentials by selected background characteristics of mothers are quite pronounced. As expected, both knowledge and use of ORS are higher among urban than among rural mothers. Levels of knowledge and use of ORS are also strongly positively related to the educational attainment of mothers and to their exposure to mass media. Both knowledge and use of ORS are higher among mothers exposed to electronic mass media than among those with no such exposure. However, without conducting a multivariate analysis, it is difficult to say whether the differences in ORS knowledge and use are due to media exposure or due to the underlying correlation between women's educational levels and media exposure.

Marked differences are observed across the states in the knowledge and ever use of ORS packets (Table 9.19). Manipur has the highest proportion of mothers knowing about and ever using ORS packets (86 and 60 per cent, respectively). Nagaland, a neighbouring state in the northeast region is at the opposite end of the spectrum with the lowest proportion of mothers knowing about and ever using ORS packets. Among the major states, the highest level of knowledge of ORS is in Delhi (74 per cent) and the lowest in Rajasthan (20 per cent). With respect to ever use of ORS packets, the highest level is observed for West Bengal (50 per cent) and the lowest again is for Rajasthan (8 per cent). In addition to Rajasthan, knowledge and use of ORS are particularly low in Madhya Pradesh and Andhra Pradesh.

Table 9.20 shows the type of treatment obtained for children who had diarrhoea during the two weeks before the survey. Sixty-one per cent of children who suffered from diarrhoea were taken to a health facility or provider. Eighteen per cent were treated with ORS packets and 19 per cent received a Recommended Home Solution with a total of 31 per cent receiving at least one of these treatments. In order to reduce dehydration due to diarrhoea, mothers are also taught to increase the

Table 9.18: Knowledge and ever use of ORS packets
Percentage of mothers with births during the four years preceding the survey who know about and have ever used ORS packets, according to selected background characteristics, India, 1992-93

Background characteristic	Know about ORS packets	Have ever used ORS packets	Number of mothers
Mother's age			
13-19	36.1	20.6	4276
20-24	44.2	25.5	13342
25-29	46.3	29.1	11183
30-34	42.1	26.7	5839
35+	34.3	22.0	3521
Residence			
Urban	55.6	32.5	8727
Rural	38.9	23.9	29434
Mother's education			
Illiterate	31.8	19.0	25062
Literate, < middle school complete	56.4	36.0	6324
Middle school complete	62.7	36.8	2717
High school and above	75.4	45.0	4059
Religion			
Hindu	41.4	24.7	30560
Muslim	46.5	30.9	5634
Christian	52.6	28.5	780
Sikh	52.9	29.6	613
Jain	64.4	31.3	115
Buddhist	52.0	30.6	2n
Other	40.9	25.9	188
Caste/tribe			
Scheduled caste	35.3	21.0	5050
Scheduled tribe	26.8	14.7	3646
Other	45.9	28.1	29465
Mother's exposure to media			
Exposed to media	55.3	32.8	18126
Watches television weekly	62.2	36.0	10185
Listens to radio weekly	55.9	33.2	14899
Visits cinema/theatre monthly	56.3	32.2	5248
Not exposed to any of the media	31.2	19.5	20036
Total	42.7	25.9	38162

Table 9.19: Knowledge and ever use of ORS packets bv state
Percentage of mothers with births during the four years preceding the survey who know about and have ever used ORS packets, according to state, India, 1992-93

State	Know about ORS packets	Have ever used ORS packets
India	42.7	25.9
North		
Delhi	74.2	45.3
Haryana	52.8	28.4
Himachal Pradesh	69.3	46.8
Jammu Region of J & K	66.3	43.9
Punjab	51.7	28.5
Rajasthan	20.2	8.3
Central		
Madhya Pradesh	24.3	9.6
Uttar Pradesh	36.4	21.4
East		
Bihar	36.3	24.3
Orissa	43.7	28.8
West Bengal	64.3	50.1
Northeast		
Arunachal Pradesh	43.8	27.7
Assam	53.2	32.1
Manipur	85.5	60.1
Meghalaya	39.5	19.8
Mizoram	74.5	39.0
Nagaland	20.1	6.1
Tripura	79.5	5'-3
West		
Goa	55.1	3'1.9
Gujarat	41.2	22.7
Maharashtra	46.7	30.9
South		
Andhra Pradesh	31.1	16.3
Karnataka	49.3	31.0
Kerala	71.3	39.8
Tamit Nadu	61.4	32.0

supply of fluids to children with diarrhoea. An increase in the supply of fluids was reported for only 14 per cent of children. Sixty-one per cent of children with diarrhoea received neither ORS/RHS treatment nor increased fluids. Thus, although many Indian mothers have gotten the message that young children with diarrhoea must be treated with oral rehydration therapy, many others remain unaware of the importance of this treatment. The findings suggest that more efforts are needed to increase the understanding of parents regarding the treatment of diarrhoea.

Differentials in the treatment of diarrhoea depend in part on the type of treatment examined. Treatment at a health facility or from a health provider is more commonly sought for children age 12-23 months, male children, children of lower order births, children in urban areas, children of more educated mothers, and children of Sikh and Muslim women. While girls with diarrhoea are less likely than boys to receive ORS packets, no such distinction is observed in the provision of RHS. A consistent positive relationship is observed between the educational level of mothers and treatment with ORS or RHS. Children in urban areas are more likely to be taken to a health facility or provider, but they are also more likely to be treated with a Recommended Home Solution or other home remedy.

It is inappropriate to reduce a child's frequency of breastfeeding or the total intake of breast milk or other fluids when a child has diarrhoea. In the NFHS, the mothers of children who suffered from diarrhoea were asked about changes in feeding practices for those children during diarrhoea. Table 9.21 provides information on feeding practices during diarrhoea for children of different ages. For a large majority of children (85 per cent), the frequency of breastfeeding remained the same or increased during the diarrhoea. In 12 per cent of the cases, however, breastfeeding was actually reduced. Moreover, intake of fluids, although maintained as usual or increased in three-quarters of the cases, was actually reduced in one-fifth of the cases. Thus, contrary to medical recommendations with regard to fluid intake during diarrhoea, a substantial number of children in India have their fluid intake reduced when they are sick with diarrhoea.

Table 9.22 summarizes the treatment patterns for cough accompanied by fast breathing, fever and diarrhoea for each state. The utilization of health services for all three conditions is generally best in the northern region (with the notable exception of Rajasthan), in the western region, and in Kerala and Karnataka. On the other hand, only about half of sick children in Rajasthan and Orissa are taken to a health facility or health provider. The use of oral rehydration therapy for children with diarrhoea is quite limited, particularly in Haryana, Gujarat, Rajasthan, Uttar Pradesh and Bihar where more than three-quarters of children who had diarrhoea were not given either ORS or RHS. Even in states where at least 70 per cent of children are taken to a health facility

Table 9.20: Treatment of diarrhoea

Among all children under four years of age who had diarrhoea in the past two weeks, the percentage taken for treatment to a health facility or provider, and the type of treatment given, according to selected background characteristics, India, 1992-43

Background characteristics	Per cent taken to a health facility or provider[1]	Oral Rehydration: Per cent given			Increased fluids	Per cent not given ORS, RHS or increased fluids	Per cent given				Number of children with diarrhoea
		ORS packets	RHS at home	Either ORS or RHS			Antibiotics	Injection	Home remedy, other	No treatment	
Child's age											
<6 months	54.4	8.6	11.0	17.0	13.7	73.0	25.8	8.6	38.0	28.1	612
6-11 months	61.7	18.9	19.7	32.7	11.8	60.4	32.4	14.9	40.7	19.3	95 8
12-23 months	65.0	20.9	20.0	34.6	15.2	57.3	32.7	17.1	45.2	16.0	1516
24-35 months	61.8	17.7	19.2	30.3	14.6	60.5	32.4	14.8	41.3	18.8	889
36-47 months	56.7	15.6	20.4	31.3	12.4	60.9	31.3	12.0	37.0	19.4	583
Sex											
Male	63.0	19.6	18.8	32.4	13.4	59.9	32.1	15.1	42.2	17.8	2386
Female	59.2	15.3	18.5	28.5	14.3	62.5	30.7	13.7	40.8	21.0	2773
Birth order											
1	64.3	19.4	17.2	31.5	14.0	60.4	32.0	15.0	43.2	18.4	1267
2-3	61.4	17.8	20.7	32.4	13.2	60.1	29.3	14.9	43.5	18.9	1854
4-5	58.6	17.7	19.5	31.0	16.1	58.5	32.8	12.9	38.0	19.4	915
6+	57.7	11.7	13.3	21.3	11.5	71.7	35.5	14.0	36.4	22.6	522
Residence											
Urban	68.7	16.9	26.4	36.8	14.4	56.5	31.9	12.2	47.5	14.2	932

Rural	59.3	17.7	16.6	29.0	13.6	62.4	31.4	15.0	40.0	20.6	3626
Mother's education											
Illiterate	58.0	15.4	14.8	25.7	13.3	65.6	31.2	14.7	38.0	22.8	3044
Lit., middle complete	66.0	20.9	22.4	36.7	12.8	55.9	28.7	13.7	47.4	15.2	799
Middle school complete	67.5	21.0	26.3	39.9	12.6	56.2	34.5	14.4	45.9	12.8	321
High school and above	70.9	24.3	34.2	48.6	21.0	41.6	36.7	13.3	52.8	6.1	394
Religion											
Hindu	60.3	17.5	17.7	29.8	13.9	61.8	31.7	15.2	40.3	20.1	3695
Muslim	66.0	16.2	22.8	32.6	13.0	59.1	33.0	12.2	44.4	16.1	629
Christian	50.3	19.9	19.5	30.0	14.9	62.3	31.9	4.4	35.2	18.6	80
Sikh	86.9	20.9	19.0	36.2	16.6	53.9	16.0	11.8	77.5	4.7	79
Buddhist	(51.0)	(21.9)	(29.8)	(46.8)	(14.6)	(48.2)	(14.3)	(9.5)	(53.4)	(33.9)	43
Other	55.7	32.5	7.3	33.7	3.3	63.8	39.6	2.7	36.0	10.8	26
Caste/tribe											
Scheduled caste	61.2	14.9	17.5	27.7	13.2	63.3	30.5	15.3	42.8	20.8	684
Scheduled tribe	51.5	20.7	16.6	30.8	12.1	62.2	24.9	12.5	36.5	28.1	426
Other	62.4	17.7	19.1	31.1	14.1	60.6	32.5	14.5	41.8	17.9	3448
Total	61.2	17.5	18.6	30.6	13.8	61.2	31.5	14.4	41.5	19.3	4558

Note: Table is based on children born in the period 1-47 months prior to the survey. Total includes 7 Jain children, who are not shown separately.

ORS: An oral rehydration solution made from a packet.

RHS: A recommended home solution of sugar, salt and water.

( ) Based on 25-49 unweighted cases.

1 Includes government/municipal hospital, private hospital/clinic, Primary Health Centre, sub-centre, doctor, or other health professional.

or provider for the treatment of diarrhoea (with the exception of West Bengal), the use of oral rehydration therapy is limited (between 33 and 45 per cent). Thus, increased efforts are necessary to promote the use of oral rehydration therapy for children who are sick with diarrhoea.

NOTES

They have received BCG, measles, and three doses of DPT and polio (excluding polio 0). Polio O was introduced only recently and because it is a vaccination given at the time of birth (whereas polio 1 is typically given at the age of six weeks), mothers may not remember whether the first dose of the polio vaccine was given just after birth or later. Therefore, the coverage of polio O reported in the NFHS may be subject to response errors.

Table 9.21: Feeding oractices during diarrhoea

Per cent distribution of children urder four years of age who had diarrhoea in the past two weeks, according to feeding practices during diarrhoea and age, India, 1992-93

	Age of the child		
Feeding practices during diarrhoea	<1 year[1]	1-3 years	Total[2]
Breastfeeding frequency[3]			
Same as usual	81.8	75.2	77.9
Increased	6.5	7.8	7.3
Reduced	9.8	14.0	12.3
Stopped	1.1	2.1	1.7
Don't know/missing	0.8	0.9	0.9
Total per cent	100.0	100.0	100.0
Number of children	1486	2200	3686
Amount of fluids given			
Same as usual	71.7	62.6	65.8
More	7.5	10.8	9.7
Less	15.1	21.9	19.6
Don't know	5.6	4.6	5.0
Total per cent	100.0	100.0	100.0
Number of children with diarrhoea	1570	2989	4558

1 Children born in the period 1-11 months prior to the survey.
2 Children born in the period 1-47 months prior to the survey.
3 Applies only to children who are still breastfed.

Table 9.22: Treatment of childhood diseases be state

Among all children under four years of age who were ill with a cough accompanied by fast breathing, fever and diarrhoea during the two weeks before the survey, the percentage taken to a health facility or provider, and among children who had diarrhoea in the past two weeks, the percentage who received either an oral rehydration solution made from a packet (ORS) or a recommended home solution (RHS), according to state, India, 1992-93.

	Percentage taken to a health facility or providers among children who were ill with:			
State	Cough accompanied by fast breathing	Fever	Diarrhoea	Among children with, diarrhoea, percentage given either ORS or RHS
India	66.3	66.8	61.2	30.6
North				
Delhi	88.0	84.8	64.7	39.4
Haryana	83.2	86.1	65.5	19.5
Himachal Pradesh	77.7	81.7	70.6	44.9
Jammu Region of J & K	77.6	71.0	70.6	44.4
Punjab	(88.1)	91.5	86.0	32.7
Rajasthan	54.3	61.9	51.3	22.7
Central				
Madhya Pradesh	61.8	64.9	64.4	33.0
Uttar Pradesh	68.3	70.7	65.7	22.7
East				
Bihar	72.9	59.7	58.5	23.0
Orissa	56.4	52.7	47.0	41.1
West Bengal	61.7	59.4	82.1	74.7
Northeast				
Arunachal Pradesh	50.0	44.2	38.1	33.3
Assam	40.7	31.8	35.8	35.2
Manipur	39.5	34.6	40.0	63.1
Meshalaya	(86.8)	59.8	66.7	40.7
Mizoram	*	35.0	31.6	24.5
Nagaland	(31.6)	33.7	11.6	24.6
Tripura	59.6	55.4	*	*
Goa	82.3	86.1	70.1	41.4
Gujarat	73.3	76.0	62.6	20.7
Maharashtra	72.6	75.4	60.9	41.7
South				
Andhra Pradesh	68.7	69.8	62.5	32.5
Karnataka	74.0	76.6	64.6	34.0
Kerala	81.3	74.1	70.6	37.8
Tamil Nadu	67.4	73.1	54.8	27.1

Note: Table is based on children born 1-47 months prior to the survey.

( ) Based on 25-49 unweighted cases.

* Percentage not shown; based on fewer than 25 unweighted cases.

1 Includes government/municipal hospital, private hospital/clinic, Primary Health Centre, sub-centre, doctor, or other health professional.

10

INFANT FEEDING AND CHILD NUTRITION

Infant feeding practices and child nutrition have significant effects on child survival, maternal health and fertility. Breastfeeding improves the nutritional status of young children and reduces morbidity and mortality. Breast milk not only provides the child with important nutrients but also protects the child against infections. The timing and type of supplementary foods introduced in the infant's diet also have significant effects on the nutritional status of the child. The duration and intensity (i.e., frequency) of breastfeeding have additional effects on the duration of postpartum amenorrhoea, birth intervals, and fertility. This chapter discusses the information collected on infant feeding, including both breastfeeding and supplementary feeding. Also included is a discussion of the nutritional status of children under four years of age as measured by the height and weight of children.

10.1 BREASTFEEDING AND SUPPLEMENTATION

The Innocenti Declaration on the Protection, Promotion and Support of Breastfeeding (1990) and the WHO Working Group on Infant Feeding (World Health Organization, 1991b) have made several recommendations on the feeding of infants and young children. These international recommendations state that infants should be given only breast milk up to 4-6 months of age. Aside from breast milk, no other foods or liquids are needed during this period. At age 4-6 months, adequate and appropriate complementary foods should be added to the infant's diet in order to provide sufficient nutrients for optimal growth. It is recommended that breastfeeding should continue, along with complementary foods, up through the second year of life or beyond. It is further recommended that a feeding bottle with a nipple should not be used at any age, for reasons having to do mainly with sanitation and the prevention of infections. In addition, the Baby Friendly Hospitals Initiative, launched by WHO, recommends the early initiation of breastfeeding, immediately after childbirth.

Several indicators of breastfeeding practices have been suggested by WHO to guide countries in the gathering of information for measuring and evaluating infant feeding practices. These indicators include the ever breastfed rate, the exclusive breastfeeding rate, the timely complementary feeding rate, the continued breastfeeding rate, and the bottle feeding rate. The *exclusive breastfeeding rate* is defined as the proportion of infants under four months who receive only breast milk. The *timely complementary feeding rate* is the proportion of infants age 6-9 months who receive both breast milk and solid or semi-solid food. The *continued breastfeeding rate through one year of age* is the proportion of children age 12-15 months who are still being breastfed. The continued breastfeeding rate through two years of age is the proportion of children age 20-23 months who are still being breastfed. The *bottle feeding rate* is the proportion of infants who are fed using a bottle with a nipple. These indicators are highlighted in the presentation of the data on breastfeeding and other feeding practices in this chapter.

In the NFHS, information on breastfeeding and supplementation was obtained from a series of questions in Section 4 of the Woman's Questionnaire. These questions pertain to births in the year of the survey and in the preceding four calendar years. The tabulations, however, are based on each woman's births in the four years prior to her date of interview. For any given woman, a maximum of three births was included in the analysis.

Table 10.1 contains information on the percentage of children ever breastfed, the timing of the initiation of breastfeeding, and the practice of squeezing the first milk from the breast before beginning breastfeeding. The results are based on 50,001 children born in the four years preceding the survey. Breastfeeding is nearly universal in India, with 95 per cent of all children having been breastfed. This is not surprising since breast milk has traditionally been the main source of nutrition for infants and young children in India. The practice of breastfeeding is high in all population subgroups, ranging from 92 to 99 per cent.

The initiation of breastfeeding immediately after childbirth is important because it benefits both the mother and the infant. As soon as the infant starts suckling at the breast, the hormone oxytocin is released, resulting in uterine contractions that facilitate the expulsion of the placenta and reduce the risk of postpartum haemorrhage. Breast milk is

Table 10.1: Initiation of breastfeeding

Per centage of all children who were ever breastfed, the percentage of last-born children who started breastfeeding within one hour and one day of birth, and percentage of last-born breastfed elildren whose mothers squeezed the first milk from the breast among children born during the four years preceding the survey, according to selected background characteristics, India, 1992-93

	Among all children:		Among last-born children:				
Background characteristic	Percentage ever breastfed	Number of children	Per cent started breastfeeding within first 1 hour of birth	Per cent started breastfeeding within 1 day of birth[1]	Number of children	Per cent of breast fed children whose mothers squeezed first milk from breast[2]	Number of children[2]
Sex of child							
Male	95.2	25541	9.4	26.3	19890	63.5	13812
Female	95.7	24460	9.6	26.4	18567	63.4	12845
Residence							
Urban	95.5	11359	11.1	32.0	8803	60.0	5929
Rural	95.4	38643	9.0	24.7	29654	64.4	20728
Mothesr's education							
Illiterate	95.4	33207	8.6	21.9	25248	64.9	17773
Lit., < middle complete	95.6	8298	10.5	31.6	6380	66.1	4187
Middle school complete	95.8	3537	12.1	37.8	2734	60.4	1800
High school and above	95.5	4959	11.6	37.9	4096	52.6	2897
Religion							
Hindu	95.3	39725	9.6	25.7	30789	63.5	20895
Muslim	95 .8	7705	7.4	24.1	5679	61.4	4141

Christian	95.8	1001	19.7	58.3	786	58.3	545
Sikh	96.9	835	4.7	25.1	622	86.8	596
Jain	98.5	143	11.1	42.1	117	60.7	90
Buddhist	96.7	353	15.4	33.3	275	53.8	257
Other	95.3	240	14.0	40.4	189	56.8	132
Caste/tribe							
Scheduled caste	94.8	6695	8.5	22.2	5027	66.2	3492
Scheduled tribe	95.6	4764	16.5	35.9	3646	64.9	2283
Other	95 .5	38543	8.8	25.9	29785	62.8	20881
Assistance at delivery							
Health professional	95.3	17146	11.7	34.8	13603	60.1	8505
Traditional birth attendant	96.4	17628	7.5	22.3	13416	68.2	9737
Other or none	95.7	14975	9.4	21.2	11319	61.4	8378
Public health facility	95.2	7309	12.8	37.2	5730	58.2	3341
Private health facility	95.5	5426	12.0	39.2	4406	54.4	2917
Own home	96.1	30796	8.5	22.6	23431	65.4	17251
Parents' home	96.0	5968	8.7	20.0	4599	67.3	3019
Other	92.0	265	5.9	23.8	205	64.2	126
Total	95 .4	50001	9.5	26.3	38457	63.5	26657

Note: Table is based on children born in the four years preceding the survey, whether living or dead at the time of interview Total includes children with missing information on place of delivery and assistance at delivery, who are not shown separately.

1 Includes children Who started breastfeeding within one hour of birth.

2 Excludes Andhra Pradesh, Himachal Pradesh, Madhya Pradesh, Tamil Nadu and West Bengal.

sufficient for newborn infants; it is not necessary to give them anything else. When the neonate is given anything else, contaminants may cause infection, leading to diarrhoea.

It is also recommended that the first breast milk should be given to the child rather than squeezed from the breast and discarded because it contains colostrum, which provides natural immunity to the child. Table 10.1 shows how soon after birth breastfeeding was initiated. This information was collected for the most recent birth of each woman who had a birth in the four years before the survey (a total of 38,457 births). For a large majority of children in India, the timing of initiation of breastfeeding is later than recommended. Only 10 per cent of children began breastfeeding within one hour of birth, and 26 per cent began breastfeeding within 24 hours of birth. The practice of squeezing the first milk from the breast is also very common in India. A majority (64 per cent) of women squeezed the first milk from the breast before they began breastfeeding their babies. This suggests the importance of launching an educational campaign to inform women about the benefits of providing the first breast milk to their children.

There is virtually no difference in the timing of initiation of breastfeeding by the sex of the child, but urban-rural differences are more substantial. Breastfeeding started within one day of birth for only one-quarter of babies in rural areas, but almost one-third of babies in urban areas. The early initiation of breastfeeding is most evident among women with more education, Christian and Jain women, and women from scheduled tribes. The early initiation of breastfeeding is also more common for children whose birth was assisted by health professionals and children born in a health facility. Even for these groups, however, no more than 4 in 10 children were first breastfeed within 24 hours of birth. This is a surprising result since health professionals should be encouraging women to breastfeed their children right from the time of birth.

In general, groups that are less likely to start breastfeeding early are more likely to squeeze the first milk from the breast before breastfeeding begins. The practice of squeezing the first milk from the breast is particularly prevalent in Sikh families and for children whose birth was assisted by a traditional birth attendant.

Table 10.2 shows state differentials in the timing of the initiation of breastfeeding and the practice of squeezing the first milk from the breast. There are substantial differentials in the timing of initiation of breastfeeding by state. The small northeastern states of Nagaland and Arunachal Pradesh come closest to meeting the international recommendations. At the other end of the spectrum, fewer than one in five children start breastfeeding the first day in Uttar Pradesh, Bihar, Maharashtra and Karnataka. In every state, the first mik is squeezed from the breast for more than two-fifths of breastfed children. This practice is most common in the predominantly Sikh state of Punjab (93 per cent), Jammu (88 per cent), and Mizoram and Orissa (79 per cent each). The practice is least evident in Arunachal Pradesh (44 per cent), and Kerala and Nagaland (49 per cent each).

Table 10.2: Initiation of breastfeeding by state

Percentage of last-born children who started breastfeeding within one hour and one day of birth and percentage of last-born breastfed children whose mothers squeezed the first milk from the breast, according to state, India, 1992-93

State	Per cent started breastfeeding within first 1 hour of birth	Per cent started breastfeeding within 1 day of birth[a]	Percentage whose mothers squeezed first milk from breast
India	4.5	26.3	63.5[b]
North			
Delhi	6.1	34.5	71.2
Haryana	2.7	43.9	57.0
Himachal Pradesh	12.2	42.3	U
Jammu Region of J & K	7.1	41.0	U
Punjab	5.3	23.7	92.9
Rajasthan	7.9	30.3	56.6
Central			
Madhya Pradesh	11.0	27.7	U
Uttar Pradesh	4.7	11.6	60.9
Bihar	1.5	11.8	60.1
Orissa	17.7	36.3	78.8
West Bengal	10.8	33.8	U
Northeast			
Arunachal Pradesh	40.6	79.8	43.7
Assam	20.0	53.2	70.3
Manipur	12.1	24.9	69.4
Meghalaya	8.3	69.1	64.4
Mizoram	29.9	68.1	78.8
Nagaland	64.3	83.8	49.3
Tripura	7.3	28.0	68.9
West			
Goa	28.8	44.1	61.9
Gujarat	14.0	25.7	57.2
Maharashtra	7.4	18.2	70.5

{Cont}.......

South			
Andhra Pradesh	20.0	27.5	U
Karnataka	5.4	18.2	61.9
Kerala	14.3	77.5	48.5
Tamil Nadu	21.8	54.5	U

Note: Table is based on children born in the four year preceding the survey, whether living or dead at the time of the interview.

U.: Not available.

a. Includes children who started breastfeeding within one hour of birth.

b. Excludes Andhra Pradesh, Himachal Pradesh, Madhya Pradesh, Tamil Nadu and West Bengal

For children currently being breastfed, mothers were asked if the child had been given other liquids or solid foods at any time during the day or night before the interview. The results are shown in Table 10.3 and Figure 10.1 according to the child's age. Children who received nothing but breast milk in the previous 24 hours are defined as being exclusively breastfed, while full breastfeeding refers to both those given only breast milk and those who received breast milk and plain water only. In India, exclusive breastfeeding is quite common for very young children, but even at age 0-1 month more than one-third of babies are given water or other supplements. On average, 51 per cent of infants under four months are given only breast milk, while 73 per cent receive full breastfeeding. The percentage of babies being exclusively breastfed drops off rapidly after the first few months of life, to less than 10 per cent for children age 8 months and older. Supplements other than plain water are given in addition to breast milk to 16 per cent of children less than 1 month of age. The percentage given supplements increases steadily to more than 80 per cent at age 11 months. Breastfeeding typically continues for long durations. A majority of children are still being breastfed at the time of their second birthday and breastfeeding continues for three years or more for more than one-quarter of children. Even at four years of age (47 months), 14 per cent of children are reported to be receiving some breast milk along with supplementary food.

Table 10.4 and Figure 10.2 show in more detail the types of food supplementation received by currently breastfeeding last-born children under four years of age during the 24 hours before the interview. The use of infant formula is rare in India. The percentage of children given infant formula increases steadily from less than 1 per cent for children under 2 months of age to a maximum of only 11 per cent at age 9 months. Overall, only 6 per cent of breastfeeding children under four years of age are given infant formula in addition to breast milk. Supplementation of

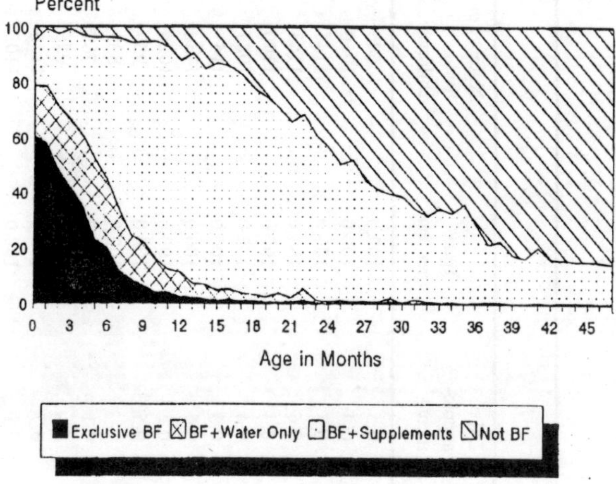

Note: BF + Supplements includes
BF + DK (Don't know) Supplements

NFHS, India, 1992-93

Figure 10.1: Distribution of Children by Breast-feeding (BF) Status According to Age

breast milk by other milk rises steadily with age to 46 per cent at age 8 months and remains fairly constant (at 45-55 per cent) in most of the older age groups. Supplementation by other liquids, such as juice or tea, rises steadily to 75 per cent at 16 months of age and remains more or less constant at older ages. Supplementation by solid or mushy food shows a rise from only 17 per cent at 6 months of age to 79 per cent by age 15 months and a slower rise thereafter to more than 90 per cent for children who are four years old. Less than one-third of infants age 6-9 months received both breast milk and solid/mushy foods, as recommended (derived from Tables 10.3 and 10.4). While 95 per cent of the infants in this age group were being breastfed, most did not receive complementary foods.

The use of a bottle with a nipple to feed children is of interest to both demographers and health personnel. Bottle feeding has a direct effect on the mother's exposure to the risk of pregnancy because the period of amenorrhoea may be shortened when breastfeeding is reduced or replaced by bottle feeding. In addition, because it is often difficult to sterilize the nipple properly, the use of feeding bottles with nipples exposes children to an increased risk of developing diarrhoea and other diseases. The use of bottles with nipples is relatively rare in India for breastfeeding children, increasing from 4 per cent in the first month

Table 10.3: Breastfeeding status by child's age

Per cent distribution of living children by breestfeeding status, according to child's age in months, India, 1992-93

Age in months	Percentage among all living children: Not breast-feeding	Exclusively breast-feeding	Breastfeeding and: Plain water only	Breastfeeding and: Supple-ments	Breastfeeding and: DK supple-ments	Total per cent	Number of living children
<1	4.9	60.5	18.2	15.9	0.5	100.0	605
1	0.7	58.0	20.5	20.4	0.4	100.0	1060
2	2.4	48.6	22.8	25.9	0.3	100.0	1141
3	0.9	41.9	24.5	32.2	0.6	100.0	1163
4	3.0	35.3	25.3	36.0	0.4	100.0	1190
5	3.8	23.2	28.9	43.7	0.4	100.0	1087
6	3.6	20.2	24.6	51.1	0.5	100.0	1157
7	4.1	11.9	21.8	61.8	0.5	100.0	1134
8	5.6	8.9	15.5	69.5	0.5	100.0	1024
9	5.3	6.8	15.2	72.1	0.5	100.0	959
10	5.1	4.4	11.5	79.0	—	100.0	839
11	7.1	4.4	7.9	80.4	0.1	100.0	767
12	12.2	2.8	8.7	76.3	—	100.0	956
13	9.6	2.5	4.9	82.3	0.7	100.0	1156
14	15.1	1.8	5.4	77.6	0.1	100.0	1108
15	13.1	1.4	3.5	81.9	0.1	100.0	1129
16	14.2	1.8	3.7	80.0	0.2	100.0	1144
17	17.2	1.2	2.8	78.4	0.3	100.0	1081
18	22.4	1.2	2.2	74.1	0.2	100.0	1064

19	25.4	0.6	1.9	71.3	0.8	100.0	954
20	29.1	0.5	3.4	66.9	0.1	100.0	907
21	34.1	0.7	1.6	63.2	0.3	100.0	865
22	31.7	1.3	4.2	62.0	0.9	100.0	740
23	39.2	0.4	1.0	58.4	1.1	100.0	749
24	43.4	—	0.8	55.0	0.8	100.0	937
25	49.7	0.4	0.9	48.5	0.6	100.0	1070
26	48.0	0.4	0.5	50.3	0.8	100.0	994
27	55.7	0.3	0.8	42.1	1.1	100.0	890
28	58.7	0.1	0.6	39.9	0.7	100.0	977
29	60.6	0.7	1.4	37.0	0.4	100.0	874
30	61.5	0.3	0.3	37.5	0.4	100.0	916
31	66.0	0.2	1.4	31.5	0.9	100.0	825
32	68.5	0.4	0.5	30.2	0.4	100.0	806
33	65.9	—	0.4	32.9	0.8	100.0	818
34	67.6	0.3	0.2	30.8	1.1	100.0	807
35	64.2	—	0.2	34.6	1.0	100.0	733
36	71.8	0.1	0.3	27.2	0.6	100.0	885
37	78.7	0.3	0.2	19.5	1.2	100.0	1101
38	77.7	0.2	0.4	21.5	0.3	100.0	1001
39	82.7	0.1	—	16.8	0.4	100.0	1051
40	83.7	—	0.2	15.3	0.8	100.0	908
41	80.0	0.2	0.2	19.2	0.6	100.0	961
42	84.2	0.1	0.1	14.5	1.1	100.0	1024
43	84.3	0.1	0.2	14.8	0.6	100.0	975
44	84.9	—	0.3	14.5	0.3	100.0	921
45	85.0	0.1	0.2	14.6	0.2	100.0	979
46	85.1	—	0.1	14.2	0.5	100.0	827
47	85.6	0.1	—	13.7	0.6	100.0	801

Note: Breastfeeding stats refers to last 24 hours. Children classified as "Breastfeeding and plain water only" receive no supplements.

DK: Don't know. — Less than 0.05 per cent.

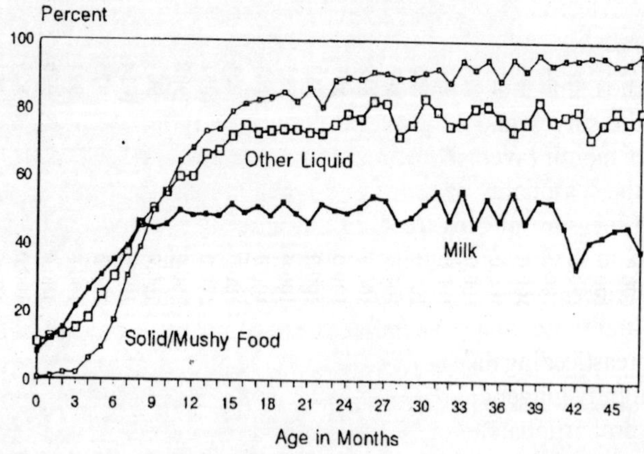

Note: Based on youngest child under age four being breastfed; Milk refers to fresh milk and tinned/powdered milk

NFHS, India, 1992-93

Figure 10.2: Percentage of Children Given Milk Other Liquid, or Solid/Mushy Food the Day before the Interview

after birth to a high of 15 per cent for children age 5-6 months, after which it declines slowly to near zero for children approaching four years of age.

The duration of breastfeeding is a widely studied indicator of breastfeeding. Several statistics describing the length of breastfeeding (the median duration of exclusive breastfeeding, full breastfeeding and breastfeeding of any kind including partial breastfeeding) are shown by selected background characteristics in Table 10.5. Also shown is the percentage of children under 6 months of age who were breastfed six or more times in the 24 hours preceding the survey interview. The median length of breastfeeding overall is slightly over two years. Supplementation begins early, however. The median length of exclusive breastfeeding is only 1.4 months, and the median length of full breastfeeding is 4.7 months. The mean length of breastfeeding (26 months) is slightly longer than the median length, reflecting the fact that some children are breastfed for very long periods of time. Estimates of both the means and the medians are based on the current proportions of children breastfeeding in each age group rather than on the mother's recall, because current status information is usually more accurate.

An alternative measure of the duration of breastfeeding is the prevalence-incidence mean, which is calculated as the "prevalence" of breastfeeding divided by its "incidence". In this case, prevalence is defined as the number of children whose mothers were breastfeeding at the time of the survey and incidence is defined as the average number of births per month (averaged over a 48-month period to overcome problems of the seasonality of births and possible reference period errors). For each measure of breastfeeding, the prevalence-incidence mean is very close to the mean calculated in the conventional manner.

Children of more "modernized" women (urban women, educated women, and those who are exposed to mass media) have shorter durations of breastfeeding than other children, but children of working women have a slightly longer duration. It should be noted that working mothers come disproportionately from rural areas where breastfeeding durations are relatively long. Male children are breastfed slightly longer than female children (25.3 months compared to 23.6 months), but the duration of exclusive breastfeeding and full breastfeeding is slightly longer for female children because male children start receiving water or supplements at an earlier age. Other groups with relatively long breastfeeding durations include scheduled tribes and children whose birth was not attended by a health professional.

In addition to the length of breastfeeding, the frequency with which mothers breastfeed can affect the duration of postpartum amenorrhoea and also the health and nutritional status of the child. There is a high intensity of breastfeeding in India. Ninety-two per cent of children under six months of age were breastfed six or more times on the day before the interview (Table 10.5). The frequency of breastfeeding is slightly lower in urban areas and for children whose mothers had received a high school education, but the differences among groups are not large.

State differentials in the duration and frequency of breastfeeding are shown in Table 10.6. The median duration of breastfeeding is exceptionally long in Tripura (34 months) and West Bengal (33 months). The shortest median durations of breastfeeding (17-18 months) are found in Goa, Tamil Nadu, Mizoram, Punjab and Meghalaya. Arunachal Pradesh is the only state in which the majority of children are exclusively breastfed for the recommended period of four months. The frequency of breastfeeding is high in every state. The percentage of children under six months of age who were breastfed six or more times the day before the interview varies from 75-76 per cent in Goa and Tamil Nadu (the same states that have the shortest median durations of breastfeeding) to 100 per cetn in Nagaland.

Table 10.4: Type of supplementation be child's age

Per centage of last-born breastfeeding children receiving food supplementation by type end percentage using a bottle with a nipple, according to child's age in months, India, 1992-93

	Percentage of breastfeeding children who are:					
	Receiving supplement					
Age in months	Infant formula	Other milk	Other liquid	Solid/ mushy food	Using bottle with a nipple	Number of breast feeding children
1	2	3	4	5	6	7
<1	0.5	8.1	10.9	0.4	4.0	575
1	1.0	12.0	12.3	0.8	7.3	1051
2	2.7	15.2	13.3	2.0	9.5	1114
3	3.9	21.2	15.0	2.0	11.5	1152
4	4.4	26.3	17.8	6.1	14.1	1152
5	6.6	30.6	24.7	9.3	15.3	1042
6	8.1	34.9	30.1	17.2	15.2	1114
7	8.3	39.3	37.3	30.2	14.5	1085
8	9.3	45.8	45.7	38.6	14.4	966
9	11.3	44.4	50.3	49.6	11.6	905
10	9.0	45.6	54.9	55.5	11.3	796
11	9.6	49.6	59.5	64.3	14.1	712
12	8.3	48.2	59.7	68.2	10.9	839
13	5.7	48.6	66.2	73.1	9.2	1043
14	5.2	48.1	67.3	73.7	7.8	939
15	5.0	51.6	71.8	77.0	6.1	981
16	7.6	49.0	74.8	81.3	7.3	980
17	6.4	50.9	72.7	82.3	5.9	892
18	5.7	48.3	73.3	83.2	4.0	825
19	6.0	52.1	73.8	84.7	5.7	707
20	5.8	48.8	73.7	81.8	4.7	643
21	7.8	46.1	72.9	85.9	5.9	568
22	4.7	51.7	72.7	80.2	4.2	503
23	6.4	50.0	75.3	88.3	6.9	448
24	4.1	49.2	78.4	89.2	2.8	524
25	3.7	50.9	77.0	88.7	5.9	533
26	4.5	54.0	82.2	90.9	3.4	509
27	4.8	53.0	81.5	90.5	5.1	387
28	4.9	46.1	71.9	89.2	4.2	397
29	4.8	48.0	75.3	89.4	3.1	342
30	3.5	51.9	83.1	90.8	2.4	351
31	4.4	55.6	79.3	92.0	4.6	274
32	8.8	47.3	75.1	87.9	5.5	250
33	3.0	55.9	76.4	94.5	3.2	275
34	3.3	45.6	80.5	91.9	1.9	253
35	3.6	53.8	81.1	94.7	3.2	255
36	2.5	47.1	77.6	88.6	2.1	244

{Cont.}.........

1	2	3	4	5	6	7
37	5.0	55.5	73.8	94.9	2.7	204
38	2.4	46.8	76.2	91.6	2.0	220
39	3.3	53.2	82.6	96.3	4.3	177
40	3.2	53.0	76.8	93.4	0.1	143
41	1.5	45.5	78.3	94.8	—	187
42	4.1	33.6	79.9	95.0	2.0	152
43	3.0	41.3	71.9	95.9	1.6	148
44	3.6	42.9	76.1	95.7	1.5	137
45	6.0	45.2	79.7	93.6	0.1	146
46	5.7	45.8	76.6	94.0	2.0	119
47	1.9	38.7	79.8	96.7	0.3	111

Note: Supplementation refers to the last 24 hours. Percentage by type of supplement among breastfeeding children may sum to more than 100.0 because children may have received more than one type of supplement.
--Less than 0.05 per cent.

The extent to which feeding practices in India conform to the international recommendations is summarized in Table 10.7. The table presents a very mixed picture of infant and child feeding practices. On the positive side, the duration of breastfeeding is relatively long and the use of feeding bottles with nipples is infrequent. On the negative side, only half of children less than four months old are exclusively breastfed and the introduction of solid or mushy food to the diet is typically much later than recommended. The timely complementary feeding rate for India as a whole is only 31 per cent. Even at one year of age (12 months), almost one-third of breastfeeding children are not receiving solid or mushy food in addition to breast milk (see Table 10.4). This poses a serious problem for the health and development of India's children, which must be urgently addressed. Effective programmes to educate parents about proper feeding practices are essential if the situation is to improve.

The statewide indicators of feeding practices shown in Table 10.7 can help to identify important emphases for educational programmes in each state. For example, Goa has extraordinarily high usage of feeding bottles (almost twice as high as any other state) and very poor achievement of the goals for exclusive breastfeeding and a long duration of breastfeeding. Punjab, Jammu and Meghalaya also have an exceptionally low proportion of children under four months of age who are exclusively breastfed. Children in Rajasthan, Bihar and Uttar Pradesh are very unlikely to be given solid or mushy food at the appropriate age.

Table 10.5: Median duration and frequency of breastfeeding, by background characteristics

Median durations of any, exclusive and full breastfeeding among children under four years and the percentage of children under six months of age who were breastfed six or more times in the 24 hours preceding the interview, by selected background characteristics, India, 1992-93.

	Median durations (months)[1]				Children under 6 months	
Background characteristic	Any breast-feeding	Exclusive breast-feeding	Full breast-feeding[2]	Number of children	Breastfed 6+ times in last 24 hours	Number of children
Sex of child						
Male	25.3	1.3	4.3	25541	91.6	3116
Female	23.6	1.6	5.1	24460	91.5	3131
Residence						
Urban	20.9	0.6	2.9	11359	86.4	1293
Rural	25.4	1.9	5.2	38643	92.9	4953
Mother s education						
Illiterate	25.9	2.1	5.8	33207	92.9	4163
Literate., < middle complete	23.4	0.7	3.4	8298	89.2	1033
Middle school complete	22.0	1.2	2.4	3537	92.3	423
High school and above	18.2	0.6	2.0	4959	85.9	628
Religion						
Hindu	25.0	1.6	4.7	39725	91.6	4892
Muslim	22.8	1.3	4.8	7705	91.2	1011
Christian	19.4	1.7	3.4	1001	89.6	135
Sikh	18.5	0.4	3.0	835	91.5	107
Jain	11.7	0.5	0.7	143	*	20
Buddhist	25.4	0.6	6.6	353	(99.0)	55
Other	23.0	1.2	4.2	240	87.1	27

Caste/tribe						
Scheduled caste	24.8	2.0	5.4	6695	92.0	893
Scheduled tribe	26.3	2.0	6.8	4764	92.5	594
Other	24.1	1.3	4.3	38543	91.3	4760
Mother s Work status						
Not working	23.6	1.3	4.5	36225	91.5	4948
Working in family farm/business	27.3	1.7	5.2	5893	91.6	581
Employed by someone else	26.2	1.9	5.4	6654	91.3	599
Self-employed	23.7	2.0	4.2	1229	94.7	119
Mother s exposure to media						
Exposed to media	22.4	0.9	3.4	23494	90.2	2802
Watches television weekly	20.4	0.7	2.6	13093	88.6	1542
Listens to radio weekly	22.5	1.2	3.5	19289	90.3	2360
Visits cinema/theatre monthly	21.5	0.8	3.1	6628	86.4	789
Not exposed to any of the media	25.9	1.9	5.9	26507	92.7	3445
Assistance at delivery						
Health professional	21.4	0.7	2.9	17146	88.0	2087
Traditional birth attendant	25.5	1.8	5.3	17628	93.0	2219
Other or none	26.3	2.3	6.0	14975	93.7	1933
Total	24.4	1.4	4.7	50001	91.6	6247
Mean for all children	26.1	3.8	6.4	NA	NA	NA
P/I for all children[3]	26.1	3.3	6.2	NA	NA	NA

Note: Total includes children with missing information on assistance at delivery, who are not shown separately.

NA: Not applicable.

() Based on fewer 25-49 unweighted cases.

* Percentage not shown; based on fewer than 25 unweighted cases.

1 Medians and means are based on current status.

2 Either exclusively breastfed or received breast milk and plain water only.

3 Prevalence-incidence mean.

Some feeding problems are universal, however. No state comes even close to achieving the recommendations for exclusive breastfeeding of children under 4 months of age or the supplementation of breast milk with solid or mushy food at age 6-9 months. These poor feeding practices are undoubtedly a factor in the nutritional deficiencies that are illustrated in the next section.

10.2 Nutritional Status of Children

One of the major contributions of the NFHS to the study of child health is the anthropometric data collected for children under four years of age. Both weight and height measurements were obtained for each child. For first phase states (Andhra Pradesh, Himachal Pradesh, Madhya Pradesh, Tamil Nadu and West Bengal), only weight was measured, because height measuring boards were not available at that timed.* The weight of each child was measured using a Salter scale, which is a hanging spring balance. For tl e measurement of height length, children under two years of age were measured lying down on an adjustable measuring board, while those age two years and above were measured in a standing position. The guidelines given in the United Nations Manual, "How to Weigh and Measure Children" (United Nations, 1986), were followed when training the field staff on measurement of the height and weight of children. Weight was measured to the nearest 100 grams. Height or length was measured to the nearest 0.1 centimetres. The data on weight and height were used to calculate three summary indices of nutritional status, which affects children's susceptibility to disease and their chances of survival. These indices are: weight-for-age, height-for-age, and weight-for-height.

The nutritional status of children calculated according to these measures is compared with the nutritional status of an international reference population that has been recommended by the World Health Organization (Dibley *et al.*, 1987a, 1987b). The use of this reference population is based on the empirical finding that well-nourished children in all population groups for which data exist follow very similar growth patterns (Martorell and Habicht, 1986). A recent scientific report from the Nutrition Foundation of India (Agarwal *et al.*, 1991) has concluded that the WHO standard is applicable to Indian children as well.

---

* The lack of height measurements for these states should not substantially bias the national estimates of heightfor-age and weight-for-height since these five states cluster closely around the national estimate of the percentage of children who are underweight (which is the only nutritional index that can be calculated for these states).

Table 10.6: Median duration and frequency of breastfeedins by state
Median durations of any exclusive and full breastfeeding among children under four years and the percentage of children under six months of age who were breastfed six or more times in the 24 hours preceding the interview by state India 1992-93

State	Median durations (months)[1]			Percentage of children urder 6months breastfed 6+ times in last 24 hours
	Any breast-feeding	Exclusive breast-feeding	Full breast-feeding[2]	
India	24.4	1.4	4.7	91.6
North				
Delhi	20.9	0.5	1.7	87.6
Haryana	23.0	0.7	2.0	90.2
Himachal Pradesh	21.7	0.7	2.6	84.9
Jammu Region of J & K	22.1	0.5	1.4	88.2
Punjab	18.4	0.4	2.6	92.7
Rajasthan	24.2	2.9	6.5	91.2
Central				
Madhya Pradesh	24.7	0.6	5.7	82.7
Uttar Pradesh	24.9	2.5	5.4	95 .5
East				
Bihar	26.6	1.5	7.5	94.9
Orissa	27.6	1.2	3.7	95.1
West Bengal	32.8	0.6	1.7	88.6
Northeast				
Arunachal Pradesh	27.8	4.0	5.1	98.8
Assam	27.8	3.1	3.6	95.5
Manipur	28.5	3.8	4.1	94.6
Meghalaya	18.4	0.5	0.5	88.6
Mizoram	18.2	1.6	5.0	97.3
Nagaland	21.2	0.7	5.4	100.0
Tripura	33.8	1.2	1.8	89.0
West				
Goa	16.5	0.4	0.6	75.2
Gujarat	19.7	0.6	5.1	95.3
Maharashtra	23.0	0.7	5.5	90.1
South				
Andhra Pradesh	26.4	2.6	4.9	88.9
Karnataka	21.4	3.2	4.6	93.9
Kerala	23.5	2.1	2.1	93.1
Tamil Nadu	16.9	1.9	2.6	75.6

1 Medians and means are based on current status.
2 Either exclusively breastfed or received breast milk and plain water only.

Table 10.7: Recommended feeding indicators
Recommended feeding indicators for children age 0-23 months by state India, 1992-93

State	Recommended feeding indicators				
	Per cent of children 0-3 months exclusively breastfed	Per cent of children 6-9 months receiving breast milk and solid/mushy food	Per cent of children 12-15 months breastfed	Per cent of children 20-23 months breastfed	Per cent of last-born children <12 months bottle fed
India	51.0	31.4	87.5	66.6	14.2
North					
Delhi	20.0	25.1	74.6	52.8	36.3
Haryana	37.5	38.5	89.0	58.3	20.0
Himachal Pradesh	36.4	39.9	80.2	54.7	24.6
Jammu Region of J & K	16.9	44.8	83.4	51.8	38.3
Punjab	3.3	37.3	77.9	40.4	27.1
Rajasthan	65.9	9.4	87.3	74.8	8.9
Central					
Madhya Pradesh	31.4	27.7	90.2	65.4	7.3
Uttar Pradesh	60.3	19.4	89.7	73.8	12.1
East					
Bihar	51.6	18.1	92.0	79.3	10.0
Orissa	45.7	30.2	91.5	78.9	14.5
West Bengal	40.0	53.6	91.9	83.6	21.7

Northeast					
Arunachal Pradesh	73.9	35.8	98.0	73.0	7.2
Assam	65.0	39.2	94.8	82.5	12.8
Manipur	70.4	50.0	89.5	61.5	7.2
Meghalaya	18.0	56.3	63.6	51.4	24.4
Mizoram	45.5	64.3	81.6	37.9	14.7
Nagaland	61.1	43.5	70.3	46.9	23.7
Tripura	47.9	65.0	98.1	74.2	29.5
West					
Goa	10.8	33.9	53.1	40.0	66.7
Gujarat	36.3	22.9	85.8	48.1	9.2
Maharashtra	37.1	25.0	85.2	62.2	11.2
South					
Andhra Pradesh	70.5	47.8	86.9	67.7	12.5
Karnataka	65.6	38.2	84.3	54.5	13.5
Kerata	59.2	69.3	84.0	61.7	26.2
Tamit Nadu	55.8	56.5	65.4	35.5	30.7

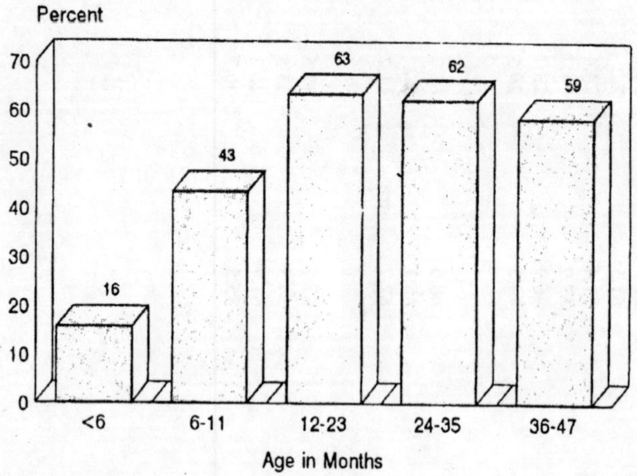

Note: Percentage of children more than 2 standard deviations below the median of the International Reference Population

NFHS, India, 1992-93

Figure 10.3 Percentage of Children Under age Four who are Underwight by Age

The three nutritional status indices are expressed in standard deviation units (z-scores) from the median for the international reference population. Children who fall more than two standard deviations below the reference median are considered to be *undernourished,* while those who fall more than three standard deviations below the reference median are considered to be *severely undernouvurished.*

Each of the indices provides somewhat different information about the nutritional status of children. The height-for-age index measures linear growth retardation among children. Children who are more than two standard deviations below the median of the reference population in terms of height-for-age are considered short for their age or *stunted.* The percentage in this category indicates the prevalence of chronic undernutrition which often leads to chronic or recurrent diarrhoea. Stunting is typically associated with inadequate food intake resulting from poor feeding practices or from the lack of sufficient food, as well as the existence of adverse environmental conditions for an extended period of time. Height-for-age, therefore, is a measure of the long-term effects of undernutrition.

The weight-for-height index measures body mass in relation to body length. Children who are more than two standard deviations below

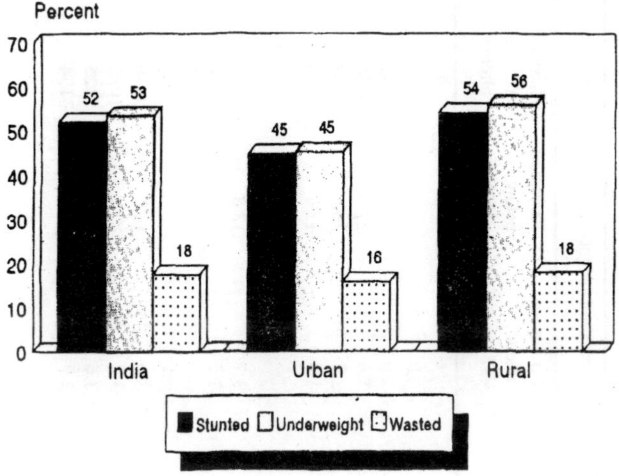

Note: *Percentage of children more than 2 standard deviations below the median of the International Reference Population*

NFHS, India, 1992-93

Figure 10.4: Undernutrition Among Children under Four Years of Age

the median of the reference population in terms of their weight-for-height are considered to be too thin or wasted. The percentage in this category indicates the prevalence of acute undernutrition. This condition is associated with the failure to receive adequate nutrition in the period immediately before the survey and may be the result of seasonal variations in food supply or recent episodes of illness (especially diarrhoea).

Weight-for-age is a composite measure which takes into account both chronic and acute undernutrition. Children who are more than two standard deviations below the reference median on this index are considered underweight.

The validity of these indices is determined by many factors, including the coverage of the population of children and accurate anthropometric measurements. In the NFHS, about 16 per cent of living children under age four were not weighed and measured, usually because the child was not at home or because the mother refused to allow the measurements to be taken. Also excluded from the analysis are children whose month and year of birth were not reported by the mother, and those with grossly improbable weight and height measurements. In addition, two of the three indices (height-for-age and weight-for-age) are sensitive to misreporting of children's ages, including heaping on preferred digits. The weight-for-height index is the only one which does not

Table 10.8: Nutritional status by demographic characteristics
Among children under four years of age, the percentage classified as undernourished according to three anehropometric indices of nutritional status, by demographic characteristics, India, 1992-93

	Weight-for-age			Height-for-age		Weight-for-height		
Demographic characteristic	Percentage below -3 SD	Percentage below -2 SD[1]	Number of children[2]	Percentage below -3 SD	Percentage below -2 SD[1]	Percentage below -3 SD	Percentage below -2 SD[1]	Number of children[3]
Child's age								
<6 months	2.8	15.6	4406	5.7	15.7	2.0	9.5	3225
6-11 months	14.1	43.3	4792	14.3	34.3	2.9	15.7	3176
12-23 months	26.3	63.4	9560	30.7 5	6.6	5.6	28.0	6945
24-35 months	25.9	62.2	8406	34.6	60.2	2.5	16.6	6033
36-47 months	21.8	58.5	8643	40.7	66.7	1.8	11.6	6204
Sex								
Male	20.2	53.3	18208	28.4	52.3	3.7	18.8	13040
Female	21.0	53.4	17599	29.4	51.7	2.6	16.1	12543
Birth order								
1	17.4	49.4	9719	24.8	48.1	3.0	16.5	6630
2-3	19.5	52.2	15209	27.3	49.8	3.2	17.4	10634
4-5	23.7	57.7	6848	32.6	56.6	3.6	19.1	5125
6+	26.8	59.8	4031	36.6	60.0	2.9	17.4	3194
Previous birth								
Interval[4]								
First birth	17.5	49.5	9762	24.8	48.1	3.0	16.5	6664

< 24 months	23.3	56.9	6106	33.1	56.9	3.7	16.3	4549
24-47 months	21.5	55.2	14713	30.4	53.9	2.9	18.0	10677
48+ months	20.7	51.5	5227	26.4	47.3	3.6	19.2	3694
Total	20.6	53.4	35807	28.9	52.0	3.2	17.5	25584

Note: Figures are for children born 1-47 months prior to the survey. Each of the indices is expressed in standard deviation units (SD) from the median of the International Reference Population. The percentages of children who are more than three and more than two standard deviation units below the median of the International Reference Population (-3SD and -2SD) are shown according to selected characteristics.

1 Also includes the children who are more than 3 standard deviations below the International Reference Population median.

2 Number of children for calculation of weight-for-age.

3 Number of children for calculation of height-for-age and weight-for-height, excluding Andhra Pradesh, Himachal Pradesh, Madhya Pradesh, Tamil Nadu and West Bengal.

4 In the case of first-born twins, both twins are counted as first births because neither has a previous birth interval.

Table 10.9: Nutritional status by background characteristics

Among children under four years of age, the percentage classified as undernourished according to three anthropometric indices of nutritional status, by selected background characteristics, India, 1992-93

Demographic characteristic	Weight-for-age			Weight-for-age		Weight-for-height		
	Percentage below -3 SD	Percentage below -2 SD[1]	Number of children[2]	Percentage below -3 SD	Percentage below -2 SD[1]	Percentage below -3 SD	Percentage below -2 SD[1]	Number of children[3]
Residence								
Urban	14.8	45.2	8464	22.0	44.8	2.9	15.8	5884
Rural	22.4	55.9	27343	30.9	54.1	3.2	18.0	19700
Mother's education								
Illiterate	24.7	59.2	22946	34.5	58.5	3.4	18.8	16639
Lit., < middle complete	16.7	50.4	6251	22.6	46.4	3.0	16.8	4260
Middle school complete	12.4	43.5	2765	17.9	39.3	2.7	14.7	1905
High school and above	7.8	30.3	3844	12.2	30.0	2.3	12.3	2780
Religion								
Hindu	21.0	53.7	28450	29.2	52.5	3.3	17.7	19897
Muslim	21.2	55.4	5440	31.4	54.5	3.0	17.2	4065
Christian	7.9	38.3	737	15.9	34.2	1.8	11.1	523
Sikh	12.6	40.2	670	13.1	34.9	2.4	17.4	656
Jain	9.6	29.9	106	12.6	25.8	0.3	6.4	78
Buddnist	22.8	54.3	262	31.7	59.5	2.0	22.2	251
Other	23.0	59.7	143	25.6	51.2	3.9	15.6	113

Caste/tribe								
Scheduled caste	23.7	57.5	4664	33.2	58.0	3.4	18.5	3347
Scheduled tribe	25.3	56.8	3203	28.8	52.8	4.1	22.0	2085
Other	19.5	52.3	27940	28.1	50.9	3.0	16.8	20152
Total	20.6	53.4	35807	28.9	52.0	3.2	17.5	25584

Note: Figures are for children born 1-47 months prior to the survey. Each of the indices is expressed in standard deviation units (SD) from the median of the International Reference Population. The percentages of children who are more than three and more than two standard deviation units below the median of the International Reference Population (-3SD and -2SD) are shown according to selected characteristics.

( ) Based on 25-49 unweighted cases.

* Percentage not shown; based on fewer than 25 unweighted cases.

1 Also includes the children who are more than 3 standard deviations below the International Reference Population median.

2 Number of children for calculation of weight-for-age

3 Number of children for calculation of height-for-age and weight-for-height, excluding Andhra Pradesh, Himachal Pradesh, Madhya Pradesh, Tamil Nadu and West Bengal.

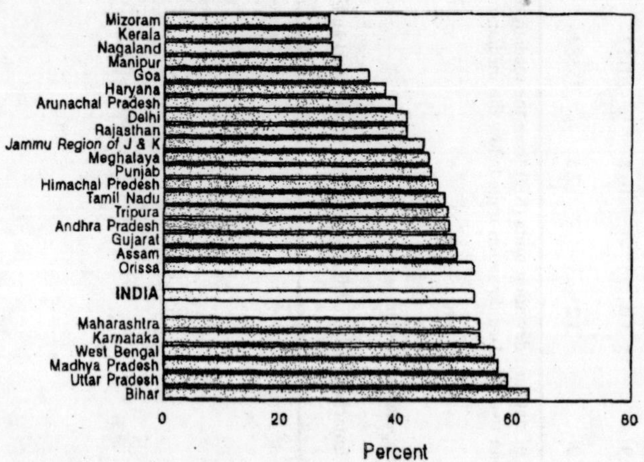

Figure 10.5: Percentage of Children Under age Four who are Underwight by Stage

depend on accurate age reporting.

Table 10.8 presents the percentage of children classified as undernourished according to weight-for-age, height-for-age, and weight-for-height by selected demographic characteristics. Both chronic and acute undernutrition are prevalent in India. Slightly more than half (53 per cent) of all children are underweight and a similar proportion (52 per cent) are stunted. The proportion of children who are severely undernourished is also notable — 21 per cent in the case of weight-for-age and 29 per cent in the case of height-for-age. Wasting is also quite evident in India, affecting more than one in every six children. These levels of undernutrition are among the highest in the world (see, for example, Sommerfelt and Stewart, 1994).

As the age of children increases, there is a marked increase in the prevalence of undernutrition in the first year of life that continues on into the second year of life and, for stunting, into the third and fourth year as well. Undernutrition is lowest in the first six months of life, when most babies are being fully breastfed. As indicated in Figure 10.3, the percentage of children who are underweight reaches its highest value (63 per cent) at age 1 year and declines slightly thereafter. The prevalence of stunting, however, continues to grow, reaching a peak of 67 per cent among three-year-old children. The prevalence of wasting, on the other hand, reaches a maximum (28 per cent) for children who are one year old and declines rapidly thereafter.

Male and female children are about equally disadvantaged nutritionally, although males are slightly more subject to wasting. Undernourishment increases somewhat with increasing birth order. Young children in families with four or more children are the most nutritionally disadvantaged. The pattern of undernourishment associated with the length of the preceding birth interval depends on the particular measure which is being examined. For the two agerelated measures, undernutrition is slightly higher for children with short birth intervals, but the opposite is true for the measure of wasting. For all three measures, however, the differentials are relatively small.

Table 10.9 shows nutritional status by selected background characteristics. All the measures indicate that undernutrition is more of a problem in rural areas than in urban areas (Figure 10.4). Even in urban areas, however, nearly half of young children are underweight and almost half are stunted. The most serious nutritional problem (wasting) is only slightly lower in urban areas than in rural areas. The differentials in undernutrition by mother's educational level are very large. Children whose mothers are illiterate are twice as likely to be underweight or stunted as children whose mothers have completed at least high school. According to these same measures, children whose mothers are illiterate are about three times as likely to be severely undernourished as those whose mothers have completed at least high school. The differentials are only half as large, but still substantial, in the case of wasting.

The other differentials in Table 10.9 are considerably smaller. Hindu, Muslim and Buddhist children are about equally likely to be undernourished. The levels of undernutrition are much lower for Christians, Sikhs and Gains. Scheduled caste and scheduled tribe children have slightly higher levels of undernutrition than other children, but the differences among these groups are generally small.

These results suggest that the mother's level of education is the most important characteristic associated with children's nutritional status. Unfortunately, a large majority of young children (65 per cent) in India have mothers who are illiterate; they are consequently at a high risk of suffering undernutrition. Programmes designed to eliminate female illiteracy are, therefore, likely to be of crucial importance for improving the nutrition status and survival of children in India. Nevertheless, it should be noted that levels of undernutrition remain unacceptably high even for children whose mothers are highly educated. This

Table 10.10: Nutritional status by state

Among children under four years of age, the percentage classified as undernourished according to three anthropometric indices of nutritional status, by state, India, 1992-93

	Weight-for-age		Height-for-age		Weight-for-height	
Demographic characteristic	Percentage below -3 SD	Percentage below -2 SD[1]	Percentage below -3 SD	Percentage below -2 SD[1]	Percentage below -3 SD	Percentage below -2 SD[1]
India	20.6	53.4	28.9	52.0	3.2	17.5
North						
Delhi	12.0	41.6	19.3	43.2	2.7	11.9
Haryana	9.0	37.9	19.3	46.7	0.6	5.9
Himachal Pradesh	12.9	47.0	U	U	U	U
Jammu Region of J & K	13.8	44.5	18.6	40.8	3.4	14.8
Punjab	14.2	45.9	15.7	40.0	2.8	19.9
Rajasthan	19.2	41.6	26.6	43.1	5.2	19.5
Central						
Madhya Pradesh	22.3	57.4	U	U	U	U
Uttar Pradesh	24.6	59.0	35.6	59.5	2.7	16.1
East						
Bihar	31.1	62.6	39.5	60.9	4.1	21.8
Orissa	22.7	53.3	25.2	48.2	3.6	21.3
West Bengal	18.4	56.8	U	U	U	U

Northeast						
Arunachal Pradesh	14.5	39.7	27.9	53.9	3.6	11.2
Assam	18.7	50.4	26.3	52.2	1.7	10.8
Manipur	7.2	30.1	16.0	33.6	1.2	8.8
Meghalaya	17.2	45.5	38.4	50.8	4.8	18.9
Mizoram	5.3	28.1	16.0	41.3	0.6	2.2
Nagaland	7.6	28.7	13.2	32.4	2.3	12.7
Tripura	18.6	48.8	21.3	46.0	0.7	17.5
West						
Goa	8.9	35.0	11.0	32.5	2.4	15.3
Gujarat	17.6	50.1	25.3	48.2	3.7	18.9
Maharashtra	21.3	54.2	23.5	48.5	4.2	20.2
South						
Andhra Pradesh	15.6	49.1	U	U	U	U
Karnataka	19.4	54.3	22.7	47.6	2.6	17.4
Kerala	6.1	28.5	9.0	27.4	1.3	11.6
Tamil Nadu	13.3	48.2	U	U	U	U

Note: Figures are for children born 1-47 months prior to the survey. Each of the indices is expressed in standard deviation units (SD) from the median of the International Reference Population. The percentages of children who are more than three and more than two standard deviation units below the median of the International Reference Population (-3SD and -2SD) are shown according to selected characteristics.

U.: Not available because children's height/length was not measured.

1 Also includes the children who are below -3 standard deviations from the International Reference Population median.

finding suggests that targeted programmes about proper feeding practices for children are necessary for parents in all segments of the population.

Variations in nutritional status by state are shown in Table 10.10 and Figure 10.5. Even in the state with the best record on nutritional status for children (Kerala), more than one-quarter of young children are underweight and more than one-quarter are stunted. Other states with relatively low levels of undernutrition are Manipur, Mizoram, Nagaland and Goa. Nutritional problems are particularly serious in Bihar and Uttar Pradesh. The problem of wasting is most evident in Bihar and Orissa, which not coincidentally have among the highest infant mortality rates in India.

11

KNOWLEDGE OF AIDS

Acquired Immune Deficiency Syndrome, or AIDS, as it is more commonly known, was first recognized in 1981. Since the beginning of the pandemic, it is estimated that over 16 million individuals throughout the world have been infected with the Human Immunodeficiency virus (HIV), which causes AIDS, and between mid-1993 and mid-1994 about 1.5 million people developed AIDS - three times as many as in the previous 12-month period (World Health Organization, 1994). The estimated total number of actual AIDS cases in adults and children since 1981 is four million, of which over 240,000 (6.0 per cent) are from Asia. A large proportion (30-50 per cent) of these infected individuals are expected to die within 5-10 years of acquiring the infection (World Health Organization, 1992). Because of the high case fatality rate and the lack of a curative treatment or vaccine, the HIV/AIDS pandemic is one of the most serious health problems in the world.

Within a few years after AIDS was first identified, its cause and mode of transmission were documented. The virus that causes AIDS may remain in a state of latency for some time without causing clinical disease. It is thought that once an individual becomes infected with the virus, he or she remains infected for life. The clinical manifestations of AIDS result primarily from critical injury to the immune system. Soon after becoming infected with HIV, some people have an acute self-limiting illness, indistinguishable from many other mild viral illnesses. After the healthy carrier state, which may last as long as 10 years (longer in some cases), most infected people progress to the full long-term clinical illness stage—the stage at which AIDS itself is contracted.

Epidemiological studies have demonstrated that the major routes of HIV transmission are sexual intercourse, intravenous injections (e.g., transfusions of HIV-contaminated blood or injections using HIV-contaminated needles) and transmission from infected mothers to unborn foetuses through the placenta. Female sex workers in India have significant levels of HIV infection, and a major route of transmission of the virus is along well-established truck routes of the country, where contact between sex workers and the drivers is common. The available evidence indicates that HIV cannot be transmitted through food, water, vectors, or casual contact. Increasingly, HIV is found in association with sexually transmitted diseases (STDs) and tuberculosis, compounding an already alarming public health problem. In urban areas of Tamil Nadu, Gujarat, Karnataka, Punjab, and West Bengal, HIV prevalence levels in STD patients are now estimated to be about 1 per cent (World Health Organization, 1994b).

India established a National AIDS Control Organization (NACO) under the Ministry of Health and Family Welfare in 1989. Prior to this, attempts were made by various nongovernmental organizations (NGOs) to raise awareness of the AIDS syndrome and implement small-scale prevention programmes, concentrating in the perceived higher-risk areas of Bombay, Calcutta, Madras, and Delhi. As the NGO work continues to make important contributions in the field of AIDS prevention, statistics compiled at the national level reveal the spread of HIV in India (based on NACO's monthly update on HIV infection in India, compiled from medical records submitted by 59 hospitals and major medical research centres throughout India).

The updates show that by June of 1988 nearly 120,000 persons from high-risk groups in India had been screened for the virus. Of these cases, 370 tested HIV-positive, and 22 of them (15 Indians and 7 foreigners) were diagnosed as having actually contracted AIDS. It was subsequently determined that 21 of these 22 AIDS cases were transmitted through sexual intercourse, and one through blood transfusion. According to another set of estimates, by 1988 16 patients (14 Indians and 2 foreigners) had died of AIDS in India (Khurana, 1989). Approximately 600,000 persons were HIV positive in India in 1992, and the number of HIV positive cases among those screened (who tend to be from high-risk groups) had shown an increase from 2.5 per 1,000 population in 1986 to 11.2 per 1,000 in 1992 (Ministry of Health and Family Welfare, 1993a).

Three-fourths of AIDS cases identified up to March, 1993, had reportedly acquired the virus through sexual intercourse, 12 per cent through blood transfusions, and 7 per cent through sharing unsterilized needles. It is estimated that if the transmission of HIV continues at the same pace, about five million persons in India will be infected by the year 2000, and the number of AIDS cases will exceed one million (Ministry of Health and Family Welfare, 1993b).

Recent estimates from the NACO monthly updates show that as of 31 March 1994 a total of 15,017 cases were confirmed HIV-positive (using the Western Blot test), out of 2,052,856 samples screened, resulting in a sero-positivity rate of 7.3 per 1,000 (National AIDS Control Organization, 1994b). The number of AIDS cases reported in India was 713 (551 males and 162 females), although according to WHO estimates, the actual number is substantially larger.

The prevalence of the HIV infection as measured in 1994 was substantially larger than in 1988, when high-risk groups were first screened. Unless serious interventions are undertaken in the area of prevention, there is great potential for a further acceleration in HIV prevalence. To summarize the recent situation in India: (1) HIV infection is rapidly spreading beyond those few areas in the country considered to be of especially high risk, and is at different epidemiological stages even within the same state; (2) the epidemic has begun to spread to the general population, mainly through heterosexual contact with those categorized as "high-risk" groups; and (3) the interaction of HIV infection with sexually transmitted diseases (STDs) and tuberculosis, both widely prevalent throughout India, presents an even more challenging public health problem. The correlation between HIV and tuberculosis may result in a resurgence of tuberculosis (56 per cent of reported AIDS cases in India have tuberculosis). Stemming STDs is essential to slowing the transmission of HIV. Fewer than 10 per cent of STD patients seek treatment from public health centres, and the quality of case management and care provided at public as well as private centres is generally low (Lal, 1994).

In 13 out of 25 states, the NFHS included a series of questions on knowledge of AIDS, which were added to the core questions used in all Indian states.* The AIDS questions enable measurement of the extent of knowledge about AIDS among women in different population subgroups, thus generating information that will be useful for planning and implementing AIDS prevention programmed Ever-married women age 13-49 were first asked if they had ever heard of an illness called AIDS. Respondents indicating knowledge of AIDS were asked further questions about the sources of their knowledge, the mechanisms of AIDS transmission, whether they believe the transmission of AIDS is preventable, and if so, their perception of the precautions a person can take to avoid AIDS.

* Because the AIDS questions were not included in 12 states, no national estimates are presented in the tables in this chapter.

11.1 Knowledge of AIDS

Table 11.1 shows the percentage of women who have heard about AIDS. In general, the knowledge that there is an illness called AIDS is very low. Even in Delhi, where considerable media attention has been focussed on AIDS, only 36 per cent of women have heard of the disease. Among the other major states where the knowledge of AIDS has been investigated (Assam, Gujarat, Maharashtra, Tamil Nadu and West Bengal), the level of knowledge is highest in Tamil Nadu, where only 23 per cent of women reported having heard about the disease. In Assam and West Bengal, less than 10 per cent of women are aware of AIDS. A relatively high proportion of women in Goa (42 per cent) have heard of AIDS. In the northeastern states, the level of knowledge varies substantially. In Mizoram and Manipur, where the incidence of AIDS is reported to be high, a large majority of women (85 and 73 per cent, respectively) reported having heard about the disease. In Arunachal Pradesh and Tripura, on the other hand, fewer than 1 in 6 women have heard of AIDS.

Table 11.1: Knowledge of Acquired Imnune Deficiency syndrome (AIDS)
Percentage of ever-married women age 13-49 who have heard about AIDS, by state, India, 1992-93

State	Percentage who have heard about AIDS
Delhi	35.8
West Bengal	9.8
Arunachal Pradesh	16.2
Assam	8.4
Manipur	72.5
Meghalaya	26.7
Mizoram	84.8
Nagaland	40.9
Tripura	13.2
Goa	41.7
Gujarat	10.6
Maharashtra	18.6
Tamil Nadu	23.4

11.2 Source of Knowledge About AIDS

As a part of the AIDS prevention programme, the Government of India has been using the mass media, especially the electronic media, to create awareness among the general public about AIDS and how to prevent its spread. In the NFHS, women who had heard about AIDS were asked about the information sources through which they came to know about AIDS. Television is the most important source of knowledge about AIDS in most states (Table 11.2). More than four-fifths of women who had heard about AIDS in Delhi, Goa and Maharashtra heard about it through the television. Television was a source of knowledge for 60-70 of women in Arunachal Pradesh, Assam, Tamil Nadu and Gujarat. The role of television in spreading the knowledge of AIDS is limited in Manipur (where radio plays a major role) and in Meghalaya and Mizoram (where the majority of women heard about AIDS through friends and relatives). In addition, newspapers are an important source of AIDS information in every state.

11.3 Misconceptions About AIDS

Misconceptions about the disease among the general public make it difficult to implement preventive measures against AIDS and to provide effective care and treatment of the persons affected with AIDS. NFHS respondents were asked if they thought that one could get AIDS from various commonly occurring social situations such as shaking hands with someone who has AIDS, hugging or kissing someone with AIDS, sharing clothing or eating utensils with someone with AIDS, or stepping on the urine or stools of a person who has AIDS. Respondents were also asked whether they thought they could get AIDS from mosquito, flea or bedbug bites. Medical professionals believe that these situations pose an extremely low risk of transmission of AIDS. Women were also asked if they thought AIDS is curable or if they thought that an AIDS vaccine exists. Results are shown in Table 11.3.

Women who have heard about AIDS have a number of misconceptions about the disease, and states differ markedly in the extent and type of misconceptions. The most common misconceptions are that AIDS can be transmitted through kissing and bug bites. Large proportions of women also believe that a person can get AIDS by sharing eating utensils or clothes with a person with AIDS or stepping on their urine or stools. Misconceptions about the transmission of AIDS through shaking hands or hugging are least widespread. In every state, the majority of women who have heard of AIDS correctly perceive that AIDS is not curable and that there is no vaccine against AIDS. Women in Maharashtra, Gujarat and Nagaland are relatively well informed about the transmission of AIDS. On the other hand, misconceptions about AIDS abound in West Bengal and Assam (where knowledge that the disease exists is lowest), as well as in Tripura.

Table 11.2: Source of knowledge about AIDS
Among women who have heard about AIDS, the percentage obtaining knowledge of AIDS from different sources, by state, India, 1992-93

State	Among those echo have heard about AIDS, percentage obtaining knowledge from:					
	Radio	Tele-vision	News-papers	Maga-zines	Friends/ relatives	Other sources
Delhi	27.9	84.0	44.7	29.4	10.2	9.4
West Bengal	20.6	59.1	54.1	11.6	20.7	8.7
Arunachal Pradesh	45.5	60.1	28.0	23.8	34.3	11.9
Assam	48.2	66.3	42.9	21.2	18.8	6.1
Manipur	62.8	22.3	20.8	4.6	54.4	28.5
Meghalaya	37.5	31.9	44.7	21.7	68.8	14.1
Mizoram	58.7	10.8	50.8	16.0	69.4	26.3
Nagaland	73.4	43.2	34.3	19.8	57.9	39.6
Tripura	44.8	53.8	40.0	11.7	22.1	20.7
Goa	35.6	82.3	45.3	20.2	22.3	13.7
Gujarat	23.1	70.5	54.8	17.0	6.9	3.9
Maharashtra	27.7	86.8	36.3	14.3	6.9	7.6
Tamil Nadu	49.5	64.3	37.1	31.1	14.2	8.2

Note: Percentages may sum to more than 100.0 because multiple responses were allowed.

11.4 Knowledge of Prevention of AIDS

The responses to an open-ended question on the precautions to be taken to avoid AIDS are shown in Table 11.4. In almost every state, wsafe sex" is spontaneously mentioned most frequently as a means of avoiding AIDS*. More than half of women in Delhi, Meghalaya, Mizoram, Goa, Maharashtra and Tamil Nadu stated that AIDS can be avoided by practising safe sex. Relatively large proportions of women also specifically mentioned the use of condoms during intercourse as a means of avoiding AIDS. In every state, other precautionary measures such as checking blood prior to transfusion, sterilizing needles/syringes before injection, and avoiding pregnancy when infected with AIDS are mentioned by less than half of women who have heard about AIDS. In several of the northeastern states, where intravenous drug use is thought to be relatively common, substantial proportions of women mention that AIDS can be avoided by sterilizing needles and syringes.

The small percentage of respondents having knowledge of AIDS, as well as the major misconceptions about transmission and prevention

* "Safe sex" was not defined for respondents, so different respondents might have had different prevention measures in mind when using that term.

Table 11.3: Misconceptions about AIDS

Among women who have heard about AIDS, the percentage having misconceptions about different ways of getting AIDS, and the percentage who think AIDS is curable or that there is a vaccine against AIDS, according to state, India, 1992-93.

	Per centage[1] who think it is possible to get AIDS from:							Percentage who think:	
State	Shaking hands with someone with AIDS	Hug-ging some-one with AIDS	Kiss-g ing some-one with AIDS	Wearing clothes of some-one with AIDS	Sharing eating utensils with someone with AIDS	Stewing on urine/ stools of someone with AIDS	Mos quito, flea, bedbug bites	AIDS is cur-able	An AIDS vaccine exists
Delhi	16.8	18.7	40.8	28.7	33.8	31.5	25.4	19.7	5.6
West Bengal	19.8	29.5	59.6	53.8	67.7	62.1	76.7	34.9	2.0
Arunachal Pradesh	25.9	31.5	56.6	41.3	46.9	42.0	57.3	25.9	16.8
Assam	32.3	39.4	58.1	57.5	66.0	69.3	66.3	32.9	9.4
Manipur	11.4	16.9	55.4	32.9	28.2	16.9	30.2	14.9	14.6
Meghalaya	22.0	17.8	52.6	70.1	55.9	35.5	70.7	8.2	3.6
Mizoram	20.4	24.6	77.3	35.8	31.8	58.0	80.0	19.4	23.8
Nagaland	5.5	10.4	45.5	20.6	18.9	22.3	24.9	9.4	8.3
Tripura	34.5	45.5	64.8	69.7	73.1	76.6	82.1	41.4	3.4
Goa	17.4	24.0	38.4	28.5	31.1	31.1	31.5	20.7	14.7
Gujarat	13.8	15.2	26.0	21.9	23.3	16.7	20.6	19.2	4.4
Maharashtra	9.4	14.7	25.8	19.5	21.3	18.1	13.2	24.1	11.5
Tamil Nadu	29.5	36.5	48.1	42.0	42.6	51.5	47.4	33.0	22.2

1 Percentages may sum to more than 100.0 since multiple responses were allowed.

Table 11.4: Knowledge about avoidance of AIDS
Among Weomen who have heard about AIDS, the percentage who believe AIDS can be avoided by various means, according to state, India, 1992-93.

	Percentage who betieve AIDS can be avoided by:				
State	Using condoms during intercourse	Practis-ing safe sex	Checking blood prior to trans-fusion	Sterilizing needles/ syringes for injections	Avoiding pregnancy when infected with AIDS
Dethi	40.1	52.0	13.0	10.7	1.3
West Bengat	35.6	42.7	16.9	6.8	4.3
Arunachal Pradesh	47.6	24.5	21.0	18.9	9.8
Assam	25.2	36.1	22.6	21.5	15.5
Manipur	18.1	48.6	6.7	24.3	9.1
Meghalaya	19.4	67.8	23.0	23.7	13.5
Mizoram	13.4	88.1	11.9	45.5	2.7
Nagaland	58.9	48.1	28.1	45.1	34.5
Tripura	29.7	35.2	13.1	13.1	-
Goa	31.9	56.0	36.4	42.0	27.3
Gujarat	32.7	32.7	14.0	10.6	5.4
Maharashtra	32.1	57.1	17.9	15.8	3.4
Tamit Nadu	14.3	70.6	5.8	6.9	0.8

Note: Percentages may sum to more than 100.0 since muttipte responses were attowed.
— Less than 0.05 per cent.

of the disease among women who have heard of the disease, indicate that public education campaigns about AIDS are very much needed in India. It will be difficult to contain the spread of AIDS unless both women and men are provided with accurate knowledge about the disease.

REFERENCES

Agarwal, K.N., D.K. Agarwal, D.G. Benakappa, S.M. Gupta, P.C. Khanduja, S.P. Khatua, K. Ramachandran, P.M. Udani and C. Gopalan, 1991, *Growth Performance of Affluent Indian Children* (Under-fives): Growth Standard for Indian Children, New Delhi: Nutrition Foundation of India.

Agarwala, S.N., 1985, *India's Population Problems*, New Delhi: Tata McGraw Hill Publishing Company.

Agrawal, A.N., 1991, *Indian Economy: Problems of Development and Planning*, New Delhi: Wiley Eastern Limited.

Arnold, Fred, 1987, The effect of sex preference on fertility and family planning: Empirical evidence, *Population Bulletin of the United Nations* 23-24:44-45.

Arnold, Fred, 1992, Sex preference and its demographic and health implications, *International Family Planning Perspectives* 18(3): 93-101.

Bairagi, Radheshyam and Ray L. Langsten. 1986. Sex preference for children and its implications for fertility in rural Bangladesh, *Studies in Family Planning* 17(6):302-307.

Basu, Alaka Malwade, 1989, Is discrimination in food really necessary for explaining sex differentials in childhood mortality?. *Population Studies* 43(2):193-210.

Basu, Alaka Malwade. 1993. Cultural influences on the timing of first births in India: Large differences that add up to little difference. *Population Studies* 47:85-95.

Bhende, Asha and Tara Kanitkar. 1994. *Principles of Population Studies.* Reprint of the fifth revised edition. Bombay: Himalaya Publishing House.

Bittles, Alan H., A.T. Eaton and L.B. Jorde. 1992. Consanguinity and fertility: A global perspective. *American Journal of Physical Anthropology*, Vol. 87, Supplement 14.

Bittles, Alan H., W.M. Mason, J. Greene and N. Appaji Rao. 1991. Reproductive behaviour and health and consanguineous marriages. *Science* 252:789-794.

Black R.E. 1984. Diarrheal Diseases and Child Mortality. In W. Henry Mosley and Lincoln C. Chen (eds.), Child Survival: Strategies for Research. *Population and Development Review*, Supplement to Volume 10.

Bruce, Judith, 1990. Fundamental elements of the quality of care: A simple framework. *Studies in Family Planning*, Vol. 21, No. 2.

Central Bureau of Health Intelligence (CBHI). 1991. *Health Information of India-1991*. New Delhi: CBHI, Directorate General of Health Services, Ministry of Health and Family Welfare.

Central Statistical Organisation (CSO). 1993. *Selected Socio-Economic Statistics for India*: 1992. New Delhi: CSO, Ministry of Planning and Programme Implementation.

Centre for Monitoring Indian Economy. 1992. *Basic Statistics Relating to the Indian Economy*, Vol. 2: States. Bombay: Centre for Monitoring Indian Economy.

Centre for Monitoring Indian Economy. 1994. *Basic Statistics Relating to the Indian Economy*. Bombay: Centre for Monitoring Indian Economy.

Cleland, John, Jane Verrall and Martin Vaessen. 1983. *Preferences for the Sex of Children and Their Influence on Reproductive Behaviour.* WFS Comparative Studies No. 27. Voorburg: International Statistical Institute.

Das Gupta, Monica. 1987. Selective discrimination against female children in rural Punjab, India. *Population and Development Review* 13(1):77-101.

Datt, Ruddar and K.P.M. Sundharam. 1995. *Indian Economy*. New Delhi: S. Chand and Company Ltd.

Deolalikar, Anil B. and Prem Vashishtha. 1992. *The Utilization of Government and Private Health Services in India*. Report prepared under the Options Project, the Futures Group, Washington, D.C.

Dibley, M.J., J.B. Goldsby, N.W. Staehling and F.L. Trowbridge. 1987a. Development of normalized curves for the international growth reference: Historical and technical considerations. *American Journal of Clinical Nutrition* 46(5):736-748.

Dibley, M.J., N.W. Staehling, P. Neiburg and F.L. Trowbridge. 1987b. Interpretation of z score anthropometric indicators derived from the international growth reference. *American Journal of Clinical Nutrition* 46(5):749-762.

Foster, Stanley. 1984. Immunizable and Respiratory Diseases and Child Mortality. In W. Henry Mosley and Lincoln C. Chen (eds.), Child Survival: Strategies for Research. *Population and Development Review*, Supplement to Volume 10.

Ghosh, Shanti. 1987. The female child in India: A struggle for survival. *Bulletin of the Nutrition Foundation of India*, Vol. 8, No. 4.

Government of India. 1946. *Report of the Health Survey and Development Committee*. Volumes I-IV. Delhi: Manager of Publications.

Government of India. 1994. *Economic Survey 1993-94*. New Delhi: Ministry of Finance, Economic Division.

Govindasamy, Pavalavalli, M. Kathryn Stewart, Shea O. Rutstein, J. Ties Boerma and A. Elisabeth Sommerfelt. 1993. *High-risk Births and Maternity Care.* DHS Comparative Studies No. 8. Columbia, Maryland: Macro International.

Goyal, R.P. 1988. *Marriage in India.* Delhi: B.R. Publishing Corporation.

Gupta, J.P. and Indira Murli. 1989. *National Review of Immunization Programrne in India.* New Delhi: National Institute of Health and Family Welfare.

Hajnal, John. 1953. Age at marriage and proportions marrying. *Population Studies* 7(2):111136.

Harrison, Kelsey A. 1990. The political challenge of maternal mortality in the Third World. *Maternal Mortality and Morbidity - A Call to Women for Action.* Special Issue, May 28.

Hobcraft, J., J. McDonald and S. Rutstein. 1983. Child-spacing effects on infant and early child mortality. *Population Index* 49(4):585-618.

Hooja, S.L. 1969. *Dowry System in India, A Case Study.* New Delhi: Asia Press.

Innocenti Declaration on the Protection, Promotion and Support of Breastfeeding. 1990. Adopted by the WHO/UNICEF policymakers' meeting on "Breastfeeding in the 1990s: A Global Initiative", 30 July - 1 August, Innocenti, Florence, Italy.

Jejeebhoy, Shireen J. 1991. Women's Roles: Health and Reproductive Behaviour. pp. 114-148 in J.K. Satia and Shireen J. Jejeebhoy (eds.), *The Demographic Challenge: A Study of Four Large Indian States.* Bombay: Oxford University Press.

Kanitkar, Tara. 1979. Development of Maternal and Child Health Services in India. In K. Srinivasan, P.C. Saxena and Tara Kanitkar (eds.), *Child in India. Bombay:* Himalaya Publishing House.

Kapadia, K.M. 1966. *Marriage and Family in India.* Calcutta: Oxford University Press.

Khan, M.E., Richard Anker, S.K. Ghosh Dastidar and Sashi Bairathi. 1989. Inequalities Between Men and Women in Nutrition and Family Welfare Services: An In-Depth Enquiry in an Indian Village. pp. 175-199 in John C. Caldwell and Gigi Santow (eds.), *Selected Readings in Cultural, Social and Behavioural Determinants of Health.* Canberra: Highland Press.

Khlat, Miriam and Muin Khoury. 1991. Inbreeding and diseases: Demographic, genetic, and epidemiologic perspectives. *Epidemiologic Reviews* 13:28 41.

Khurana, Pushpa. 1989. *AIDS - Humanity's Gravest Challenge.* New Delhi: Hind Pocket Books.

Kosambi, D.D. 1981. *The Culture and Civilization of Ancient India in Historical Outline.* New Delhi: Vikas Publishing House.

Lal, Shiv. 1994. HIV Infection in India: Valuable Pointers. *CARC Calling, Bulletin of the Centre for AIDS Research and Control, Bombay,* Vol.7, No. 2.

Lightbourne, Robert E. and Alphonse L. MacDonald. 1982. *Family Size Preferences.* WFS Comparative Studies No.14. Voorburg: International Statistical Institute.

Loaiza, Edilberto. 1995. Sterilization regret in the Dominion Republic: Looking for quality-of care issues. *Studies in Family Planning* 26(1): 39-48.

MacDonald, Paul C. and Jack A. Pritchard. 1980. *Williams Obstetrics.* Sixteenth Edition. New York: Appleton-Century-Crofts.

Martorell, R. and J.P. Habicht. 1986. Growth in Early Childhood in Developing Countries. pp. 241-262 in Frank Falkner and J.M. Tanner (eds.), *Human Growth: A Comprehensive Treatise,* Vol. 3. New York: Plenum Press.

Miller, Barbara D. 1981. *The Endangered Sex: Neglect of Female Children in Rural North India.* Ithaca, New York: Cornell University Press.

Ministry of Health and Family Welfare (MOHFW). 1978. *Manual for Health Worker* (Female), Volume 1. New Delhi: MOHFW.

Ministry of Health and Family Welfare (MOHFW). 1989. *Family Welfare Programme in India, Year Book, 1987-88.* New Delhi: Department of Family Welfare, MOHFW.

Ministry of Health and Family Welfare (MOHFW). 1991. *Family Welfare Programme in India, Year Book, 1989-90.* New Delhi: Department of Family Welfare, MOHFW.

Ministry of Health and Family Welfare (MOHFW). 1992a. *Family Welfare Programme in India, Year Book 1990-91.* New Delhi: Department of Family Welfare, MOHFW.

Ministry of Health and Family Welfare (MOHFW). 1992b. *Module for Health Workers.* New Delhi: National Child Survival and Safe Motherhood Programme, MOHFW.

Ministry of Health and Family Welfare (MOHFW). 1993a. *National AIDS Control Programme in India - Country Scenario: An Update.* New Delhi: National AIDS Control Organization, MOHFW.

Ministry of Health and Family Welfare (MOHFW). 1993b. *Annual Report 1992-93.* New Delhi: Department of Family Welfare, MOHFW.

National AIDS Control Organization. 1994: AIDS Update. *CARC Calling, Bulletin of the Centre for AIDS Research and Control, Bombay,* Vol.7, No. 2.

Nutrition Foundation of India. 1993. *NFI Bulletin,* Vol.14, No.4.

Office of the Registrar General. 1982. *Sample Registration System.* 1970-75. New Delhi: Office of the Registrar General.

Office of the Registrar General. 1985 *Sample Registration System 1981.* New Delhi: Office of Registrar General.

Office of the Registrar General. 1992. *Sample Registration System 1989.* New Delhi: Office of the Registrar General.

Office of the Registrar General. 1993a. *Sample Registration System: Fertility and Mortality Indicators 1991*. New Delhi: Office of the Registrar General.

Office of the Registrar General. 1993b. *Sample Registration System: Fertility and Mortality Indicators 1990*. New Delhi: Office of the Registrar General.

Office of the Registrar General. 1994. *Sample Registration System: Fertility and Mortality Indicators 1992*. New Delhi: Office of the Registrar General.

Office of the Registrar General and Census Commissioner. 1972. *Census of India, 1971, Series 1, India, Paper 2 of 1972, Religion. New Delhi:* Office of the Registrar General and Census Commissioner.

Office of the Registrar General and Census Commissioner. 1974. *Census of India, 1971, Series1, India, Part II-A(ii), Union Primary Census Abstract*. New Delhi: Office of the Registrar General and Census Commissioner.

Office of the Registrar General and Census Commissioner. 1976. *Census of India, 1971, Series1, India, Part II-C(ii), Social Cultural Tables*. New Delhi: Office of the Registrar General and Census Commissioner.

Office of the Registrar General and Census Commissioner. 1983. *Census of India, 1981, Series1, Part VII-B (ii), The Physically Handicapped: Report and Tables*. New Delhi: Office of the Registrar General and Census Commissioner.

Office of the Registrar General and Census Commissioner. 1984a. *Census of India, 1981, Series-1, India, Paper-4 of 1984, Household Population by Religion of Head of Household*. New Delhi: Office of the Registrar General and Census Commissioner.

Office of the Registrar General and Census Commissioner. 1984b. *Census of India, 1981, Series-1, India, Paper-2 of 1984, General Population and Population of Scheduled Castes and Scheduled Tribes*. New Delhi: Office of the Registrar General and Census Commissioner.

Office of the Registrar General and Census Commissioner. 1984c. *Census of India, 1981, Series-1, India, Paper-5 of 1984, Age Tables Based on 5 Per cent Sarnple Data*. New Delhi; Office of the Registrar General and Census Commissioner.

Office of the Registrar General and Census Commissioner. 1987. *Census of India, 1981, Series1, India, Part IV-A(ii), Social Cultural Tables*. New Delhi: Office of the Registrar General and Census Commissioner.

Office of the Registrar General and Census Commissioner. 1988. *Census of India, 1981, Series1, Part XII, Census Atlas, National Volume*. New Delhi: Office of the Registrar General and Census Commissioner.

Office of the Registrar General and Census Commissioner. 1992. *Census of India, 1991, Series1, India, Paper-2 of 1992, Final Population Totals, Brief Analysis of Primary Census Abstract*. New Delhi: Office of the Registrar General and Census Commissioner.

Office of the Registrar General and Census Commissioner. 1995. *Census of India, 1991, Series1, India, Paper I of 1995, Religion.* New Delhi: Office of the Registrar General and Census Commissioner.

Operations Research Group. 1990. *Family Planning Practices in India: Third All India Survey.* Baroda: Operations Research Group.

Park, Chai Bin and Nam Hoon Cho. 1995. Consequences of son preference in a low fertility society: Imbalance of the sex ratio at birth in Korea. *Population and Development Review* 21 :59. 84

Park, J.E. and K. Park. 1989. *Textbook of Preventive and Social Medicine.* Twelfth Edition. Jabalpur: M/S Banarsidas Bhanot Publishers.

Population Reference Bureau. 1994. *World Population Data Sheet 1994.* Population Reference Bureau, Washington, D.C.

Population Research Centre, CRRID. 1993. *People's Perception and Reproductive Behaviour in North West India: An Interdisciplinary Field Study of Eight Districts in Haryana, Himachal Pradesh and Uttar Pradesh.* Chandigarh: Centre for Research in Rural and Industrial Development.

Prabhu, P.H. 1963. *Hindu Social Organization*, Fourth Edition. Bombay: Popular Prakashan.

Premi, Mahendra K. 1991. *India's Population: Heading Towards a Billion - An Analysis of 1991 Census Provisional Results.* New Delhi: B.R. Publishing Corporation.

Preston, Samuel H. 1990. Mortality in India. pp. 81-86 in International Union for the Scientific Study of Population (IUSSP), *International Population Conference, New Delhi, 1989,* Vol. 4. Liege: IUSSP.

Ramachandran, Prema. 1992. Need of organization of antenatal and intrapartum care in India. *Demography India* 21(2): 179-193.

Rao, P.S.S. and S.G. Inbaraj. 1977. Inbreeding in Tamil Nadu, South India. *Social Biology* 24:281-288.

Rao, P.S.S., S.G. Inbaraj and G. Jesudian. 1972. Rural-urban differentials in consanguinity. *Journal of Medical Genetics* 9:174-178.

Rastogi, S.R. and Raj Kumari. 1988. *Study of Family Welfare and MCH Programme in Azamgarh District.* Lucknow: Population Research Centre, Lucknow University.

Rastogi, S.R. and Raj Kumari. 1992. Son Preference and Effectiveness of the Family Welfare Programme in Uttar Pradesh. pp. 165-179 in R.N. Patil (ed.), *Health, Environment and Population.* New Delhi: Ashish Publishing House.

Renou, Louis. 1959. *The Civilization of Ancient India.* Calcutta: Susil Gupta (India) Private Ltd.

Roberts, P.E. 1967. *History of British India.* London: Oxford University Press.

Roychoudhury, A.K. 1976. Incidence of inbreeding in different states of India. *Demography India* 5: 108-119.

Rutstein, Shea Oscar. 1984. *Infant and Child Mortality: Levels, Trends, and Demographic Differentials*. Revised edition. WFS Comparative Studies No. 43. Voorburg: International Statistical Institute.

Rutstein, Shea Oscar and George T. Bicego. 1990. Assessment of the Quality of Data Used to Ascertain Eligibility and Age in the Demographic and Health Surveys. In *An Assessment of DHS-I Data Quality*. DHS Methodological Reports No. l. Columbia, Maryland: Institute for Resource Development/Macro Systems Inc.

Sanghvi, L.D. 1966. Inbreeding in India. *Eugenics Quarterly* 13:291-301.

Shryock, Henry S. and Jacob S. Siegel. 1980. *The Methods and Materials of Demography*, Volume 1 (fourth edition, revised). Washington, D.C.: U.S. Bureau of the Census.

Sommerfelt, A. Elisabeth and M. Kathryn Stewart. 1994. *Children's Nutritional Status*. DHS Comparative Studies No. 12. Calverton, Maryland: Macro International.

Stempbridge, H. Jasper. 1963. *The World: A General Regional Geography*. London: Oxford University Press.

Sullivan, Jeremiah M., Shea Oscar Rutstein, and George T. Bicego. 1994. *Infant and Child Mortality*. DHS Comparative Studies No. 15. Calverton, Maryland: Macro International.

Thorthwaite, C.W. 1933. The climates of the earth. *Geographic Review*, 33:433-440.

United Nations. 1955. *Methods of Appraisal of Quality of Basic Data for Population Estimates*. New York: United Nations.

United Nations. 1986. *How to Weigh and Measure Children: Assessing the Nutritional Status of Young Children in Household Surveys*. Department of Technical Co-operation for Development and Statistical Office, United Nations. New York: United Nations.

United Nations Secretariat. 1988. Sex differentials in survivorship in the developing world: Levels, regional patterns and demographic determinants. *Population Bulletin of the United Nations* 25:51-64.

Verma, Ravi K., T.K. Roy and P.C. Saxena. 1994. *Quality of Family Welfare Services and Care in Selected Indian States*. Bombay: International Institute for Population Sciences.

Westoff, Charles F. and Luis Hernando Ochoa. 1991. *Unmet Need and the Demand for Family Planning*. DHS Comparative Studies No.5. Columbia, Maryland: Macro International.

World Health Organization. 1991a. *Maternal Mortality: A Global Factbook*. Geneva: World Health Organization.

World Health Organization. 1991b. *Indicators for Assessing Breast-feeding Practices: Report of an Informal Meeting*, 11-12 June, Geneva. Geneva: World Health Organization.

World Health Organization. 1992. *AIDS in Africa: A Manual for Physicians.* Geneva: World Health Organization.

World Health Organization. 1994a. *Care of Mother and Baby at the Health Centre: A Practical Guide.* Geneva: Maternal Health and Safe Motherhood Programme, Division of Family Health.

World Health Organization. 1994b. *Global AIDS News: The Newsletter of the World Health Organization Global Programme on AIDS*, No. 3.

World Health Organization and UNICEF. 1978. *Primary Health Care: Report of the International Conference on Primary Health Care, Alma Ata, USSR, 6-12 September 1978.* Geneva: World Health Organization.

World Health Organization-UNICEF. 1992. Low Birth Weight: *A Tabulation of Available Information.* Geneva: World Health Organization.